Practical Pediatric Imaging

Editor

EDWARD Y. LEE

RADIOLOGIC CLINICS OF NORTH AMERICA

www.radiologic.theclinics.com

Consulting Editor
FRANK H. MILLER

July 2017 • Volume 55 • Number 4

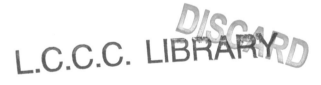

ELSEVIER

1600 John F. Kennedy Boulevard • Suite 1800 • Philadelphia, Pennsylvania, 19103-2899

http://www.theclinics.com

RADIOLOGIC CLINICS OF NORTH AMERICA Volume 55, Number 4
July 2017 ISSN 0033-8389, ISBN 13: 978-0-323-53152-8

Editor: John Vassallo (j.vassallo@elsevier.com)
Developmental Editor: Donald Mumford

Radiologic Clinics of North America (ISSN 0033-8389) is published bimonthly by Elsevier Inc., 360 Park Avenue South, New York, NY 10010-1710. Months of issue are January, March, May, July, September, and November. Periodicals postage paid at New York, NY and additional mailing offices. Subscription prices are USD 474 per year for US individuals, USD 831 per year for US institutions, USD 100 per year for US students and residents, USD 551 per year for Canadian individuals, USD 1062 per year for Canadian institutions, USD 680 per year for international individuals, USD 1062 per year for international institutions, and USD 315 per year for Canadian and international students/residents. To receive student and resident rate, orders must be accompanied by name of affiliated institution, date of term and the signature of program/residency coordinatior on institution letterhead. Orders will be billed at individual rate until proof of status is received. Foreign air speed delivery is included in all *Clinics* subscription prices. All prices are subject to change without notice. **POSTMASTER:** Send address changes to *Radiologic Clinics of North America*, Elsevier Health Sciences Division, Subscription Customer Service, 3251 Riverport Lane, Maryland Heights, MO63043. **Customer Service: Telephone: 1-800-654-2452** (U.S. and Canada); **1-314-447-8871** (outside U.S. and Canada). **Fax: 1-314-447-8029. E-mail: journalscustomerservice-usa@elsevier.com (for print support); journalsonlinesupport-usa@elsevier.com (for online support).**

Reprints. For copies of 100 or more of articles in this publication, please contact the Commercial Reprints Department, Elsevier Inc., 360 Park Avenue South, New York, New York 10010-1710. Tel.: +1-212-633-3874; Fax: +1-212-633-3820; E-mail: reprints@elsevier.com.

Radiologic Clinics of North America also published in Greek Paschalidis Medical Publications, Athens, Greece.

Radiologic Clinics of North America is covered in *MEDLINE/PubMed (Index Medicus), EMBASE/Excerpta Medica, Current Contents/Life Sciences, Current Contents/Clinical Medicine, RSNA Index to Imaging Literature, BIOSIS, Science Citation Index,* and *ISI/BIOMED.*

Printed in the United States of America.

Contributors

CONSULTING EDITOR

FRANK H. MILLER, MD
Chief, Body Imaging Section and Fellowship
Program; Medical Director of MRI; Professor,
Department of Radiology, Northwestern
University Feinberg School of Medicine,
Chicago, Illinois

EDITOR

EDWARD Y. LEE, MD, MPH
Chief, Division of Thoracic Imaging, Associate
Professor, Department of Radiology;
Pulmonary Division, Department of Medicine,
Boston Children's Hospital, Harvard Medical
School, Boston, Massachusetts

AUTHORS

TAHIYA SALEM ALYAFEI, MD
Program Director of Pediatric
Radiology Fellowship, Consultant Pediatric
Imaging-HMC, Clinical Imaging Department,
Hamad General Hospital, Hamad Medical
Corporation, Doha, Qatar

JOO CHO, MD
Diagnostic Radiology Fellow, Department of
Radiology, Boston Children's Hospital,
Harvard Medical School, Boston,
Massachusetts

WINNIE C.W. CHU, MD, FRCR
Professor of Radiology, Department of Imaging
and Interventional Radiology, Prince of Wales
Hospital, The Chinese University of Hong
Kong, Shatin, NT, Hong Kong SAR, China

JOSEPH T. DAVIS, MD
Medical Instructor, Department of Radiology,
Duke University Medical Center, Durham,
North Carolina

MICHAEL GEORGE, MD, MFA
Diagnostic Radiology Fellow, Department of
Radiology, Boston Children's Hospital,
Harvard Medical School, Boston,
Massachusetts

VICTOR M. HO-FUNG, MD
Assistant Professor, Department of Radiology,
Children's Hospital of Philadelphia, Perelman
School of Medicine, University of
Pennsylvania, Philadelphia, Pennsylvania

ANASTASIA L. HRYHORCZUK, MD
Assistant Professor, Department of Pediatric
Radiology, Floating Hospital for Children at
Tufts Medical Center, Boston, Massachusetts

JEFFREY L. KONING, MD
Chief Diagnostic Radiology Fellow,
Department of Radiology, Boston Children's
Hospital, Harvard Medical School, Boston,
Massachusetts

NEHA S. KWATRA, MD
Instructor, Department of Radiology, Boston Children's Hospital, Harvard Medical School, Boston, Massachusetts

BERNARD F. LAYA, MD, DO
Professor of Radiology, Head, Institute of Radiology, St. Luke's Medical Center-Global City, Taguig City, Philippines

EDWARD Y. LEE, MD, MPH
Chief, Division of Thoracic Imaging, Associate Professor, Department of Radiology; Pulmonary Division, Department of Medicine, Boston Children's Hospital, Harvard Medical School, Boston, Massachusetts

MARK C. LISZEWSKI, MD
Assistant Professor, Division of Pediatric Radiology, Department of Radiology, Montefiore Medical Center, Albert Einstein College of Medicine, Bronx, New York

VICTORIA M. PARENTE, MD
Assistant Professor, Department of Pediatrics, Duke University Medical Center, Durham, North Carolina

JEANNETTE M. PEREZ-ROSELLO, MD
Assistant Professor of Radiology, Department of Radiology, Boston Children's Hospital, Harvard Medical School, Boston, Massachusetts

GRACE S. PHILLIPS, MD
Associate Professor, Department of Radiology, Seattle Children's Hospital, University of Washington School of Medicine, Seattle, Washington

RICARDO RESTREPO, MD
Voluntary Professor at Florida International University School of Medicine, Chief, Pediatric Interventional Radiology Section, Department of Radiology, Nicklaus Children's Hospital, Miami, Florida

JULIA RISSMILLER, MD
Assistant Professor, Department of Pediatric Radiology, Floating Hospital for Children at Tufts Medical Center, Boston, Massachusetts

ASHA SARMA, MD
Diagnostic Radiology Fellow, Department of Radiology, Boston Children's Hospital, Harvard Medical School, Boston, Massachusetts

GARY R. SCHOOLER, MD
Assistant Professor, Department of Radiology, Duke University Medical Center, Durham, North Carolina

SHREYA SOOD, MD
Assistant Professor, Department of Pediatric Radiology, Floating Hospital for Children at Tufts Medical Center, Boston, Massachusetts

A. LUANA STANESCU, MD
Assistant Professor, Department of Radiology, Seattle Children's Hospital, University of Washington School of Medicine, Seattle, Washington

ABBEY J. WINANT, MD, MFA
Instructor, Department of Radiology, Boston Children's Hospital, Harvard Medical School, Boston, Massachusetts

EDWARD YANG, MD, PhD
Instructor, Department of Radiology, Boston Children's Hospital, Harvard Medical School, Boston, Massachusetts

ALI YIKILMAZ, MD
Chief, Department of Radiology, Associate Professor of Radiology, Goztepe Research and Training Hospital, Istanbul Medeniyet University Medical School, Istanbul, Turkey

MATTHEW A. ZAPALA, MD, PhD
Assistant Professor of Clinical Radiology, Pediatric Radiology Section, Department of Radiology and Biomedical Imaging, Benioff Children's Hospital, University of California, San Francisco, San Francisco, California

EVAN J. ZUCKER, MD
Clinical Assistant Professor of Radiology, Department of Radiology, Lucile Packard Children's Hospital, Stanford University School of Medicine, Stanford, California

Contents

For general radiologists, congenital brain malformations pose substantial challenges in terms of recognition, description, and classification. This review describes a practical approach to imaging and classifying the most common supratentorial brain malformations. It begins with a discussion of embryology and optimal imaging technique and then summarizes distinguishing imaging features for several major categories of cerebral malformation, including holoprosencephaly, gray matter heterotopia, lissencephaly/pachygyria, focal cortical dysplasia, polymicrogyria, and cobblestone malformation. The importance of identifying abnormalities in the corpus callosum and basal ganglia is also discussed, both for detection and characterization of cerebral malformations.

The imaging evaluation of the neonate in respiratory distress has been described since the most early days of pediatric radiology but advances in diagnosis and treatment have changed the patient population presenting with these conditions and altered the imaging findings. In this article, the range of conditions that cause neonatal respiratory distress is depicted, including congenital lung malformations and lung disease in both preterm and full-term infants. An updated approach to the imaging of these conditions is reviewed, with a focus on changes that have resulted from advances in treatment and diagnosis.

Cough and fever in infants and children are frequent but nonspecific symptoms. Several usual differential diagnoses are under consideration and imaging is often necessary to help arrive at an accurate diagnosis and ensure proper management. A broad spectrum of underlying disorders may be present. Radiologists must remain cognizant of the potential for immune dysfunction and underlying structural abnormalities. A clear understanding of up-to-date imaging evaluation recommendations and characteristic imaging features can assist radiologists and clinicians in arriving at the most accurate diagnosis in a timely manner and help ensure proper management and necessary follow-up imaging assessment.

This article focuses on commonly encountered primary lung, airway, mediastinal, and chest wall neoplasms that occur in the pediatric population. Although primary pediatric thoracic neoplasms are rare, imaging is critical in their diagnostic work-up. An overview of the latest imaging techniques specific to evaluate these pediatric thoracic neoplasms is presented across the spectrum of modalities from radiography to PET/MR imaging. In addition, the characteristic imaging appearances of these pediatric primary thoracic neoplasms are discussed with an emphasis on what the radiologist needs to know in routine clinical practice.

Anatomic variants are common incidental findings in pediatric chest imaging and can be mistaken for true underlying pathology, sometimes resulting in unnecessary additional imaging evaluation or invasive procedures. Clear understanding of the imaging characteristics and clinical significance of anatomic thoracic variants is important for accurate diagnosis and avoidance of unnecessary intervention. This article provides an up-to-date review of anatomic variants in the pediatric chest to increase knowledge and aide in timely, correct diagnosis.

The cyanotic congenital heart diseases are a rare and heterogeneous group of disorders, often requiring urgent neonatal management. Although echocardiography is the mainstay for imaging, continued technological advances have expanded the role for computed tomography and magnetic resonance imaging, helping to limit invasive cardiac catheterization. In this article, the authors review the broad spectrum of cyanotic congenital heart disease, focusing on the utility of advanced noninvasive imaging modalities while highlighting key clinical features and management considerations.

Neonatal gastrointestinal emergencies are caused by a diverse set of primarily congenital entities that may affect the upper or lower gastrointestinal tracts, and occasionally both. Although a diagnosis can sometimes be made on prenatal imaging, more commonly patients present after birth and require prompt diagnosis to facilitate timely treatment. Imaging plays a central role in the accurate diagnosis of these entities and typically consists of an initial abdominal series followed by either an upper gastrointestinal series or contrast enema. The authors review the most common neonatal gastrointestinal emergencies and provide a step-by-step approach to the accurate imaging diagnosis.

Recent developments regarding the treatment of pediatric liver tumors have significantly improved patient care. Stimulated by collaboration between international pediatric groups, advances have been made in surgical techniques, transplantation options, and chemotherapy schemas. In light of this progress, clear understanding of the state-of-the-art imaging evaluation of hepatobiliary tumors has become even more integral to the effective management of children with hepatic neoplasms. The unique imaging features of hepatic neoplasms in the pediatric population, when coupled with supportive demographic data and laboratory findings, can lead to accurate diagnosis and proper treatment of hepatobiliary tumors.

Pediatric Urinary System Neoplasms: An Overview and Update

Michael George, Jeannette M. Perez-Rosello, Ali Yikilmaz, and Edward Y. Lee

Pediatric urinary system neoplasms are a diverse group of tumors that frequently overlap in their clinical and radiologic features. By contrast, the histopathologic classification and treatment of these entities have become increasingly refined, resulting in improved outcomes, with the overall survival of Wilms tumors now exceeding 90%. Significantly, many contemporary protocols rely on radiologic diagnosis in the absence of tissue confirmation. This review article provides up-to-date clinical, epidemiologic, and imaging findings of pediatric urinary system neoplasms and their mimics frequently encountered in daily clinical practice.

Musculoskeletal Traumatic Injuries in Children: Characteristic Imaging Findings and Mimickers

Victor M. Ho-Fung, Matthew A. Zapala, and Edward Y. Lee

Musculoskeletal traumatic injuries in children demonstrate characteristic imaging findings. The physis is the most susceptible structure to traumatic injury. The periosteum in children plays a key role in rapid bone healing and stability. The main complications of fractures in children are premature physeal closure, potential limb length discrepancy, and angular deformities. Understanding the normal bone growth, healing, and complications of pediatric fractures is crucial for appropriate imaging diagnosis. This article discusses currently available imaging modalities with up-to-date techniques, underlying mechanisms, and characteristic imaging findings of musculoskeletal traumatic injuries and mimickers encountered in daily clinical practice.

Practical Indication-Based Pediatric Nuclear Medicine Studies: Update and Review

Neha S. Kwatra, Asha Sarma, and Edward Y. Lee

Pediatric nuclear medicine imaging presents unique challenges and requires a thorough understanding of the patients' developmental stages and physiology to optimize study protocols. This article provides an overview of the current practice of diagnostic pediatric nuclear medicine, including the common clinical applications and imaging protocol considerations.

Practical Imaging Evaluation of Foreign Bodies in Children: An Update

Bernard F. Laya, Ricardo Restrepo, and Edward Y. Lee

Foreign bodies (FBs) may be unintentionally ingested, inhaled, or inserted into a body cavity or tissue, or may be due to traumatic or iatrogenic injury. They are frequently detected in clinical practice and emergency rooms. Early detection and prompt management are mandatory to avoid severe and life-threatening complications. Imaging plays an important role in confirming the presence and characterization of the FB, and its relationship with any affected organs. This article reviews commonly encountered FBs with regard to incidence, risk factors, mechanisms of entry, clinical presentation, associated complications, and typical imaging appearance in children.

Although pediatric tumors are largely sporadic in cause, continued advancements in science have elucidated a growing body of tumors that are associated with syndromes. Early identification of these syndromic disorders associated with developing tumors can alter the course of disease and potentially save lives. Medical imaging has a pivotal role in screening surveillance, diagnosis, and management of these tumors. Understanding characteristic manifestations of these syndromes is important to optimize image utilization. This article discusses clinically important syndromes associated with pediatric tumors with brief overview of the background, genetics, and clinical features. Diagnosis, imaging, management, and treatment are also reviewed.

PROGRAM OBJECTIVE

The objective of the *Radiologic Clinics of North America* is to keep practicing radiologists and radiology residents up to date with current clinical practice in radiology by providing timely articles reviewing the state of the art in patient care.

TARGET AUDIENCE

Practicing radiologists, radiology residents, and other health care professionals who provide patient care utilizing radiologic findings.

LEARNING OBJECTIVES

Upon completion of this activity, participants will be able to:
1. Review normal thoracic anatomic variants in pediatric imaging.
2. Discuss updates in imaging for pediatric and neonatal emergencies.
3. Recognize developments in the imaging of pediatric tumors.

ACCREDITATION

The Elsevier Office of Continuing Medical Education (EOCME) is accredited by the Accreditation Council for Continuing Medical Education (ACCME) to provide continuing medical education for physicians.

The EOCME designates this enduring material for a maximum of 15 *AMA PRA Category 1 Credit*(s)™. Physicians should claim only the credit commensurate with the extent of their participation in the activity.

All other healthcare professionals requesting continuing education credit for this enduring material will be issued a certificate of participation.

DISCLOSURE OF CONFLICTS OF INTEREST

The EOCME assesses conflict of interest with its instructors, faculty, planners, and other individuals who are in a position to control the content of CME activities. All relevant conflicts of interest that are identified are thoroughly vetted by EOCME for fair balance, scientific objectivity, and patient care recommendations. EOCME is committed to providing its learners with CME activities that promote improvements or quality in healthcare and not a specific proprietary business or a commercial interest.

The planning committee, staff, authors and editors listed below have identified no financial relationships or relationships to products or devices they or their spouse/life partner have with commercial interest related to the content of this CME activity:
Tahiya Salem Alyaefi, MD; Joo Cho, MD; Winnie C.W. Chu, MD, FRCR; Joseph T. Davis, MD; Anjali Fortna; Michael George, MD, MFA; Victor M. Ho-Fung, MD; Anastasia Hryhorczuk, MD; Jeffrey L. Koning, MD; Neha S. Kwatra, MD; Bernard F. Laya, MD, DO; Edward Y. Lee, MD, MPH; Mark C. Liszewski, MD; Victoria M. Parente, MD; Jeannette Perez-Rosello, MD; Grace S. Phillips, MD; Ricardo Restrepo, MD; Julia Rissmiller, MD; Asha Sarma, MD; Gary R. Schooler, MD; Shreya Sood, MD; A. Luana Stanescu, MD; Karthik Subramaniam; John Vassallo; Katie Widmeier; Amy Williams; Abbey J. Winant, MD, MFA; Ali Yikilmaz, MD; Matthew A. Zapala, MD, PhD; Evan J. Zucker, MD.

The planning committee, staff, authors and editors listed below have identified financial relationships or relationships to products or devices they or their spouse/life partner have with commercial interest related to the content of this CME activity:
Edward Yang, MD, PhD is a consultant/advisor for CorticoMetrics, LLC.

UNAPPROVED/OFF-LABEL USE DISCLOSURE

The EOCME requires CME faculty to disclose to the participants:
1. When products or procedures being discussed are off-label, unlabelled, experimental, and/or investigational (not US Food and Drug Administration [FDA] approved); and
2. Any limitations on the information presented, such as data that are preliminary or that represent ongoing research, interim analyses, and/or unsupported opinions. Faculty may discuss information about pharmaceutical agents that is outside of FDA-approved labelling. This information is intended solely for CME and is not intended to promote off-label use of these medications. If you have any questions, contact the medical affairs department of the manufacturer for the most recent prescribing information.

TO ENROLL

To enroll in the PET Clinics Continuing Medical Education program, call customer service at 1-800-654-2452 or sign up online at http://www.theclinics.com/home/cme. The CME program is available to subscribers for an additional annual fee of USD $315.

METHOD OF PARTICIPATION

In order to claim credit, participants must complete the following:

1. Complete enrolment as indicated above.
2. Read the activity.
3. Complete the CME Test and Evaluation. Participants must achieve a score of 70% on the test. All CME Tests and Evaluations must be completed online.

CME INQUIRIES/SPECIAL NEEDS

For all CME inquiries or special needs, please contact elsevierCME@elsevier.com.

RADIOLOGIC CLINICS OF NORTH AMERICA

Preface
Practical Pediatric Imaging

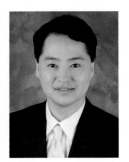

Edward Y. Lee, MD, MPH
Editor

In recent years, the breadth and scope of pediatric imaging continue to rapidly expand. A substantial portion of pediatric radiology is still practiced by general radiologists, whose expertise, however, may not be related to pediatric imaging. Therefore, the main focus of this issue of the *Radiologic Clinics of North America* is to respond to this need for an up-to-date review of the constantly expanding and changing field of pediatric imaging for practicing general radiologists to stay current.

The present issue is a collection of thirteen up-to-date review articles related to pediatric imaging. As the guest editor for this issue, I have selected topics that are considered to be practical in daily clinical practice and need to be mastered by radiologists to provide optimal management of pediatric patients with various congenital and acquired disorders. An additional goal of this issue is to close the knowledge gap in imaging evaluation of children that presently exists in various practices so that a uniform standard of care for pediatric patients can be achieved.

I had the great privilege and pleasure of working with highly experienced and talented contributing authors—all of whom are experts or rising stars in the field of pediatric imaging. Their invaluable efforts and extraordinary expertise have helped create a resource of information that should facilitate the improved understanding of often complex pediatric disorders. I would also like to thank my colleagues at Boston Children's Hospital for their encouragement; John G. Vassallo and his colleagues at Elsevier for their administrative and editorial assistance; and my family for their constant encouragement and support.

Edward Y. Lee, MD, MPH
Division of Thoracic Imaging
Departments of Radiology and Medicine
Boston Children's Hospital and
Harvard Medical School
300 Longwood Avenue
Boston, MA 02115, USA

E-mail address:
Edward.Lee@childrens.harvard.edu

Radiol Clin N Am 55 (2017) xiii
http://dx.doi.org/10.1016/j.rcl.2017.02.015
0033-8389/17/© 2017 Published by Elsevier Inc.

A Practical Approach to Supratentorial Brain Malformations
What Radiologists Should Know

Edward Yang, MD, PhD[a],*, Winnie C.W. Chu, MD, FRCR[b],
Edward Y. Lee, MD, MPH[a]

KEYWORDS

- Brain malformation • Holoprosencephaly • Callosal dysgenesis • Lissencephaly • Pachygyria
- Focal cortical dysplasia • Polymicrogyria • Cobblestone malformation

KEY POINTS

- The number of genetically elucidated brain malformations has dramatically increased in recent years. However, a morphologic approach based on an understanding of embryology remains essential to correctly recognizing these malformations and placing them in a mechanistic context.
- Errors in hemispheric cleavage and neuronal migration/organization explain the most common cerebral malformations encountered in clinical practice.
- Cerebral malformations frequently co-occur with abnormalities in the deep gray matter structures, corpus callosum, and overall brain size. These associated features help narrow the differential diagnosis.

INTRODUCTION

Congenital brain malformations are a major contributor to neurodevelopmental disability potentially manifesting as epilepsy, cerebral palsy, developmental delay, or as part of a broader genetic syndrome.[1–5] Therefore, brain malformations should be considered a focal point in the imaging evaluation of children with developmental delay and seizure, along with evidence of prior injury and metabolic disorders. Even in general radiology practice, these malformations are encountered periodically on obstetric imaging or as an incidental finding, making a basic understanding of brain malformations essential to all radiologists.

Correct classification of brain malformations is critical in guiding the appropriate work-up for these pediatric patients and setting expectations for prognosis. This classification can be particularly challenging for supratentorial malformations, which can have overlapping morphologic features or multiple abnormalities. To complicate the matter further, an enormous body of work has defined the genetic etiologies of many brain malformations over the past several years, making brain malformations an increasingly intimidating subject even for those who deal with such malformations routinely.[1,6]

In this review, a practical approach to supratentorial brain malformations is discussed based on a standard framework used by pediatric neurologists and neuroradiologists.[7] Fundamental to this approach is an understanding of the embryologic steps necessary to create the morphologically normal brain and optimal imaging technique for recognizing structural abnormalities, both of which are reviewed. Once this foundation is established,

[a] Department of Radiology, Boston Children's Hospital, Harvard Medical School, 300 Longwood Avenue, Boston, MA 02115, USA; [b] Department of Imaging and Interventional Radiology, The Chinese University of Hong Kong, Prince of Wales Hospital, 30-32 Ngan Shing Street, Shatin, NT, Hong Kong SAR, China
* Corresponding author.
E-mail address: Edward.Yang@childrens.harvard.edu

Radiol Clin N Am 55 (2017) 609–627
http://dx.doi.org/10.1016/j.rcl.2017.02.005
0033-8389/17/© 2017 Elsevier Inc. All rights reserved.

major categories of supratentorial brain malformation can be placed into a mechanistic context, including disorders of hemispheric cleavage (ie, holoprosencephaly [HPE]) and disorders of neuronal migration/organization (eg, gray matter heterotopia, lissencephaly/pachygyria, cortical dysplasia, polymicrogyria [PMG], and cobblestone malformation). Although nonspecific, callosal abnormalities also deserve discussion along with these supratentorial malformations due to their frequency in supratentorial brain malformations and their role as a sentinel sign for more widespread abnormalities. Finally, the issues of specificity that arise once a particular cerebral malformation is identified are briefly discussed.

EMBRYOLOGIC CONSIDERATIONS

The morphologically normal supratentorial brain or cerebrum has several obvious features. To begin with, there are 2 cerebral hemispheres of equal size separated by the interhemispheric fissure as well as the falx cerebri and joined by the major interhemispheric commissural tract, the corpus callosum, which suspends the septum pellucidum at the midline. In each cerebral hemisphere, there is an orderly arborization of the cerebral white matter peripherally. Overlying the subcortical white matter, there is cortical gray matter 2 mm to 4 mm thick, which is sharply defined from the white matter and seemingly uniform in thickness in any one region.[8] Although not visible on standard MR imaging, the cortex has 6 histologically recognizable layers.

This complex morphology of the cerebral hemispheres arises through embryologic transformations that far exceed what can be summarized briefly. But for the purpose of this article, the embryogenesis of the cerebral hemispheres can be viewed schematically as a series of steps (Fig. 1).[7,9,10] The first step is folding of the neural tube and closure of the tube at each end near the fourth week postconception, a process known as neurulation. By the 6th week, 2 separate vesicles arise from the primitive neuronal matrix at the anterior neural tube setting the stage for 2 separate cerebral hemispheres (ie, hemispheric separation). Between the 6th week and 16th week, neuronal precursor proliferation occurs deep within the cerebral hemispheres in the ventricular zone and subventricular zone, the ventricular zone representing what is later recognized as germinal matrix on imaging.[11–13] These neuronal precursors then undergo neuronal migration by moving radially outward between 8 weeks and 24 weeks postconception, populating the cortex with neurons and eventually organizing into 6 layers. As this migration occurs, there is also crossing of fiber tracts at sites of acquired fusion in the midline. Although initially at the anterior midline, the largest of these commissures, the corpus callosum, fuses with the hippocampal commissure located slightly posterior, and it progressively expands posteriorly between weeks 13 to 20 (discussed later).[14]

By the end of this schematized process through the 24th week postconception, the brain still has a primitive appearance with only minimal gyral convolution (see Fig. 1F–H), and the process described above omits certain key details, such as the presence of tangential as well as radial/centrifugal migration of neurons.[15,16] Nonetheless, the steps described above set the basic architectural plan for the brain and can explain the congenital brain malformations, described later. During the remainder of fetal life (24+ weeks), the brain assumes dramatically greater size/weight and increasing gyral complexity.[9] These later transformations, however, build on the foundation established earlier in gestation.

IMAGING TECHNIQUES

High-quality brain MR imaging is essential for an accurate analysis of brain malformations. Although a variety of technical parameters can provide good results,[17] pediatric patients at the authors' hospital for whom a structural brain abnormality is suspected (eg, medically intractable epilepsy) are imaged on a 3T MR instrument with a 32-channel or 64-channel head coil according to the imaging protocol, summarized in Box 1. This protocol includes isotropic (0.9-mm) T1-weighted and fluid-attenuated inversion recovery (FLAIR) MR imaging as well as high-resolution T2-weighted MR imaging in the axial and coronal planes, as shown in Fig. 2. Magnetization prepared T1-weighted MR imaging at isotropic resolution beautifully depicts gray-white matter interfaces with any regional abnormality easily compared with multiple cortical ribbons seen elsewhere in the same slice. The volumetric FLAIR MR imaging accentuates subtle signal abnormalities (cortical as well as white matter) that can indicate a cortical dysplasia; some institutions supplement this sequence with magnetization transfer imaging.[18] Finally, diffusion-weighted MR imaging can complement other imaging sequences in characterizing suspected gray matter heterotopias because heterotopias should follow gray matter sequences on all sequences, including diffusion-weighted sequences.

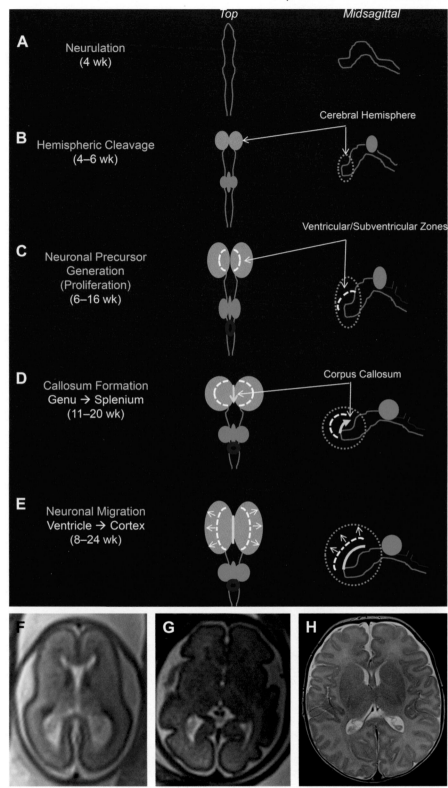

Fig. 1. Schematic for normal brain embryogenesis depicted from dorsal (top) and lateral (midsagittal) perspectives. Note: gestational age is greater than postfertilization age by 2 weeks. (*A*) Neurulation. After gastrulation and induction of the neural plate, the neural plate fuses at the dorsal midline by 4 weeks postfertilization to create a neural tube that defines the neuraxis (red) from brain to spinal cord. (*B*) Hemispheric separation. By 4 weeks to 6 weeks postfertilization, 2 discrete vesicles form defining the right and left cerebral hemisphere,

---

Box 1
Standard structural malformation (epilepsy) protocol (whole-brain coverage for all sequences)

3T MR imaging

32-channel or 64-channel head coil

Sagittal T1-weighted MPRAGE or IR-SPGR at isotropic resolution

Sagittal T2-weighted SPACE FLAIR or T2-weighted CUBE FLAIR at isotropic resolution

Coronal T2-weighted (0.4 mm × 0.5 mm × 2.5 mm skip 0 mm)

Axial T2-weighted (0.4 mm × 0.5 mm × 2.5 mm skip 0 mm)

Axial FLAIR (0.6 mm × 0.6 mm × 4 mm skip 1 mm)

Simultaneous multislice diffusion tensor imaging (35 directions, 1.5 mm × 1.5 mm × 2 mm skip 0 mm)

Pulsed arterial spin-labeled perfusion

Abbreviations: IR-SPGR, inversion recovery spoiled gradient echo; MPRAGE, magnetization prepared rapid acquisition gradient echo; SPACE, sampling perfection with application optimized constraints using different flip angle evolution.

ABNORMALITIES OF HEMISPHERIC CLEAVAGE

Alobar, Semilobar, and Lobar Holoprosencephaly

The HPEs are a group of disorders whose hallmark is fusion of the hemispheres across the midline and deficiency of the midline structures, reflecting failure of the hemispheric cleavage process, described previously. Classic HPEs disproportionately affect the ventral forebrain and exist in a spectrum of severity where alobar is the most severe, lobar is the least severe, and semilobar is somewhere in the middle.[19] The causes of these classic HPEs are myriad and include maternal factors, aneuploidies, and single-gene causes.[20–23]

Alobar HPE is characterized by complete lack of hemispheric separation. As a result, there is continuity of brain parenchyma across the midline with absence of the corpus callosum, falx cerebri, and septum pellucidum (**Fig. 3**A–C). Instead of 2 cerebral hemispheres and lateral ventricles, there is a thin saucer-shaped lobe of brain tissue enclosing a monoventricle without distinct temporal or frontal horns; frequently, the ventricle decompresses into a dorsal cyst. The abnormal fusion of the hemispheres usually involves the deep gray matter, resulting in an unusually small or absent third ventricle. As has long been appreciated,[24] facial anomalies (ie, hypotelorism, single maxillary central incisor, and facial clefting) are associated with HPE and tend to track with severity of the HPE. Therefore, such facial anomalies are more frequently associated with alobar HPE. Other accompanying abnormalities may occur with alobar as well as semilobar/lobar HPE, including azygous anterior cerebral arteries and absence of the olfactory apparatus.[19]

As less severe forms of HPE, semilobar and lobar HPEs demonstrate partial cleavage of the hemispheres posteriorly and dorsally. As a result, midline structures are partially formed, and there is proportionately greater formation of a normal ventricular system as well as hemispheric separation. For the more severe semilobar form, this partial separation results in some rudimentary posterior corpus callosum and definition of the temporal horns (**Fig. 3**D–F). Although the distinction between lobar and semilobar is somewhat arbitrary, lobar HPE is usually accepted for HPE with definition of at least the posterior half of the corpus callosum, the frontal/temporal horns,

---

depicted as gray ovals. (*C*) Neuronal precursor proliferation. From weeks 6 to 16, neuronal precursors proliferate in the ventricular and subventricular zones (dashed white lines deep in each hemisphere) to produce the neurons, which will eventually invest the gray matter. (*D*) Callosum formation. Between weeks 11 to 20, neurons cross the midline through the rudimentary corpus callosum increasing its posterior extent (*yellow arrow*). (*E*) Neuronal migration/organization. During weeks 8 to 24, neuronal precursors migrate radially outward (*white arrows*) to populate the cortex and eventually organize into 6 distinct cortical layers. (*F–H*) Gyral maturation. Axial T2-weighted imaging of the brain at 20 weeks postconception (*F*), at 28 weeks postconception (*G*), and at term (*H*). Although the brain at 20 weeks and even 28 weeks lacks the gyral complexity (and also the size that is not well appreciated) of the brain at term, the basic morphology of the brain has already been determined at midgestation by the events schematically depicted (*A–E*).

and the hippocampi (**Fig. 3G–I**).[25] For both semi-lobar and lobar HPEs, the ventral forebrain remains abnormally fused often with involvement of the deep gray matter structures,[26] and this fusion of the deep gray matter is also critical in recognizing a newly described mild HPE variant confined to the subcallosal ventral forebrain known as septopreoptic HPE (**Fig. 3J–L**).[27] Septopreoptic HPE fails to meet enrollment criteria for many historical HPE studies due to the sparing of the frontal cortex and presence (in some instances) of a fully formed septum pellucidum as well as corpus callosum.[28] It shares, however, many of the maxillofacial abnormalities seen in the other HPEs.

Middle Interhemispheric Variant of Holoprosencephaly

Unlike the classic HPE variants, described previously, middle interhemispheric variant (MIV) HPE (also called syntelencephaly) features a predominance of fusion in the dorsal forebrain.[29] Therefore, basal ganglia fusion is rare (although thalamic/midbrain fusion is still reported), and instead there is midline fusion of the dorsal fronto-parietal lobes. As a result, there is segmental disruption of the corpus callosum at the sites of fusion (ie, body of the callosum, sparing the genu/splenium) rather than the anterior-predominant disruption seen with classic HPEs,

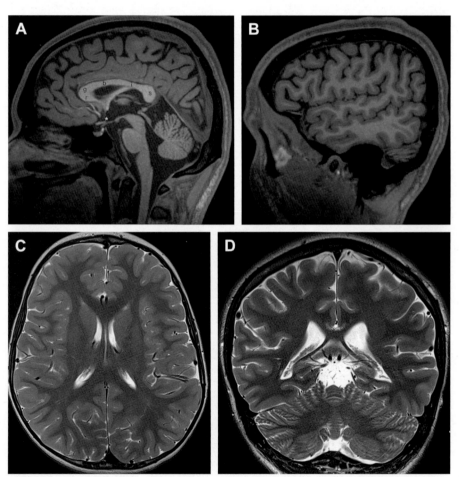

Fig. 2. Morphologically normal 3T brain MR image from a 17-year-old boy undergoing evaluation for generalized seizures. (*A*) The midsagittal T1-weighted sequence depicts the rostrum (r), genu (g), body (b), isthmus (i), and splenium (s) segments of a fully formed and normal-thickness corpus callosum. Note that the infundibular recess (*asterisk*) is sharply outlined by cerebrospinal fluid consistent with absence of deep gray matter (eg, hypothalamic) fusion anomalies. (*B*) A parasagittal T1-weighted image sharply defines gray-white matter interfaces with uniform gyral frequency and cortical thickness in any 1 region. The presence of multiple gray-white matter interfaces in 1 image slice facilitates comparison of any region of the brain to other regions of the brain. (*C, D*) Axial T2-weighted (*C*) and coronal T2-weighted (*D*) images of the brain confirm separation of the hemispheres in general and the deep gray matter specifically as suggested on the midsagittal T1-weighted image. They also depict the uniform gyral frequency, cortical thickness, and sharp gray-white matter differentiation seen on the parasagittal T1-weighted image.

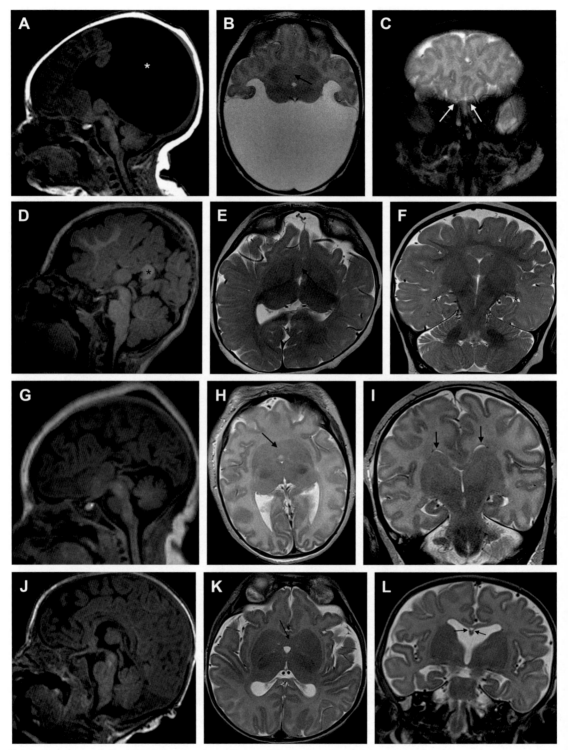

Fig. 3. Spectrum of classic HPE. As disorders of ventral induction, the classic HPEs share failure of cleavage of the ventral forebrain but have varying degrees of cleavage of the dorsal/posterior forebrain. This concept is illustrated (in order of decreasing severity) by infants with alobar (A–C), semilobar (D–F), lobar (G–I), and septopreoptic (J–L) HPE using sagittal T1-weighted (A, D, G, J), axial T2-weighted images through the deep gray matter (B, E, H, K), and coronal T2-weighted images (C, F, I, L). In alobar HPE (A–C), there is an undivided cerebrum enclosing a monoventricle frequently in communication with a dorsal cyst (asterisk [A]). There is no falx/callosum/septum pellucidum, and the deep gray matter structures are fused (arrow [B]). Often, the olfactory apparatus are absent

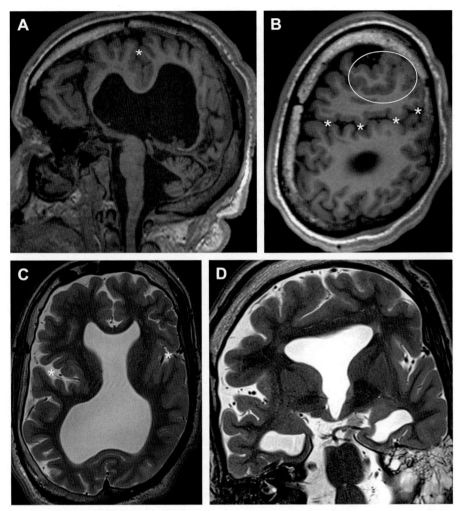

Fig. 4. MIV HPE in a 17-year-old boy with intellectual disability and cerebral palsy. Sagittal T1-weighted (*A*), axial T1-weighted (*B*), axial T2-weighted (*C*), and coronal T2-weighted (*D*) images demonstrate continuity of the dorsal frontoparietal lobes across the midline, where there is absence of a falx and segmental disruption of the normal corpus callosum. As a result, there is continuity of the sylvian fissures across the midline (*asterisks [A–C]*). In contrast to the classic HPEs described earlier (see **Fig. 3**), the anterior and posterior interhemispheric fissure and the ventral forebrain (basal ganglia) are normally cleaved (*C, D*) despite the segmental fusion at the dorsal frontoparietal junction. MIV HPE is unique among the HPEs for the high reported prevalence of cortical malformations, a point illustrated by frontal PMG in this case (*circle [B]*). The posterior pituitary bright spot is not visualized in this patient (*A*), but he has no clinical endocrine deficiencies.

although the septum pellucidum is still absent (**Fig. 4**). Along the cerebral convexities, MIV HPE is also recognizable for rotation of the sylvian fissures into the coronal plane and continuity side-to-side over the vertex. Unlike the other forms of HPE, MIV HPE is reported to have a very high co-occurrence of migrational abnormalities, mandating close attention to the cerebral cortex

---

(*arrows [C]*). In semilobar HPE (*D–F*), there is rudimentary separation of the posterior hemispheres by a posterior falx and short posterior callosum (*asterisk [D]*). The temporal horns (*asterisks [F]*) may be formed but not the frontal horns. The frontal lobes and the basal ganglia remain fused (*arrow [E]*). In lobar HPE (*G–I*), this partitioning of the hemispheres is more complete with at least half the posterior corpus callosum being formed along with the frontal horns (*arrows [I]*). The deep gray matter remains abnormally fused (*arrow [H]*), however. In septopreoptic HPE, the deep gray matter structures are also fused (*arrow [K]*), but, unlike the other classic HPEs, a rudimentary septum pellucidum is identifiable (*arrows [L]*) and the corpus callosum is fully formed.

in patients where this diagnosis is suggested. Although the difference in location of fused brain suggests genetic/mechanistic differences in MIV HPE versus classic HPEs, a monozygotic twin pregnancy (ie, same mutation) has been documented with MIV HPE in 1 and alobar HPE in the other twin so these distinctions may not be as biologically different as believed.[30] In any event, the morphologic distinction of MIV HPE is nonetheless important because this group of patients has lower endocrine and movement disorder morbidity than seen with other HPEs (spasticity and developmental delay are still significant problems).[31,32]

Septo-optic Dysplasia

Septo-optic dysplasia is a clinical syndrome featuring optic pathway hypoplasia and hypothalamic-pituitary axis deficiencies. It is discussed in this section because it sometimes enters the differential diagnosis in a case of HPE due to the absence of the septum pellucidum as well as associated optic nerve hypoplasia, pituitary hypoplasia/ectopia, and (sometimes) malformed olfactory apparatus. The imaging features are otherwise quite distinct from HPE, however, in that the hemispheres are fully cleaved, and, unlike classic HPEs, there is schizencephaly or polymicrogyria in up to half of cases.[33,34] It is important to acknowledge that this clinico-radiologically defined group of pediatric patients is diverse, with some evidence of both environmental as well as genetic etiologies.[35,36] Additionally, it should also be recognized that some clinically diagnosed cases of septo-optic dysplasia may nonetheless have a septum pellucidum.[37,38] A typical septo-optic dysplasia case is shown in **Fig. 5**.

CALLOSAL ABNORMALITIES

Although common in congenital brain malformations as a group,[39–41] particular types of corpus callosum abnormalities do not generally segregate with specific classes of brain malformations with the exception of the posterior-sparing callosal dysgenesis, described previously.[42] Nonetheless, callosal abnormalities appropriately receive a great deal of emphasis when screening the brain for structural abnormalities because the 5 segments of the corpus callosum are superbly depicted by midsagittal MR imaging sequences (see **Fig. 2A**), providing a sensitive means of detecting abnormalities in the corpus callosum. These callosal abnormalities are sometimes the first or only clue that a patient's brain is structurally abnormal, focusing attention on the potential for additional abnormalities. Therefore, it is worth considering callosal abnormalities as a group.

As suggested in **Fig. 1**, the corpus callosum develops after hemispheric cleavage from the neural tube and overlaps with the process of radial neuronal migration. This sequence is not surprising because the nerve fibers that cross the interhemispheric fissure and form the corpus callosum must themselves migrate across the midline. Although historically described as developing by stepwise crossing of fibers in a largely anterior-to-posterior fashion (genu then body, isthmus, splenium, and finally rostrum), current understanding is that 3 distinct commissures are present at approximately the 13th week postconception near an anterior structure above the foramen of Monro called the lamina reunions[14]: the anterior commissure, the hippocampal commissure/posterior callosum, and the anterior corpus callosum where the anterior callosum is actually the last to form. By the 14th week, the anterior and posterior callosum fuse creating the template for all remaining callosal fibers, but the callosum is short. This rudimentary callosum then lengthens/thickens into a recognizable 5-segment corpus callosum by the twentieth week, driven by the disproportionate enlargement of the frontal lobes and their crossing fibers into the preexisting callosum, effectively pushing the splenial segment posteriorly. As a result, underdevelopment of the callosum results in truncation posteriorly. Two exceptions to this tendency to grow posteriorly include the HPEs, discussed previously, as well as very rare cases of segmental dysgenesis of the corpus callosum (ie, failure of fusion of the anterior and posterior callosum, leading to a missing segment of callosum).

Dysgenesis or hypogenesis of the corpus callosum refers to incomplete formation of the 5 segments of the corpus callosum and resultant foreshortening of anteroposterior (AP) dimension. On the other hand, callosal hypoplasia refers to abnormal thickness of a corpus callosum, which has normal AP dimension.[42] The most severe form of dysgenesis, agenesis, is recognizable by absence of the corpus callosum, absence of a normal septum pellucidum, absence of the cingulate gyrus, under-rotation of the hippocampi, prominence of the posterior lateral ventricles (colpocephaly), parallel configuration of the lateral ventricles in the axial plane, steer-horn shape of the frontal horns in the coronal plane, a high-riding third ventricle, and redirection of white matter tracts along the medial aspect of the lateral ventricles (Probst bundles).[25] A more attenuated phenotype is present with partial agenesis of the corpus callosum (eg, parallel configuration of the

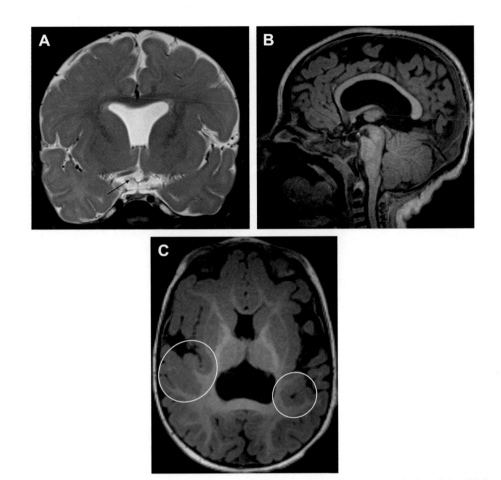

Fig. 5. Septo-optic dysplasia in a 9-month-old boy with optic nerve hypoplasia. Coronal T2-weighted (*A*), sagittal T1-weighted (*B*), and axial T1-weighted (*C*) images of the brain demonstrate absence of the septum pellucidum in the presence of a fully formed corpus callosum. Optic hypoplasia, olfactory hypoplasia, and abnormalities of the pituitary gland are also common in septoptic dysplasia—in this case, there is radiographic hypoplasia of the right optic nerve (*arrow* [*A*]). Although bearing some superficial similarity to HPE due to the lack of a septum pellucidum, a major point of distinction from HPE is the full separation of the cerebral hemispheres in septo-optic dysplasia, including of the ventral forebrain. Also in distinction from classic HPE, there is a high incidence of cortical malformations, such as schizencephaly and PMG. In this case, extensive perisylvian and frontal PMG are present (perisylvian PMG circled [*C*]).

lateral ventricles and colpocephaly but presence of the septum for dysgenesis restricted to the posterior callosum). Hypoplasia does not typically share the features of callosal dysgenesis and must be distinguished from volume loss secondary to injury. When in doubt whether hypoplasia or dysgenesis is present (eg, thinning of the splenium), reference measurements are available for normal children that can bring some quantitative rigor to a visual assessment.[43,44] The spectrum of callosal abnormalities is depicted in **Fig. 6.**

ABNORMALITIES OF NEURONAL MIGRATION

Although the remaining supratentorial brain malformations to be discussed have a wide diversity of morphologic appearances, they can be regarded as deviations from the schematically outlined process of radial migration shown in **Fig. 1.** As discussed below, aberrant neuronal migration can be insufficient or excessive, focal or global.

Gray Matter Heterotopia

Gray matter heterotopia are foci of neurons inappropriately arrested between the origin of neuron migration (subependymal or periventricular regions, corresponding to germinal matrix and subventricular zones, respectively) and their normal destination (ie, cortex). This arrested migration has been attributed to genetic defects in

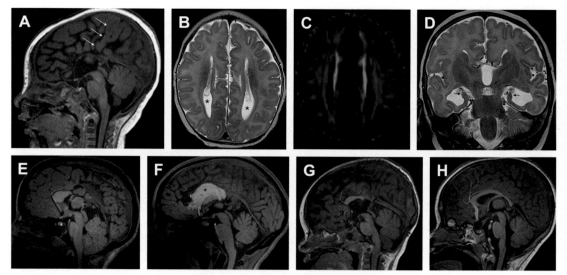

Fig. 6. Spectrum of callosal abnormalities. Complete agenesis of the corpus callosum with absence of the anterior/hippocampal commissures (tricommissural callosal agenesis) in a 4-month-old boy with microcephaly is depicted using sagittal T1-weighted (A), axial T2-weighted (B), color fractional anisotropy maps from diffusion tensor imaging (C), and coronal T2-weighted images (D). As depicted in (A), the third ventricle is high riding and there is no distinct cingulate gyrus/sulcus due to absence of the corpus callosum. Instead, the gyral folds (eg, arrows [A]) radiate uninterrupted from the vertex down to the third ventricle. Associated ventricular dysmorphology is present, including a parallel configuration of the ventricles (B, D) and dilation of the atria of the lateral ventricles or colpocephaly (asterisks [B]). Accompanying structural abnormalities include redirection of Probst bundles along medial walls of the lateral ventricles (medial green fibers [C]) and underrotation of the hippocampi (arrows [D]). Hypogenesis or partial agenesis of the corpus callosum refers to arrested elongation of the corpus callosum from its starting point near the roof of the third ventricle. As a result, the callosum is variably foreshortened in the AP dimension, as demonstrated by midsagittal T1-weighted images from 12-year-old, 5-year-old, and 14-month-old patients with varying degrees of callosal foreshortening (E–G). As illustrated by these cases, the formed segments are often dysmorphic and may have accompanying abnormalities (eg, pericallosal lipoma [asterisk (F)]). Unlike hypogenesis, callosal hypoplasia refers to normal AP length and formation of the callosal segments with abnormal thickness. An example of callosal (splenial) hypoplasia from a 5-year-old boy with developmental delay is shown (H).

structural proteins necessary for radial migration and possibly to focal insults.[6,45] Gray matter heterotopia are classified according to location: periventricular (ie, at the ventricular margin, also called subependymal), subcortical (nodular and curvilinear forms), and transmantle.[46] Of these categories, the most commonly encountered as well as the best understood type of gray matter heterotopia is periventricular nodular heterotopia (PVNH). Genetically defined forms of PVNH are known to occur as multifocal masslike conglomerates of gray matter—for example, in association with posterior fossa anomalies (eg, mega cisterna magna), hyperextensibility, and congenital cardiac disease in female patients (ie, FLNA mutations) or with microcephaly (ie, ARGEF2 mutations).[6,47,48]

The hallmark of PVNH is nodular soft tissue, which follows gray matter on all sequences (T1-weighted, T2-weighted, and diffusion).[49,50] Therefore, nodular foci with signal characteristics different from gray matter elsewhere should prompt skepticism of gray matter heterotopia as an explanation with few exceptions.[51,52] Location of the heterotopias has been shown to have some importance. For instance, unilateral and posterior (trigonal/temporal) PVNH are known to have an association with additional cortical malformations in up to half of cases, the posterior PVNH also notable for high association with callosal and posterior fossa anomalies (eg, cerebellar hypoplasia and mega cisterna magna).[45,53] Reductions in white matter volume are frequent across all PVNH subgroups.[45] Although historically PVNH has been associated with extremely high rates of epilepsy, there is some evidence of decreased neurologic morbidity for individuals with less extensive PVNH.[46] Also, it has been the authors' experience that small PVNH foci may be incidentally detected in neurologically normal individuals during routine clinical work (eg, in patients referred for trauma). Examples of PVNH and their differentiation from other causes of ependymal nodularity are shown in **Fig. 7A–G.**

Although the clinical significance and genetic basis of PVNH are well documented, the other forms of gray matter heterotopia (nodular subcortical, curvilinear subcortical, and transmantle) are much less well understood.[54,55] In the authors' experience, subcortical nodular gray matter heterotopia are most commonly encountered in pediatric patients with developmental delay, and curvilinear subcortical gray matter heterotopia most commonly encountered in pediatric patients with multiple congenital anomalies or callosal dysgenesis (eg, some forms of callosal agenesis with interhemispheric cysts are associated with subcortical gray matter heterotopia[56]). Also by clinical experience, transmantle cortical dysplasia is often encountered in the setting of cortical malformations, such as PMG. The imaging characteristics are similar, however, to PVNH despite the differences in location apart from prominent perivascular spaces in the curvilinear form of subcortical heterotopia. Examples of subcortical and transmantle heterotopia are shown in **Fig. 7H–J.**

Lissencephaly/Pachygyria/Subcortical Band Heterotopia

Where PVNH represents a focal disturbance in neuronal migration, lissencephaly, pachygyria, and subcortical band heterotopia (SBH) represent a more diffuse disturbance of neuronal migration. The hallmark of lissencephaly, pachygyria, and SBH is a thick zone of cortical/subcortical gray matter with varying degrees of gyral simplification. Even before current genetic understanding united them mechanistically, these entities were understood to exist on a spectrum where the most severe form, lissencephaly, features complete lack of normal sulcation (agyria); pachygyria (incomplete lissencephaly) features undersulcation with broadened/rudimentary gyri; and the least severe form, SBH, demonstrates the presence of some normal sulcation with a subcortical layer of heterotopic gray matter.[57,58] Histologically, lissencephaly and pachygyria reflect abnormal layering of the cortex where the cortex has 2 to 4 layers rather than the normal 6 layers, and high-resolution MR imaging can sometimes distinguish a cell-sparse

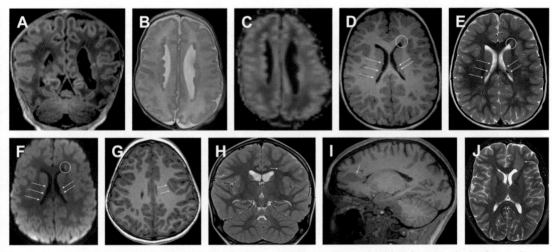

Fig. 7. Gray matter heterotopias depicted by location. PVNH in a 7-month-old girl with valvular heart disease, developmental delay, and a *FLNA* mutation (*A–C*) as well as a 4-year-old boy with tuberous sclerosis (*D–F*). In periventricular gray matter heterotopia, islands of gray matter signal are found near the ependymal origin of neuronal precursor cells. In the case of the patient with an *FLNA* mutation (*A–C*), there is multifocal studding of the ependymal surface by gray matter nodules. In the case of the tuberous sclerosis patient (*D–F*), there is a solitary gray matter heterotopion in the left frontal horn (*circles*). In both cases, the gray matter heterotopia follow gray matter signal on coronal/axial T1-weighted (*A, D*), axial T2-weighted (*B, E*), and diffusion-weighted imaging (*C, F*) regardless of myelination stage. The signal characteristics of gray matter heterotopia allow differentiation from other causes of ependymal nodularity. For example, the subependymal nodules of tuberous sclerosis (*arrows [D–F]*) are readily differentiated from the gray matter signal in the left frontal periventricular nodular heterotopion (*circles [D–F]*) due to their dissimilarity from gray matter on multiple sequences. Additional sites of gray matter heterotopia include subcortical gray matter heterotopia (axial T1-weighted [*arrows (G)*] and coronal T2-weighted [*arrow (H)*]), from a 4-year-old girl with developmental delay) and transmatle heterotopia (in sagittal T1-weighted [*arrow (I)*] and axial T2-weighted [*arrow (J)*] images from a 19-year-old girl with neurofibromatosis type 2).

layer separating the outer cortex from cortical layers arrested over a wide zone in the white matter.[59,60]

On the other hand, the more normal gyration in SBH has been shown to reflect a normal 6-layer cortex separated by a well-defined gap of radiographically normal white matter from a thick heterotopic layer of neurons in the subcortical white matter.[61–63] Therefore, the histologic basis of the unusually thick cortical/subcortical gray matter differs in lissencephaly/pachygyria and SBH. The exact location along the lissencephaly/pachygyria/SBH spectrum depends on both the specific genetic cause as well as the percentage of brain tissue expressing aberrant gene product:

fractional involvement by mutations (mosaic mutations) have less severe imaging/clinical phenotypes than those mutations found in every cell (germline mutations).[64,65] Finally, certain gene mutations are known to produce anterior-predominant lissencephaly (eg, the doublecortin gene, DCX) whereas others produce posterior-predominant lissencephaly (eg, the LIS1 gene).[6] These concepts are illustrated in Fig. 8 by sexual dimorphism associated with mutations in the DCX gene, which is located on the X chromosome: there is anterior pachygyria in a male patient (see Fig. 8A–B) with a DCX mutation (single copy is mutated) and less severe anterior-predominant SBH in a female patient (see Fig. 8C–D) with a

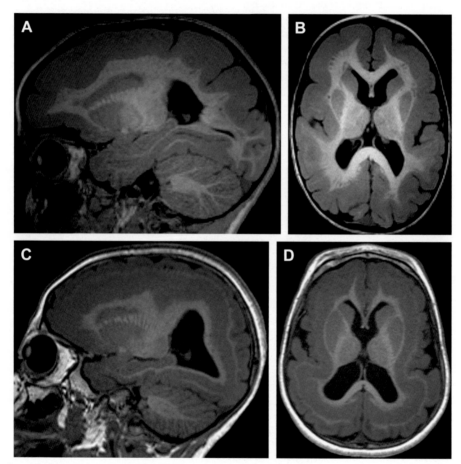

Fig. 8. Pachygyria (incomplete lissencephaly) in an 18-month-old boy (A, B) and SBH in a 25-month-old girl (C, D). In pachygyria, there is failure to form a normal 6-layer cortex with resultant cortical thickening and broadening of gyri as seen on the provided sagittal T1-weighted (A) and axial T1-weighted (B) images. SBH is a more attenuated phenotype where abnormal heterotopic neurons accumulate underneath a cortex with more normal thickness and gyration. As seen on the sagittal T1-weighted (C) and axial T1-weighted (D) images from the shown example, there is a thick band of arrested/heterotopic gray matter underneath the simplified cortical ribbon separated by normal-appearing white matter. Both of these patients had a mutation in the doublecortin gene DCX located on the X chromosome, explaining the attenuated phenotype (SBH) usually seen in female patients who have 1 normal and 1 abnormal copy of the gene. In both the pachygyria and SBH for doublecortin mutations, the cortical malformation is most severe anteriorly; an AP gradient is also seen in other genetic causes of pachygyria.

DCX mutation (1 of 2 *DCX* copies are mutated with disease expression partly governed by X-linked inactivation).

Focal Cortical Dysplasia

Focal cortical dysplasia (FCD) is defined as an area of cortical disorganization where FCD I features disruption of normal cortical lamination and columnar organization; FCD II features dysplastic neurons and microscopic foci of neuronal heterotopia in the white matter; and FCD III consists of collision lesions of FCD I and another epileptic lesion (eg, mesial temporal sclerosis, cavernoma, or ganglioglioma).[66] FCD I and FCD II can be conceptualized as microscopic smearing of normal neuronal precursors en route to the cortex, for FCD IIs which are better understood at a molecular level, probably with co-occurrence of abnormal proliferation based on emerging evidence for underlying somatic mutations.[67–71] Detection of FCDs has outsized importance in pediatric patients with refractory epilepsy because FCDs are highly epileptogenic (difficult to manage by medication) and are found in up to 75% of medically refractory epilepsy cases considered for resection, and identification of FCD before surgery dramatically improves seizure freedom.[72–74]

On imaging, the FCDs share loss (blurring) of the normally crisp gray-white matter interface with or without associated signal abnormality. In cases of FCD I, these abnormalities may be subtle and in some instances a radiographically recognizable abnormality may not be found.[73,75] For FCD IIs, up to half of FCD IIa and almost all FCD IIb lesions feature a so called transmantle sign (signal increase widest at the cortex and tapering toward the ventricular margin), an anatomic configuration that recapitulates normal dispersion of neuronal precursors as they transit from subventricular/ventricular zones to the cortex.[73,74,76] The resemblance of the transmantle sign to cortical tubers of tuberous sclerosis is not a coincidence: tubers are histologically related to FCD IIb,[77] and the *TSC* genes are involved in the same signaling pathways implicated in FCD II.[6] Imaging features of FCDs are illustrated in **Fig. 9A–F.** Although generally static in appearance once myelination is mature,[78,79] occasional follow-up imaging is entirely reasonable for suspected FCDs that lack a transmantle sign because the differential for cortically based signal increase includes infiltrating gliomas.

Polymicrogyria

In PMG, neuronal precursors arrive at the cortex but do not organize normally. Therefore, most experts consider this malformation a disorder of cortical organization rather than one of migration,[7] but it is discussed with disorders where the cortical migration itself is aberrant. Although some investigators use differing histologic criteria (eg, whether to include transpial neuronal migration as seen in cobblestone malformations), it is generally agreed that there is abnormal fusion of the outer cortical layer (layer I, the molecular layer), and as a result there is buckling of the cortical surface that produces the increased gyral frequency that is a hallmark of PMG.[80–82] A wide range of genetic mutations and environmental insults (eg, ischemia and cytomegalovirus infection) has been implicated in PMG.[6,83,84]

The most common pattern of PMG is perisylvian PMG, with diffuse or unilateral PMG the second most common depending on the case series. In regions affected by PMG, there is abnormally increased gyral frequency with loss of normal surface anatomy (eg, absence/distortion of normal sylvian fissure in perisylvian PMG). With inadequate resolution, PMG can be mistaken for pachygyria (ie, thickened cortex), although this error is infrequently encountered with modern high-field MR imaging systems and isotropic imaging. With 7T imaging, prominent cortical veins may be identified within areas of PMG, as is the case histologically, and different morphologic categories of PMG (coarse, delicate, and sawtooth) begin to approximate one another.[85] Gray-white matter interfaces remain sharply defined to the extent that gyral frequency can be adequately resolved, a point also illustrated by high field 7T imaging. Examples of PMG are shown in **Fig. 10.**

Cobblestone Malformation

The cerebral cortex is bounded by the pia mater with an intervening basement membrane. Should migrating neurons fail to stop at the basement membrane, they continue through the pia and spill into the subarachnoid space.[86] This overmigration leads to the so-called cobblestone malformation (once known as type II lissencephaly, reflecting historical confusion between this entity and classic or type I lissencephaly, discussed earlier). A large number of structural proteins involved in adherence of the neuronal cell membrane to the basement membrane have been implicated in cobblestone malformation.[6] Perhaps the best known cause is mutation involving the dystroglycan complex anchoring neuronal cytoskeleton to the extracellular matrix, which produces clinical syndromes with central nervous system and muscle phenotypes (ie, muscle-eye-brain disease, Walker-Warburg syndrome, and Fukuyama muscular dystrophy).[87]

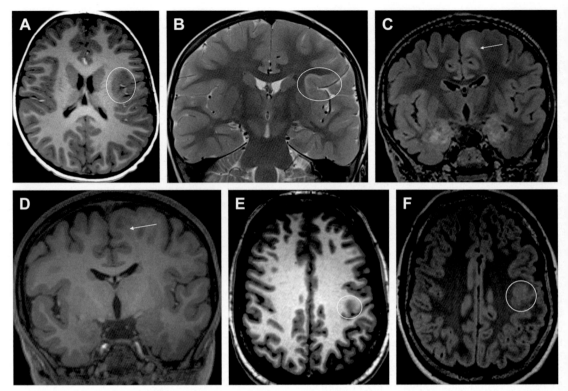

Fig. 9. FCD type I in a 3-year-old boy with focal right upper extremity motor seizures (*A, B*). An axial T1-weighted image (*A*) demonstrates thickening and indistinctness of the left frontal operculum and insular cortical ribbon (*circle* [*A*]). The same area demonstrates cortical T2-weighted hyperintensity on a coronal T2-weighted image (*circle* [*B*]). FCD type IIb in a 6-year-old girl with epileptic encephalopathy (*C, D*). Coronal FLAIR (*C*) and coronal T1-weighted (*D*) images demonstrate a left frontal transmantle sign (*arrow*) with cortical/subcortical signal increase that tapers to a point in the periventricular white matter. This is a specific sign for type IIb FCD and the tubers of tuberous sclerosis with which they share a microscopic similarity in appearance. FCD type IIb in an 18-year-old boy with longstanding focal right-sided motor seizures (*E, F*). Axial T1-weighted (*E*) and axial FLAIR (*F*) images demonstrate indistinctness of the left precentral gyrus (*circle*). The absence of a discernible transmantle sign in this case is a reminder that FCD IIb may have a variety of radiographic presentations.

As shown in **Fig. 11**, the cerebral cortex in these patients appears thick and nodular on high-resolution imaging with subcortical islands of gray matter and subcortical white matter dysmyelination (ie, inappropriate FLAIR/T2-weighted hyperintensity for age).[25] Accompanying abnormalities may include a kinked dysmorphic brainstem, distortion/hypoplasia and microcystic change of the cerebellum, callosal hypoplasia, cephaloceles, and eye abnormalities (eg, microphthalmia and persistent hyperplastic primary vitreous). With time, it has become apparent that the cortical nodularity of the cobblestone malformations can present in a manner indistinguishable from PMG (ie, increased gyral frequency and nodular appearance of the cortex).[88,89] Additional imaging features are usually present for the many known mimics, however, such as abnormal basal ganglia fusion in tubulinopathies (discussed later)

or dysmyelination for *GPR56*-related cobblestone malformation.[88,90]

SPECIFICITY IN SUPRATENTORIAL BRAIN MALFORMATIONS

Once a specific supratentorial brain malformation has been suggested, referring physicians naturally have an interest in a differential diagnosis that includes specific genetic causes. Although that degree of specificity can be challenging, even for subspecialists who deal with brain malformations on a daily basis, some helpful clues can be gleaned from additional imaging findings, including abnormal brain size, basal ganglia anomalies, brainstem/cerebellar abnormalities, and callosal dysgenesis. This concept of integrating all imaging findings to suggest a specific diagnosis is familiar to most radiologists from

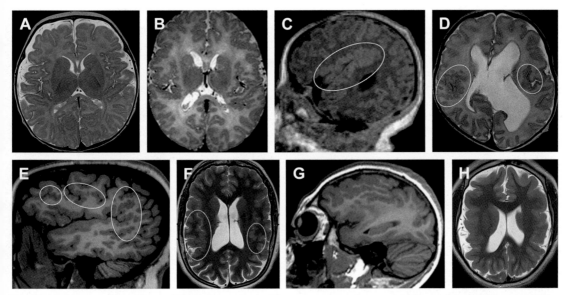

Fig. 10. Various manifestations of PMG. Compared with a normal newborn axial T2-weighted MR imaging (*A*), a newborn with macrocephaly (*B*) demonstrates diffuse increase in gyral frequency typical of PMG. Right parasagittal T1-weighted (*C*) and axial T2-weighted (*D*) images in another newborn with prenatally diagnosed partial agenesis of the corpus callosum demonstrates obscuration of the normal sylvian fissures by perisylvian PMG (right greater than left [*circles* (*C*, *D*)]). Right parasagittal T1-weighted (*E*) and axial T2-weighted (*F*) images from a 17-year-old boy with focal seizures demonstrate thicker/coarser increase in gyral frequency in areas of PMG (*circles* [*E*, *F*]), reflecting mature myelination and thickening of the cortex compared with the earlier neonatal cases. An 11-year-old boy with microcephaly, global developmental delay, and spastic quadraparesis demonstrates extensive frontoparietal PMG on sagittal T1-weighted (*G*) and axial T2-weighted (*H*) images. The polymicrogyria in this case is finer than the case in the 17 year old (*E–F*) but is still easily recognizable, particularly because of the loss of normal surface anatomy (eg, obscuration of the sylvian fissures [*H*]).

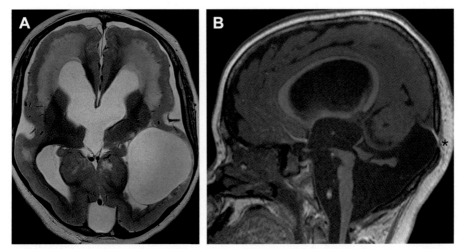

Fig. 11. Cobblestone malformation in a 10-year-old boy with Walker-Warburg syndrome (*A–B*). Axial T2-weighted image (*A*) demonstrates irregular cortical thickening with tiny centrifugal tongues of gray matter extending from the white matter. The white matter volume is low and the white matter that is present demonstrates diffuse T2-weighted hyperintensity (dysmyelination). The sagittal T1-weighted image (*B*) demonstrates marked thinning of the brainstem and cerebellar hypoplasia. A defect from a repaired occipital cephalocele is visible (*asterisk* [*B*]). Although some forms of cobblestone malformation may simulate polymicrogyria, the presence of dysmyelination and additional syndromic clinical findings (eg, muscle weakness and eye anomalies) allow for radiographic and clinical differentiation of most cobblestone malformations from PMG.

cytomegalovirus infection where PMG is found in the setting of microcephaly, calcifications, parenchymal cysts, and cerebellar hypoplasia.[91] It also applies, however, to genetic causes. For example, tubulin dimers assemble into microtubules necessary for radial neuronal migration. Therefore, it is unsurprising that lissencephalies and radiographic PMG (shown to be cobblestone malformation in pathology series) are found in mutations affecting several tubulin genes.[92] These tubulinopathies can be frequently recognized by the high prevalence of basal ganglia fusion (ie, fusion of the caudate to the ipsilateral lentiform nucleus), callosal dysgenesis, cerebellar dysplasia, and microcephaly.[93,94] The finding of basal ganglia fusion is sufficiently distinctive that it has led to recognition of abnormal gyral patterns in some tubulinopathies, which do not meet imaging criteria for PMG or pachygyria.[95,96]

Although neuronal precursor proliferation is treated as a schematically separate process in **Fig. 1**, it is also important to note that there is a linkage between neuronal proliferation (brain size) and neuronal migration abnormalities. This concept has been illustrated in several genetically defined microcephalies where cortical malformations have been encountered.[97,98] Conversely, large brains with PMG or dysplastic megalencephaly (the broader term for hemimegalencephaly featuring disorganized brain with histologic resemblance to FCD type IIb) can suggest mutations affecting proliferative gene products in the PTEN/AKT/mTOR signaling pathway.[99] In addition to obvious macrocephaly, these megalencephaly syndromes may have additional clinical findings, such as polydactyly and skin lesions (eg, capillary malformations).

SUMMARY

In this brief up-to-date review, malformations of the supratentorial brain are outlined from the perspective of the embryologic processes required to create the morphologically normal cerebrum and the malformations that result from errors in these processes. These processes include hemispheric cleavage (HPE) and neuronal migration/organization (gray matter heterotopia, lissencephaly/pachygria spectrum, FCD, PMG, and cobblestone malformations). Even though a specific diagnosis is usually not possible to suggest, this practical approach allows for sufficient phenotypic specificity such that neurologists can order appropriate gene panels and direct the care of patients. Although understanding of the genetics of supratentorial brain malformations is certain to evolve further, the basic patterns of dysmorphology described will continue to provide a basis for understanding pediatric patients with congenital brain malformations far into the future.

REFERENCES

1. Olson H, Yang E, Poduri A. Epileptogenic cerebral cortical malformations. 4th Edition. In: Pellock JM, Nordli DR, Sankar R, et al, editors. Pellock's pediatric epilepsy. New York: Demos Medical; 2016. p. 111–43.
2. Wu YW, Croen LA, Shah SJ, et al. Cerebral palsy in a term population: risk factors and neuroimaging findings. Pediatrics 2006;118(2):690–7.
3. Griffiths PD, Batty R, Warren D, et al. The use of MR imaging and spectroscopy of the brain in children investigated for developmental delay: what is the most appropriate imaging strategy? Eur Radiol 2011;21(9):1820–30.
4. Moeschler JB, Shevell M, Committee on Genetics. Comprehensive evaluation of the child with intellectual disability or global developmental delays. Pediatrics 2014;134(3):e903–18.
5. Verity C, Firth H, French-Constant C. Congenital abnormalities of the central nervous system. J Neurol Neurosurg Psychiatr 2003;74(Suppl 1):i3–8.
6. Guerrini R, Dobyns WB. Malformations of cortical development: clinical features and genetic causes. Lancet Neurol 2014;13(7):710–26.
7. Barkovich AJ, Guerrini R, Kuzniecky RI, et al. A developmental and genetic classification for malformations of cortical development: update 2012. Brain 2012;135(Pt 5):1348–69.
8. Fischl B, Dale AM. Measuring the thickness of the human cerebral cortex from magnetic resonance images. Proc Natl Acad Sci U S A 2000;97(20):11050–5.
9. Ten Donkelaar HJ, Lammens M, Renier W, et al. Development and developmental disorders of the cerebral cortex. Chapter 10. In: Ten Donkelaar HJ, Lammens M, Hori A, editors. Clinical neuroembryology. Germany: Springer-Verlag; 2010. p. 429–518.
10. Ten Donkelaar HJ, Van der Vliet T. Overview of the development of the human brain and spinal cord. Chapter 1. In: Ten Donkelaar HJ, Lammens M, Hori A, editors. Clinical neuroembryology. Germany: Springer-Verlag; 2010. p. 1–45.
11. Kostovic I, Vasung L. Insights from in vitro fetal magnetic resonance imaging of cerebral development. Semin Perinatol 2009;33(4):220–33.
12. Lui JH, Hansen DV, Kriegstein AR. Development and evolution of the human neocortex. Cell 2011;146(1):18–36.
13. Glenn OA, Barkovich AJ. Magnetic resonance imaging of the fetal brain and spine: an increasingly important tool in prenatal diagnosis, part 1. AJNR Am J Neuroradiol 2006;27(8):1604–11.
14. Raybaud C. The corpus callosum, the other great forebrain commissures, and the septum

pellucidum: anatomy, development, and malformation. Neuroradiology 2010;52(6):447–77.

15. Ten Donkelaar HJ, Lammens M, Cruysberg RM, et al. Development and developmental disorders of the forebrain. Chapter 9. In: Ten Donkelaar HJ, Lammens M, Hori A, editors. Clinical neuroembryology. Germany: Springer-Verlag; 2010. p. 345–428.

16. Kolasinski J, Takahashi E, Stevens AA, et al. Radial and tangential neuronal migration pathways in the human fetal brain: anatomically distinct patterns of diffusion MRI coherence. Neuroimage 2013;79:412–22.

17. Gaillard WD, Chiron C, Cross JH, et al. Guidelines for imaging infants and children with recent-onset epilepsy. Epilepsia 2009;50(9):2147–53.

18. Vezina LG. MRI-negative epilepsy: protocols to optimize lesion detection. Epilepsia 2011;52(Suppl 4): 25–7.

19. Hahn JS, Barnes PD. Neuroimaging advances in holoprosencephaly: Refining the spectrum of the midline malformation. Am J Med Genet C Semin Med Genet 2010;154C(1):120–32.

20. Miller EA, Rasmussen SA, Siega-Riz AM, et al. Risk factors for non-syndromic holoprosencephaly in the National Birth Defects Prevention Study. Am J Med Genet C Semin Med Genet 2010;154C(1):62–72.

21. Solomon BD, Rosenbaum KN, Meck JM, et al. Holoprosencephaly due to numeric chromosome abnormalities. Am J Med Genet C Semin Med Genet 2010;154C(1):146–8.

22. Mercier S, Dubourg C, Belleguic M, et al. Genetic counseling and "molecular" prenatal diagnosis of holoprosencephaly (HPE). Am J Med Genet C Semin Med Genet 2010;154C(1):191–6.

23. Haas D, Muenke M. Abnormal sterol metabolism in holoprosencephaly. Am J Med Genet C Semin Med Genet 2010;154C(1):102–8.

24. Demyer W, Zeman W, Palmer CG. The face predicts the brain: diagnostic significance of median facial anomalies for Holoprosencephaly (Arhinencephaly). Pediatrics 1964;34:256–63.

25. Barkovich AJ, Raybaud CA. Congenital malformations of the brain and skull. Chapter 5. In: Barkovich AJ, Raybaud CA, editors. Pediatric neuroimaging. Philadelphia: Wolters Kluwer; 2012. p. 367–568.

26. Simon EM, Hevner R, Pinter JD, et al. Assessment of the deep gray nuclei in holoprosencephaly. AJNR Am J Neuroradiol 2000;21(10):1955–61.

27. Hahn JS, Barnes PD, Clegg NJ, et al. Septopreoptic holoprosencephaly: a mild subtype associated with midline craniofacial anomalies. AJNR Am J Neuroradiol 2010;31(9):1596–601.

28. Marcorelles P, Laquerriere A. Neuropathology of holoprosencephaly. Am J Med Genet C Semin Med Genet 2010;154C(1):109–19.

29. Simon EM, Hevner RF, Pinter JD, et al. The middle interhemispheric variant of holoprosencephaly. AJNR Am J Neuroradiol 2002;23(1):151–6.

30. Nakayama J, Kinugasa H, Ohto T, et al. Monozygotic twins with de novo ZIC2 gene mutations discordant for the type of holoprosencephaly. Neurology 2016; 86(15):1456–8.

31. Levey EB, Stashinko E, Clegg NJ, et al. Management of children with holoprosencephaly. Am J Med Genet C Semin Med Genet 2010;154C(1):183–90.

32. Lewis AJ, Simon EM, Barkovich AJ, et al. Middle interhemispheric variant of holoprosencephaly: a distinct cliniconeuroradiologic subtype. Neurology 2002;59(12):1860–5.

33. Barkovich AJ, Fram EK, Norman D. Septo-optic dysplasia: MR imaging. Radiology 1989;171(1): 189–92.

34. Miller SP, Shevell MI, Patenaude Y, et al. Septo-optic dysplasia plus: a spectrum of malformations of cortical development. Neurology 2000;54(8): 1701–3.

35. Webb EA, Dattani MT. Septo-optic dysplasia. Eur J Hum Genet 2010;18(4):393–7.

36. Mellado C, Poduri A, Gleason D, et al. Candidate gene sequencing of LHX2, HESX1, and SOX2 in a large schizencephaly cohort. Am J Med Genet A 2010;152A(11):2736–42.

37. Riedl S, Vosahlo J, Battelino T, et al. Refining clinical phenotypes in septo-optic dysplasia based on MRI findings. Eur J Pediatr 2008;167(11):1269–76.

38. Signorini SG, Decio A, Fedeli C, et al. Septo-optic dysplasia in childhood: the neurological, cognitive and neuro-ophthalmological perspective. Dev Med Child Neurol 2012;54(11):1018–24.

39. Glass HC, Shaw GM, Ma C, et al. Agenesis of the corpus callosum in California 1983-2003: a population-based study. Am J Med Genet A 2008; 146A(19):2495–500.

40. Hetts SW, Sherr EH, Chao S, et al. Anomalies of the corpus callosum: an MR analysis of the phenotypic spectrum of associated malformations. AJR Am J Roentgenol 2006;187(5):1343–8.

41. Schell-Apacik CC, Wagner K, Bihler M, et al. Agenesis and dysgenesis of the corpus callosum: clinical, genetic and neuroimaging findings in a series of 41 patients. Am J Med Genet A 2008;146A(19): 2501–11.

42. Edwards TJ, Sherr EH, Barkovich AJ, et al. Clinical, genetic and imaging findings identify new causes for corpus callosum development syndromes. Brain 2014;137(Pt 6):1579–613.

43. Garel C, Cont I, Alberti C, et al. Biometry of the corpus callosum in children: MR imaging reference data. AJNR Am J Neuroradiol 2011;32(8):1436–43.

44. Harreld JH, Bhore R, Chason DP, et al. Corpus callosum length by gestational age as evaluated by fetal MR imaging. AJNR Am J Neuroradiol 2011; 32(3):490–4.

45. Gonzalez G, Vedolin L, Barry B, et al. Location of periventricular nodular heterotopia is related to the

malformation phenotype on MRI. AJNR Am J Neuroradiol 2013;34(4):877–83.

46. Barkovich AJ, Kuzniecky RI. Gray matter heterotopia. Neurology 2000;55(11):1603–8.

47. Parrini E, Ramazzotti A, Dobyns WB, et al. Periventricular heterotopia: phenotypic heterogeneity and correlation with Filamin A mutations. Brain 2006; 129(Pt 7):1892–906.

48. Sheen VL, Ganesh VS, Topcu M, et al. Mutations in ARFGEF2 implicate vesicle trafficking in neural progenitor proliferation and migration in the human cerebral cortex. Nat Genet 2004;36(1):69–76.

49. Barkovich AJ, Kjos BO. Gray matter heterotopias: MR characteristics and correlation with developmental and neurologic manifestations. Radiology 1992;182(2):493–9.

50. Smith AS, Weinstein MA, Quencer RM, et al. Association of heterotopic gray matter with seizures: MR imaging. Work in progress. Radiology 1988;168(1):195–8.

51. Kang SY, Han YM, Choi K, et al. Neurological picture. Transient high-intensity signal of heterotopia on DWI in an epilepsy patient. J Neurol Neurosurg Psychiatr 2012;83(10):1017–8.

52. Yilmaz U, Papanagiotou P, Roth C, et al. Peri-ictal restricted diffusion in heterotopic gray matter assessed by MRI. Neurology 2012;79(12):1300.

53. Mandelstam SA, Leventer RJ, Sandow A, et al. Bilateral posterior periventricular nodular heterotopia: a recognizable cortical malformation with a spectrum of associated brain abnormalities. AJNR Am J Neuroradiol 2013;34(2):432–8.

54. Barkovich AJ. Subcortical heterotopia: a distinct clinicoradiologic entity. AJNR Am J Neuroradiol 1996;17(7):1315–22.

55. Barkovich AJ. Morphologic characteristics of subcortical heterotopia: MR imaging study. AJNR Am J Neuroradiol 2000;21(2):290–5.

56. Barkovich AJ, Simon EM, Walsh CA. Callosal agenesis with cyst: a better understanding and new classification. Neurol 2001;56(2):220–7.

57. Dobyns WB, Truwit CL. Lissencephaly and other malformations of cortical development: 1995 update. Neuropediatrics 1995;26(3):132–47.

58. Fry AE, Cushion TD, Pilz DT. The genetics of lissencephaly. Am J Med Genet C Semin Med Genet 2014;166C(2):198–210.

59. Barkovich AJ, Koch TK, Carrol CL. The spectrum of lissencephaly: report of ten patients analyzed by magnetic resonance imaging. Ann Neurol 1991; 30(2):139–46.

60. Landrieu P, Husson B, Pariente D, et al. MRI-neuropathological correlations in type 1 lissencephaly. Neuroradiology 1998;40(3):173–6.

61. Forman MS, Squier W, Dobyns WB, et al. Genotypically defined lissencephalies show distinct pathologies. J Neuropathol Exp Neurol 2005;64(10):847–57.

62. Mai R, Tassi L, Cossu M, et al. A neuropathological, stereo-EEG, and MRI study of subcortical band heterotopia. Neurology 2003;60(11):1834–8.

63. Bahi-Buisson N, Souville I, Fourniol FJ, et al. New insights into genotype-phenotype correlations for the doublecortin-related lissencephaly spectrum. Brain 2013;136(Pt 1):223–44.

64. Jamuar SS, Lam AT, Kircher M, et al. Somatic mutations in cerebral cortical malformations. N Engl J Med 2014;371(8):733–43.

65. Poduri A, Evrony GD, Cai X, et al. Somatic mutation, genomic variation, and neurological disease. Science 2013;341(6141):1237758.

66. Blumcke I, Thom M, Aronica E, et al. The clinicopathologic spectrum of focal cortical dysplasias: a consensus classification proposed by an ad hoc Task Force of the ILAE diagnostic methods commission. Epilepsia 2011;52(1):158–74.

67. Baulac S, Ishida S, Marsan E, et al. Familial focal epilepsy with focal cortical dysplasia due to DEPDC5 mutations. Ann Neurol 2015;77(4):675–83.

68. D'Gama AM, Geng Y, Couto JA, et al. Mammalian target of rapamycin pathway mutations cause hemimegalencephaly and focal cortical dysplasia. Ann Neurol 2015;77(4):720–5.

69. Jansen LA, Mirzaa GM, Ishak GE, et al. PI3K/AKT pathway mutations cause a spectrum of brain malformations from megalencephaly to focal cortical dysplasia. Brain 2015;138(Pt 6):1613–28.

70. Lim JS, Kim WI, Kang HC, et al. Brain somatic mutations in MTOR cause focal cortical dysplasia type II leading to intractable epilepsy. Nat Med 2015;21(4):395–400.

71. Mirzaa GM, Campbell CD, Solovieff N, et al. Association of MTOR mutations with developmental brain disorders, including megalencephaly, focal cortical dysplasia, and pigmentary mosaicism. JAMA Neurol 2016;73(7):836–45.

72. Jobst BC, Cascino GD. Resective epilepsy surgery for drug-resistant focal epilepsy: a review. JAMA 2015;313(3):285–93.

73. Lerner JT, Salamon N, Hauptman JS, et al. Assessment and surgical outcomes for mild type I and severe type II cortical dysplasia: a critical review and the UCLA experience. Epilepsia 2009;50(6):1310–35.

74. Palmini A, Holthausen H. Focal malformations of cortical development: a most relevant etiology of epilepsy in children. Handb Clin Neurol 2013;111:549–65.

75. Hong SJ, Bernhardt BC, Schrader DS, et al. Whole-brain MRI phenotyping in dysplasia-related frontal lobe epilepsy. Neurology 2016;86(7):643–50.

76. Colombo N, Tassi L, Deleo F, et al. Focal cortical dysplasia type IIa and IIb: MRI aspects in 118 cases proven by histopathology. Neuroradiology 2012;54(10):1065–77.

77. Becker AJ, Urbach H, Scheffler B, et al. Focal cortical dysplasia of Taylor's balloon cell type: mutational analysis of the TSC1 gene indicates a pathogenic relationship to tuberous sclerosis. Ann Neurol 2002;52(1):29–37.

78. Yogi A, Hirata Y, Karavaeva E, et al. DTI of tuber and perituberal tissue can predict epileptogenicity in tuberous sclerosis complex. Neurology 2015;85(23): 2011–5.

79. Peters JM, Prohl AK, Tomas-Fernandez XK, et al. Tubers are neither static nor discrete: Evidence from serial diffusion tensor imaging. Neurology 2015; 85(18):1536–45.

80. Judkins AR, Martinez D, Ferreira P, et al. Polymicrogyria includes fusion of the molecular layer and decreased neuronal populations but normal cortical laminar organization. J Neuropathol Exp Neurol 2011;70(6):438–43.

81. Squier W, Jansen A. Polymicrogyria: pathology, fetal origins and mechanisms. Acta Neuropathol Commun 2014;2:80.

82. Jansen AC, Robitaille Y, Honavar M, et al. The histopathology of polymicrogyria: a series of 71 brain autopsy studies. Dev Med Child Neurol 2016;58(1): 39–48.

83. Barkovich AJ. MRI analysis of sulcation morphology in polymicrogyria. Epilepsia 2010;51(Suppl 1):17–22.

84. Leventer RJ, Jansen A, Pilz DT, et al. Clinical and imaging heterogeneity of polymicrogyria: a study of 328 patients. Brain 2010;133(Pt 5):1415–27.

85. De Ciantis A, Barkovich AJ, Cosottini M, et al. Ultra-high-field MR imaging in polymicrogyria and epilepsy. AJNR Am J Neuroradiol 2015;36(2): 309–16.

86. Devisme L, Bouchet C, Gonzales M, et al. Cobblestone lissencephaly: neuropathological subtypes and correlations with genes of dystroglycanopathies. Brain 2012;135(Pt 2):469–82.

87. Sparks S, Quijano-Roy S, Harper A, et al. Congenital muscular dystrophy overview. In: Pagon RA, Adam MP, Ardinger HH, et al, editors. Seattle (WA): Gene Reviews(R); 1993.

88. Bahi-Buisson N, Poirier K, Boddaert N, et al. GPR56-related bilateral frontoparietal polymicrogyria: further evidence for an overlap with the cobblestone complex. Brain 2010;133(11):3194–209.

89. Jaglin XH, Poirier K, Saillour Y, et al. Mutations in the beta-tubulin gene TUBB2B result in asymmetrical polymicrogyria. Nat Genet 2009;41(6):746–52.

90. Luo R, Yang HM, Jin Z, et al. A novel GPR56 mutation causes bilateral frontoparietal polymicrogyria. Pediatr Neurol 2011;45(1):49–53.

91. Manara R, Balao L, Baracchini C, et al. Brain magnetic resonance findings in symptomatic congenital cytomegalovirus infection. Pediatr Radiol 2011; 41(8):962–70.

92. Bahi-Buisson N, Cavallin M. Tubulinopathies overview. In: Pagon RA, Adam MP, Ardinger HH, et al, editors. Seattle (WA): Gene Reviews(R); 1993.

93. Bahi-Buisson N, Poirier K, Fourniol F, et al. The wide spectrum of tubulinopathies: what are the key features for the diagnosis? Brain 2014;137(Pt 6): 1676–700.

94. Oegema R, Cushion TD, Phelps IG, et al. Recognizable cerebellar dysplasia associated with mutations in multiple tubulin genes. Hum Mol Genet 2015; 24(18):5313–25.

95. Mutch CA, Poduri A, Sahin M, et al. Disorders of microtubule function in neurons: imaging correlates. AJNR Am J Neuroradiol 2016;37(3):528–35.

96. Whitman MC, Andrews C, Chan WM, et al. Two unique TUBB3 mutations cause both CFEOM3 and malformations of cortical development. Am J Med Genet A 2016;170A(2):297–305.

97. Alcantara D, O'Driscoll M. Congenital microcephaly. Am J Med Genet C Semin Med Genet 2014;166C(2): 124–39.

98. Seltzer LE, Paciorkowski AR. Genetic disorders associated with postnatal microcephaly. Am J Med Genet C Semin Med Genet 2014;166C(2):140–55.

99. Mirzaa GM, Poduri A. Megalencephaly and hemimegalencephaly: breakthroughs in molecular etiology. Am J Med Genet C Semin Med Genet 2014; 166C(2):156–72.

Respiratory Distress in Neonates
Underlying Causes and Current Imaging Assessment

Mark C. Liszewski, MD[a],*, A. Luana Stanescu, MD[b],
Grace S. Phillips, MD[b], Edward Y. Lee, MD, MPH[c,d]

KEYWORDS

- Neonatal • Respiratory distress • Pulmonary • Preterm • Full-term • Congenital lung malformations

KEY POINTS

- Respiratory distress in the newborn can be caused by a variety of underlying conditions, and appropriate management depends on accurate and timely imaging and diagnosis.
- Imaging and pathologic features of congenital lung malformations often overlap and lesions are best considered on a spectrum, with each lesion demonstrating various degrees of parenchymal, airway, and vascular involvement.
- The leading cause of morbidity and mortality among premature infants remains surfactant deficiency disorder (previously known as hyaline membrane disease or respiratory distress syndrome) but advances in treatment, including prenatal glucocorticoids and exogenous surfactant, have altered the classic radiographic findings of surfactant deficiency disorder.
- Advances in treatment have resulted in a change in the radiographic features of chronic lung disease of prematurity (previously known as bronchopulmonary dysplasia). Though certain radiographic features are typical for chronic lung disease of prematurity, current diagnostic criteria for chronic lung disease of prematurity are based solely on clinical criteria.
- The congenital surfactant dysfunction disorders are a rare group of genetic diseases that lead to abnormal production and/or function of surfactant in the lungs and produce typical, though nonspecific imaging findings.

INTRODUCTION

Respiratory distress is among the most common clinical indications for imaging the newborn. A variety of underlying conditions can cause respiratory distress in the neonate, and familiarity with the imaging appearance of each of these conditions is essential to timely diagnosis and appropriate management. In this article, current imaging techniques and modalities are described and the most commonly encountered neonatal lung diseases are discussed, including congenital

Disclosure Statement: The authors have nothing to disclose.
[a] Division of Pediatric Radiology, Department of Radiology, Montefiore Medical Center, Albert Einstein College of Medicine, 111 East, 210th Street, Bronx, NY 10467, USA; [b] Department of Radiology, Seattle Children's Hospital, University of Washington School of Medicine, 4800 Sand Point Way Northeast, Seattle, WA 98105, USA; [c] Division of Thoracic Imaging, Department of Radiology, Boston Children's Hospital, Harvard Medical School, 300 Longwood Avenue, Boston, MA 02115, USA; [d] Pulmonary Division, Department of Medicine, Boston Children's Hospital, Harvard Medical School, 300 Longwood Avenue, Boston, MA 02115, USA
* Corresponding author.
E-mail address: mliszews@montefiore.org

Radiol Clin N Am 55 (2017) 629–644
http://dx.doi.org/10.1016/j.rcl.2017.02.006
0033-8389/17/

lung malformations and lung abnormalities in pre-term infants, as well as full-term infants.

IMAGING MODALITIES AND TECHNIQUES
Radiography

Chest radiographs are the primary imaging modality used in the assessment of the newborn with respiratory distress. In many cases, the management of neonates relies only on chest radiographs without the use of other imaging modalities. Chest radiographs are relatively inexpensive, easy to obtain, and use a very low amount of radiation, making them an ideal initial test to evaluate many neonatal lung diseases. Radiation doses can be further minimized through shielding and proper coning of images.[1,2]

Most chest radiographs performed in neonates are obtained portably and consist of a single anterior-posterior (AP) view with the child in a supine position. In certain scenarios, a lateral view may be useful to localize a finding. AP lateral decubitus views may be used in select cases, such as to visualize layering pleural effusion or to better assess a suspected pneumothorax. Though chest radiographs are an indispensable tool, they do not provide the same anatomic detail as computed tomography (CT) or MR imaging, and these may be indicated to further evaluate a finding seen on chest radiograph.

Fluoroscopy

Fluoroscopy can be useful to evaluate dynamic disease processes that change throughout the respiratory cycle but its role in neonatal respiratory distress is limited to a few scenarios. Fluoroscopy may be used to evaluate diaphragmatic motion in cases of suspected diaphragmatic paralysis or eventration, though ultrasound is often preferred due to its portability and lack of radiation.[3] Airway fluoroscopy may be performed in cases of suspected tracheobronchomalacia to evaluate for large airway collapse during expiration.[4]

Ultrasound

In recent years, ultrasound has received increasing attention as a tool in the evaluation of lung disease, though inherent physical properties of the chest, including acoustic shadowing from air-filled lung and ribs, often impede ultrasound's diagnostic utility in the thorax. Despite these limitations, ultrasound can be very useful in selected scenarios.[5] When chest radiograph demonstrates a completely opacified hemithorax, ultrasound can help differentiate pleural fluid from pulmonary parenchymal disease.[5] Doppler ultrasound can assess for anomalous vasculature in cases of suspected pulmonary sequestration.[5] Real-time, cine, and M-mode ultrasound imaging are the preferred methods for assessing diaphragmatic motion in cases of suspected paralysis and eventration, and can be helpful in the evaluation of congenital diaphragmatic hernia.[3,6–9] The aerated lung can even be assessed in selected scenarios through analysis of B-lines, the comet-tail artifacts that are produced when the sound beam interacts with the interlobular septa at the pleural surface. Increased B-lines have been reported in transient tachypnea of the newborn (TTN) and surfactant deficiency,[10,11] though these entities are more commonly diagnosed and managed using chest radiography alone.

Computed Tomography

CT has the ability to produce cross-sectional images with excellent anatomic detail, making it a powerful tool in the evaluation of many thoracic diseases. CT uses ionizing radiation to produce images, and every effort should be made to use low-dose pediatric protocols and limit unnecessary CT scans, particularly in neonates who are inherently more sensitive to the effects of radiation than adults.[12–15] Alternative modalities that use less or no ionizing radiation, such as radiography, ultrasound, and MR imaging, should always be considered before performing CT. After considering these factors, CT is often the best imaging modality to assess many neonatal lung diseases given its excellent anatomic detail and is lower susceptibility to artifacts. The addition of intravenous contrast is often indicated to better evaluate the mediastinal structures and vasculature.

MR Imaging

MR imaging has received much attention due to its ability to generate images without the use of ionizing radiation, though its role in the evaluation of respiratory distress in the newborn is limited. Cost, availability, and physical properties of the lung, including low signal-to-noise ratio, respiratory and cardiac motion, and signal dephasing at air-tissue interphases, limit the routine use of chest MR imaging in neonates. Despite these limitations, MR imaging with MR angiography (MRA) may be used as a first-line alternative to CT in several specific conditions, including pulmonary sequestration, pulmonary artery hypoplasia, pulmonary vascular anomalies, partial or total anomalous pulmonary venous return, and vascular rings and sling.[16,17] Small-bore and modified MR imaging scanners have been used in research settings to evaluate changes of chronic lung disease of prematurity (previously known as bronchopulmonary dysplasia [BPD]) in neonates,[18,19] though these techniques are not yet widely available in the clinical setting. Chest MR imaging using hyperpolarized gas (^{3}He or ^{129}Xe) as an inhaled contrast agent has the potential to quantify changes in lung microstructure, and has been studied in older children with a past history of chronic lung disease of prematurity[20] but has not been studied in the neonatal period.[21]

Nuclear Medicine

Nuclear medicine does not play a major role in the routine evaluation of most causes of neonatal respiratory distress. Pulmonary ventilation-perfusion (V/Q) scans, in which the pulmonary distribution of an inhaled radiotracer (eg, ^{99m}Tc-labeled diethylenetriamine penta-acetic acid [DTPA], ^{133}Xe, or Technegas) and an injected radiotracer (eg, 99mTc-labeled macroaggregated albumin) are imaged can be useful in certain diseases. For example, V/Q scans have been used to assess pulmonary hypoplasia in patients with history of congenital diaphragmatic hernia.[22–24] V/Q scans can provide information about severity and abnormalities in regional lung function in chronic lung disease of prematurity.[25,26] Perfusion scintigraphy can also be useful to determine differential pulmonary perfusion in cases of congenital heart disease, pulmonary hypoplasia, and scimitar syndrome,[27,28] and can be used to quantify right-to-left shunts.[27]

SPECTRUM OF UNDERLYING PULMONARY CAUSES OF NEONATAL RESPIRATORY DISTRESS
Congenital Lung Malformations

Congenital lung malformations are a group of developmental lesions involving the lung parenchyma, airway, and/or pulmonary vasculature. Symptoms are variable and can range from no symptoms to progressive respiratory distress requiring surgical intervention. The 3 most common congenital lung malformations detected in the neonate are congenital pulmonary airway malformation (CPAM), pulmonary sequestration, and congenital lobar overinflation (CLO). There is considerable overlap between these entities and they can be best considered as lesions on a spectrum with each lesion demonstrating various degrees of parenchymal, airway, and vascular involvement.[29–31] The classic radiographic and pathologic features of these lesions are discussed in the following sections and imaging findings are summarized in **Table 1**.

Congenital pulmonary airway malformation

CPAMs, previously known as cystic adenomatoid malformations, are congenital macrocystic or microcystic lung lesions that are associated with an abnormal bronchial tree and bronchiolar overgrowth.[32,33] Typically, CPAMs are associated with normal pulmonary vascular anatomy (**Fig. 1**), though pathologic features of CPAM are seen in 29% to 33% of pulmonary lesions with abnormal systemic arterial supply (**Figs. 2 and 3**) and up to 50% of lobar emphysemas.[31,34,35] Several different classification systems have been proposed to categorize CPAM lesions. Though no classification scheme is universally accepted, the system proposed by Stocker and colleagues in 1977[36] and updated in 2001[37] is often used. In this classification system, type 1 lesions are composed of 1 or more cysts measuring greater than 2 cm, type 2 lesions are composed of 1 or more cysts measuring less than 2 cm, and type 3 lesions appear as solid masses macroscopically but contain microcysts on pathologic analysis. Stocker also describes type 0 lesions (acinar dysplasia, which is incompatible with life) and type 4 lesions (large peripherally located lung cysts sometimes associated with pneumothorax), though these lesions are controversial.[38–43]

The clinical presentation of CPAM varies. With increased prenatal imaging, an increasing number of lesions are currently detected incidentally during routine fetal ultrasound (see **Fig. 2**). Some lesions cause no symptoms, whereas others cause varying degrees of respiratory distress soon after birth, particularly when large.[43–45] Lesions may present later in life due to superinfection or rarely due to development of associated malignancy.[43] Approximately half of type 2 lesions are associated with additional congenital anomalies, including cardiovascular malformations, extralobar pulmonary sequestration, tracheoesophageal fistula, renal agenesis, intestinal atresia, and congenital diaphragmatic hernia.[43,46]

The imaging appearance of CPAM depends on the type. Lesions with macroscopic cystic components (types 1 and 2) are typically filled with fetal lung fluid at birth and fluid partially or completely clears from the cysts in the first few days of life.[32] Initial chest radiographs typically demonstrate a dense lung lesion that becomes less dense as fetal lung fluid clears. CT and MR imaging demonstrate a cyst or cysts within the lung parenchyma, containing air and/or fluid.[29,32] Lesions composed of microscopic cysts (type 3) appear as solid masses macroscopically and, therefore, will appear as dense lung lesions on radiographs and as solid enhancing masses on CT and MR imaging.[29,32] When CPAMs present later in life with

Table 1
Imaging findings of congenital lung malformations

Congenital Lung Malformation	Imaging Findings	Pearls and Pitfalls
Congenital pulmonary airway malformation (CPAM)		
Stocker type 0[a]	Atretic large airways and lungs	Type 0 CPAM lesions can be only seen in prenatal ultrasound or MR imaging
Stocker type 1[a]	1 or more cysts measuring >2 cm	In type 1 and 2 CPAM lesions initial CXR typically demonstrates a dense lung lesion that becomes less dense as fetal lung fluid clears
Stocker type 2[a]	2 or more cysts <2 cm	
Stocker type 3[a]	Both imaging-wise and macroscopically solid mass composed of microcysts on pathologic analysis	
Stocker type 4[a]	Large peripherally located lung cysts sometimes associated with pneumothorax	Type 3 CPAM lesions remain dense because they are macroscopically solid masses
		On imaging studies, pleuropulmonary blastoma type 1 (pure cystic lesion) has similar imaging appearance to type 1, 2, and 4 CPAM lesions
		When CT or MR imaging is performed, contrast-enhanced CTA or MRA technique should always be used to evaluate for systemic arterial supply, seen in so-called hybrid lesions
Pulmonary sequestration	Cystic or solid lung mass Systemic arterial supply seen on US, CT or MR imaging Intralobar: venous drainage to pulmonary veins Extralobar: venous drainage to systemic pulmonary vein	Frequently detected during prenatal ultrasound Contrast-enhanced CTA or MRA are recommended in cases of suspected sequestration Most often occur in the lower lobes, left>right Extralobar sequestration may be intrathoracic or extrathoracic 3D volume rendered CT images can increase the diagnostic accuracy and confidence level for correctly identifying small anomalous vessels in patients with pulmonary sequestration
Congenital lobar overinflation (CLO)	Serial CXRs after birth first show an opacified lobe that becomes lucent and then hyperexpands LUL>RML>RUL>RLL & LLL	AKA congenital lobar emphysema Hyperexpansion often causes significant mass effect that may result in significant respiratory distress and necessitate lobectomy

Abbreviations: 3D, 3-dimensional; AKA, also known as; CTA, CT angiography; CXR, chest radiograph; LLL, left lower lobe; LUL, left upper lobe; MRA, MR Angiography; RLL, right lower lobe; RML, right middle lobe; RUL, right upper lobe.
[a] Per the classification system described in: Stocker J. The respiratory tract. In: Stocker JT, Dejner LP, editors. Pediatric pathology. 2nd edition. Philadelphia: Lippincott, Williams & Wilkins; 2001. p. 466–73.

superinfection, chest radiographs typically demonstrate consolidation with air-fluid levels, and CT or MR imaging demonstrate cystic lung lesions containing air-fluid levels and a thick enhancing irregular wall.[29,32,33] Typically, CPAMs have a conventional pulmonary vascular anatomy but attention to vascular supply is essential because a proportion of CPAMs have a systemic arterial supply (so-called hybrid lesions; see

Figs. 2 and 3).[34,35] Therefore, CT or MR imaging should be performed with contrast and CT angiography (CTA) or MRA techniques should be used.

Pulmonary sequestration
Pulmonary sequestration is typically defined as a disconnected bronchopulmonary mass or cyst with an anomalous arterial supply.[47] There are 2 types of sequestration that are commonly

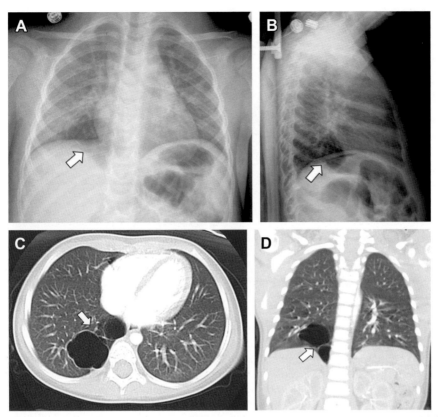

Fig. 1. A 2-year-old-boy with type 1 congenital pulmonary airway malformation (CPAM). Frontal (*A*) and lateral (*B*) chest radiographs demonstrate an air-filled multicystic lesion (*arrows*) in the right lower lobe. Axial (*C*) and coronal (*D*) lung window CT images show the lesion (*arrows*) is composed of multiple large air-filled cysts.

described: intralobar and extralobar. Intralobar sequestration is typically characterized by abnormal lung tissue that does not communicate with the tracheobronchial tree, has an arterial supply from the aorta or one of its branches, has venous drainage to the pulmonary vein, and shares a 1 visceral pleural covering with the adjacent normal lung.[29,32,33] Extralobar sequestration is also characterized by abnormal lung tissue that does not communicate with the tracheobronchial tree and has an arterial supply from the aorta or one of its branches. Extralobar sequestration differs from intralobar sequestration in that its venous drainage is to a systemic vein and its pleural covering is separate from the adjacent lung.[29,32,33] Extralobar sequestration is most often located within the lower

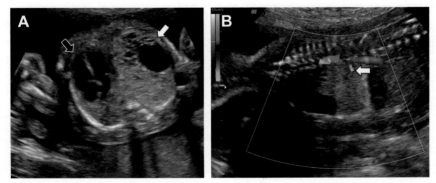

Fig. 2. A 22-week-old fetus with congenital pulmonary airway malformation (CPAM) and bronchopulmonary sequestration (hybrid lesion). (*A*) Grayscale prenatal ultrasound shows a multicystic mass (*white arrow*) in the left lung displacing the heart (*black arrow*) to the right. (*B*) Color Doppler ultrasound image demonstrates a feeding systemic artery (*arrow*) arising from the aorta.

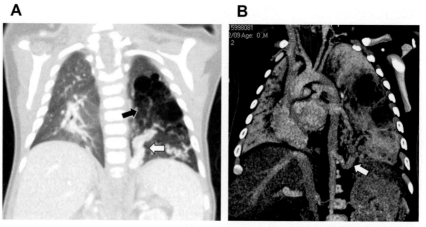

Fig. 3. A 5-month-old boy with congenital pulmonary airway malformation (CPAM) and bronchopulmonary sequestration (hybrid lesion) (same patient as **Fig. 2**). (*A*) Coronal image from contrast-enhanced CT angiography (CTA) demonstrates an air-filled multicystic lesion within the left lung (*black arrow*) with a large feeding systemic artery (*white arrow*). (*B*) Three-dimensional (3D) volume-rendered CT image shows the systemic feeding artery (*arrow*) arising from the aorta.

lung but can occur below the diaphragm or within the mediastinum. The traditional description of pulmonary sequestration has shortcomings and many lesions do not fit the strict definition. For example, lesions may have an abnormal arterial supply but normal tracheobronchial connection.[48] These issues have led some to propose alternative classification systems[34,38,49] but the terms intralobar and extralobar sequestration seem deeprooted despite their inherent limitations.

Pulmonary sequestration is frequently detected incidentally during prenatal ultrasound as a pulmonary mass with anomalous systemic arterial supply (see **Fig. 2**).[44] At birth, most pulmonary sequestrations are asymptomatic and appear as a lung mass within a lower lobe, on the left side more often than the right side.[29] Postnatal chest ultrasound with Doppler imaging may demonstrate a lung mass with an anomalous systemic arterial vascular supply.[5] Contrast-enhanced CTA or MRA are recommended in cases of suspected sequestration.[17,29] Extralobar sequestration typically appears as a solid enhancing mass with systemic arterial and venous circulation that may be intrathoracic or extrathoracic. Intralobar sequestration typically appears as a cystic lung lesion with variable aeration (due to collateral air drift), arterial supply from the aorta or one of its branches, and venous drainage to a pulmonary vein (see **Fig. 3**; **Fig. 4**).[32] Intralobar sequestration can present later in life with superinfection and chest radiograph and CT may demonstrate increased consolidation and air-fluid levels within a pre-existing lesion.[29,32]

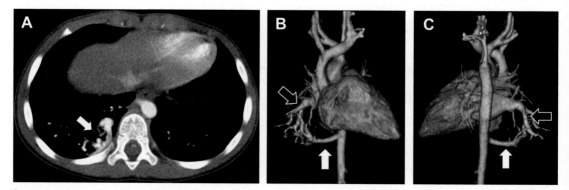

Fig. 4. A 21-month-old boy with intralobar bronchopulmonary sequestration. (*A*) Axial contrast-enhanced CT demonstrates a heterogeneous lesion in the right lower lobe containing large abnormal vessels (*arrow*). (*B, C*) 3D volume-rendered CT images show systemic feeding artery (*white arrows*) arising from the aorta and venous drainage (*black arrows*) to the pulmonary veins and left atrium.

Congenital lobar overinflation

CLO, also known as congenital lobar emphysema, is a lung lesion characterized by hyperexpansion of a lobe of the lung. The primary defect in CLO is bronchial obstruction due to compression from an external structure or intrinsic narrowing. The lung distal to the obstruction becomes hyperinflated. Mass effect from the hyperinflated lobe can result in significant symptoms, typically presenting within the first 6 hours of life. CLO affects certain lobes more frequently; from most to least: left upper lobe, right middle lobe, right upper lobe, right or left lower lobes.[50]

CLO produces a classic appearance on serial chest radiographs. The initial radiograph performed immediately after birth typically shows an opacified lobe due to entrapped fetal lung fluid. As the fluid clears, the lobe becomes more lucent and demonstrates progressive hyperinflation. Hyperinflation often continues to increase and causes mass effect on the mediastinum and diaphragm (**Fig. 5**A). Mass effect is frequently accompanied by worsening respiratory distress, requiring lobectomy. If clinically stable, preoperative CT is generally indicated to define the lobar anatomy before lobectomy (**Fig. 5**B, C).[29] Classically, CLO is associated with conventional vascular anatomy.

Lung Abnormalities in Preterm Infants

Advances in neonatal intensive care over the past 50 years have led to greatly improved survival rates for infants born before term. The leading cause of morbidity and mortality among premature infants is respiratory distress due to insufficient surfactant production. Complications of surfactant deficiency disorder, including pulmonary interstitial emphysema (PIE) and chronic lung disease of prematurity, can further contribute to morbidity and mortality in this patient group. The radiographic and pathologic features of these entities are discussed in the following sections and imaging findings are summarized in **Table 2**.

Surfactant deficiency disorder, hyaline membrane disease, or respiratory distress syndrome

Surfactant deficiency disorder, also known as hyaline membrane disease or respiratory distress syndrome (RDS), is primarily a disease of premature infants. Surfactant deficiency disorder occurs when immature type II pneumocytes are unable to produce sufficient surfactant to support normal lung function. In the healthy state, surfactant reduces surface tension within alveoli and is essential to normal alveolar expansion. Hyaline membranes, which contain necrotic cells, fibrin, and plasma transudate, form within the alveoli of the surfactant-deficient lung and further impair oxygenation. Antenatal corticosteroids (which accelerate surfactant production) and exogenous surfactant have improved survival among premature children.[51] Mechanical ventilation is often required to treat patients with surfactant deficiency disorder but efforts are focused on reducing barotrauma because this is a major cause of morbidity through air-leak phenomena and increased risk of chronic lung disease of prematurity.

Chest radiographs in untreated surfactant deficiency disorder typically demonstrate low lung volumes with diffuse homogenous granular opacities (**Fig. 6**). This classic appearance is altered by the administration of exogenous surfactant. After surfactant, granular opacities and lung hypoinflation may uniformly improve, asymmetrically decrease, or show no change.[52] Surfactant is often administered before the first radiograph, so even initial chest radiographs may not demonstrate the classic pattern of surfactant deficiency disorder. Asymmetric improvement can produce radiographic findings similar to neonatal pneumonia or meconium aspiration, and correlation with clinical history is essential in these cases.[51] Surfactant deficiency disorder is typically managed using radiographs alone, and other imaging modalities are rarely used.

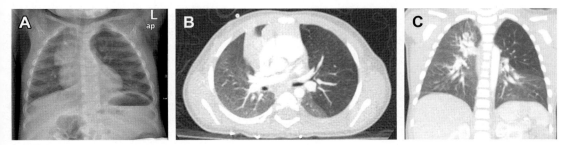

Fig. 5. A 9-month-old girl with left upper lobe congenial lobar overinflation (CLO). (*A*) Frontal chest radiograph demonstrates hyperlucent left upper lobe with mild mass effect on the mediastinum. Axial (*B*) and coronal (*C*) contrast-enhanced CT images show hyperlucent left upper lobe.

Table 2
Imaging findings of the most common lung abnormalities in preterm infants

Lung Abnormality	Imaging Findings	Pearls and Pitfalls
Surfactant deficiency disorder, hyaline membrane disease, or respiratory distress syndrome (RDS)	Low lung volumes with diffuse homogenous granular opacities After surfactant granular opacities may uniformly improve, asymmetrically decrease, or show no change	Initial CXR may not demonstrate the classic pattern of surfactant deficiency disorder because surfactant is often administered before the first radiograph is obtained CXR may show asymmetric improvement after surfactant is administered and can appear similar to neonatal pneumonia or meconium aspiration
Pulmonary interstitial emphysema (PIE)	CXR: bubbly and/or linear lucencies CT: line-and-dot pattern due to interstitial air surrounding the bronchovascular bundles	Most common in mechanically ventilated patients with surfactant deficiency disorder Surfactant given to treat surfactant deficiency disorder can cause localized acinar overdistention that may mimic PIE
Chronic lung disease of prematurity or bronchopulmonary dysplasia (BPD)	Coarse reticular opacities, cystic lucencies and hyperexpansion	New diagnostic criteria for BPD are based solely on clinical features, and do not include radiographic features

Pulmonary interstitial emphysema

PIE is a condition that occurs when air ruptures through the bronchoalveolar junctions and dissects into the pulmonary interstitium.[53] PIE occurs most commonly in mechanically ventilated patients with surfactant deficiency disorder but can also occur in meconium aspiration syndrome (MAS) or neonatal pneumonia. PIE may be accompanied by additional air-leak phenomena, including pneumothorax, pneumomediastinum, pneumopericardium, and pneumoperitoneum.

Chest radiographs in PIE typically demonstrate bubbly or linear lucencies with morphology different from air-bronchograms or normal air within alveoli (**Fig. 7**).[54,55] PIE may be focal, diffuse, unilateral or bilateral.[55] If PIE persists for longer than 1 week, it is termed persistent PIE (PPIE) (see **Fig. 7C**). The involved lung can enlarge and cause mass effect.

Other entities can occasionally mimic the appearance of PIE on chest radiographs. Exogenous surfactant given to treat surfactant deficiency disorder can cause localized acinar overdistention that produces an appearance of bubbly lucencies that may mimic PIE.[51] In this scenario, consideration of the child's clinical condition is essential: patients with PIE tend to decompensate and patients with acinar distention from exogenous surfactant tend to improve.[51] Localized PPIE can mimic CPAM and CLO on chest radiographs but prior imaging studies typically demonstrate a characteristic pattern of PIE in the same region.[53] If the diagnosis of PPIE is unclear, CT may be performed and demonstrate interstitial air surrounding the bronchovascular

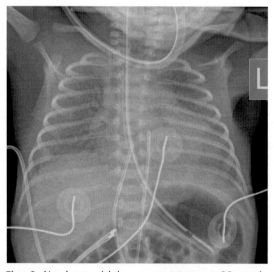

Fig. 6. Newborn girl born premature at 28 weeks gestation with surfactant deficiency disorder. Frontal chest radiograph demonstrates diffuse bilateral hazy pulmonary opacities and low lung volumes.

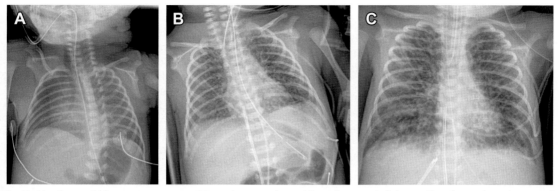

Fig. 7. Newborn girl born premature at 29 weeks gestation with surfactant deficiency disorder and persistent pulmonary interstitial emphysema (PIE) (PPIE). (*A*) Chest radiograph at day 1 of life shows diffuse bilateral hazy pulmonary opacities of surfactant deficiency disorder. (*B*) Chest radiograph at day 2 of life demonstrates new bilateral bubbly and linear lucencies that do not conform to the shape of air-bronchograms, compatible with PIE. (*C*) Chest radiograph at day 9 of life shows persistent bubbly and linear lucencies of PIE, compatible with PPIE.

bundles, producing a line-and-dot pattern.[55–57] Bubbly lucencies in PIE can also mimic lucencies seen in chronic lung disease of prematurity, and consideration of the time course and patient age are essential to differentiate these entities. PIE generally occurs as an acute event during the first week of life, whereas imaging findings of chronic lung disease of prematurity tend to appear gradually around the second and third week.[58]

Presence of PIE should be reported to neonatal intensive care unit (NICU) staff immediately because patients will often be changed from conventional mechanical ventilation to high-frequency oscillatory ventilation.[56] Most PIE responds to conservative management and resolves spontaneously. A minority of cases persist, leading to PPIE. Most PPIE is managed conservatively. A small number of cases of PPIE require surgical resection due to mass effect.[56] CT is often indicated in these cases to aid surgical planning.[55–57]

Chronic lung disease of prematurity or bronchopulmonary dysplasia

Though many patients with surfactant deficiency disorder completely recover, a subset of patients develops persistent pulmonary disease called chronic lung disease of prematurity, also known as BPD. Northway and colleagues[59] first described this condition in 1967, describing 4 stages of BPD occurring in a subset of patients with surfactant deficiency disorder and treated with mechanical ventilation. In the classic BPD described by the investigators, chest radiographs evolve from findings of surfactant deficiency disorder in the first days of life to diffuse bilateral opacities that are slowly replaced by coarse reticular opacities, cystic lucencies, and hyperexpansion beginning around day 10 and progressing beyond 1 month of age (**Fig. 8**). Pathologically, chronic lung disease of prematurity is characterized by emphysema, atelectasis,

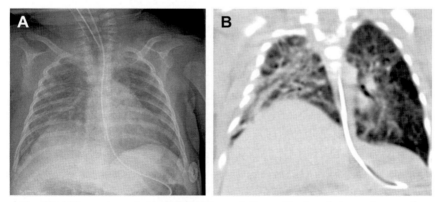

Fig. 8. A 3-month-old girl born premature at 26 weeks gestation with chronic lung disease of prematurity. (*A*) Chest radiograph shows bilateral coarse interstitial opacities, atelectasis, and right hemidiaphragm elevation due to right lung volume loss. (*B*) Coronal lung window CT image demonstrates bilateral ground glass opacities, septal thickening, and atelectasis that are greater on the right with right hemidiaphragm elevation.

smooth muscle hypertrophy, and pulmonary fibrosis. Patients with chronic lung disease of prematurity have persistent respiratory distress requiring continued respiratory treatment ranging from supplemental oxygen to long-term mechanical ventilation.

There have been many changes in the treatment of surfactant deficiency disorder and chronic lung disease of prematurity since the original 1967 description by Northway and colleagues.[59] These changes include antenatal glucocorticoid therapy, exogenous surfactant, use of lower oxygen concentrations, and less harmful ventilation techniques. This has resulted in survival of larger numbers of infants who have low and extremely low birth weight, many of whom go on to develop chronic lung disease requiring long-term respiratory support. The imaging features of chronic lung disease in this group often differ from the original findings described by Northway and colleagues,[59] leading to the term *the new BPD*. For example, early chest radiographs in extremely premature infants may only demonstrate mild perihilar opacities and fine granularity in a pattern termed immature lung[60] but subsequent radiographs often demonstrate typical features of BPD, including coarse interstitial opacities, cystic lucencies, and hyperexpansion.[51,53] Because the radiographic features in these patients often differ from those originally described by Northway and colleagues,[59] the National Institute of Child Health and Human Development's National Heart, Lung, and Blood Institute Workshop developed new diagnostic criteria for BPD that are based solely on clinical features and do not include a consideration of the radiographic findings because they did not increase the established diagnostic sensitivity or specificity.[61,62] This workshop recommended continued use of the term BPD, though many now prefer the term chronic lung disease of prematurity given the evolution of the disease since the original description by Northway and colleagues.[59]

Treatment of chronic lung disease of prematurity is supportive. Oxygen toxicity and barotrauma are major risk factors for developing chronic lung disease of prematurity[63]; therefore, high supplemental oxygen concentrations and positive pressure ventilation are limited as much as possible. Inhaled bronchodilators may be used for temporary symptom relief, though they do not improve long-term outcomes.[63,64] Systemic corticosteroids can improve lung function but are reserved for only the most severe cases due to serious potential side effects, including neurologic dysfunction.[65–67]

Lung Abnormalities in Full-Term Infants

A variety of conditions may lead to respiratory distress in full-term newborns, often leading to NICU admission. Conditions range from rare genetic diseases, such as congenital surfactant dysfunction disorders, to more common conditions, including TTN, MAS, and infection. The radiographic and pathologic features of these entities are discussed in the following sections and imaging findings are summarized in **Table 3**.

Congenital surfactant dysfunction disorders

The surfactant dysfunction disorders are a rare group of genetic diseases that lead to abnormal production and/or function of surfactant in the lungs, and can cause respiratory distress in the newborn. Several mutations have been identified, including mutations in genes for surfactant protein B (**Fig. 9**), surfactant protein C, adenosine triphosphate (ATP)-binding cassette transporter protein, thyroid transcription factor-1, and granulocyte-macrophage colony-stimulating factor–Rα.[68–72]

Patients affected with surfactant dysfunction disorder are typically born at term with respiratory distress. Symptoms may range from mild to severe. Chest radiograph typically shows bilateral patchy or diffuse hazy opacities.[73–75] Findings on CT may include ground-glass opacities, consolidation, and interlobular septal thickening.[73–76] Definitive diagnosis can be established with genetic testing. Some cases are related to yet-unknown genetic mutations and, in these cases, biopsy is required for diagnosis.

Transient tachypnea of the newborn

TTN is a condition caused by retained fetal fluid within the lung after birth, resulting in respiratory distress. Fetal lung liquid is cleared through the airway, lymphatic channels, and capillaries.[51] Clearance is promoted by adrenergic stimulation that occurs during the normal vaginal birth process.[77–80] Therefore, TTN is more common among infants born by cesarean section or precipitous vaginal delivery.[81,82] Retained fluid in TTN is located within the alveoli, pulmonary interstitium, and enlarged lymphatics. This distribution is very similar to the distribution of fluid in pulmonary edema; therefore, the imaging findings are similar.

Chest radiographs obtained soon after birth typically show perihilar interstitial opacities, indistinct pulmonary markings, and small pleural effusions (**Fig. 10**). Lung volumes may be normal or increased. Symptoms are usually mild and typically resolve by days 2 to 3 of life. Chest radiographs also typically normalize during this time period.

Table 3
Imaging findings of the most common lung abnormalities in full-term infants

Lung Abnormality	Imaging Findings	Pearls and Pitfalls
Surfactant dysfunction disorders	CXR: bilateral patchy or diffuse hazy opacities CT: ground-glass opacities, consolidation, and interlobular septal thickening	Entities include surfactant protein B and C deficiency, ATP-binding cassette transporter protein deficiency, thyroid transcription factor-1 deficiency, granulocyte-macrophage colony-stimulating factor–Rα deficiency Definitive diagnosis is established with genetic testing or biopsy
Transient tachypnea of newborn (TTN)	CXR soon after birth: Perihilar interstitial opacities, indistinct pulmonary markings, and small pleural effusions. Lung volumes may be normal or increased. Aeration improves on CXR after 2–3 d	Caused by retained fetal fluid within the lung after birth Clearance of fluid is promoted by adrenergic stimulation that occurs during the normal vaginal birth process Therefore, TTN is more common after cesarean section or precipitous vaginal delivery
Meconium aspiration syndrome (MAS)	Hyperinflation with asymmetric irregular opacities Pneumothorax in 10%–40% Pleural effusion in 10%–20%	Exogenous surfactant may be given to replace surfactant that has been chemically inactivated by meconium Affected neonates are at higher risk for pneumonia and imaging findings are similar to neonatal pneumonia, therefore patients are often treated with antibiotics
Pulmonary infection	Most commonly, bilateral alveolar opacities Findings may be identical to RDS or TTN CXR can be normal	Fever is not typical, temperature instability is more common May be difficult to differentiate neonatal pneumonia from other entities based on imaging findings alone, therefore patients are often treated presumptively with antibiotics

Abbreviation: ATP, adenosine triphosphate.

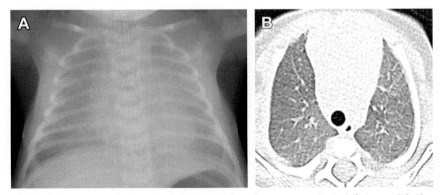

Fig. 9. A 26-day-old girl born at full term with congenital surfactant protein B deficiency. (*A*) Chest radiograph demonstrates diffuse bilateral hazy pulmonary opacities. (*B*) Axial lung window CT image shows diffuse ground glass opacity throughout bilateral lungs.

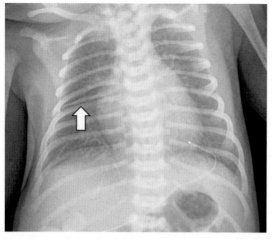

Fig. 10. A 3-hour-old full-term boy born via cesarean section with transient tachypnea of newborn (TTN). Frontal chest radiograph demonstrates bilateral pulmonary interstitial opacities and trace fluid (*arrow*) in the minor fissure.

Meconium aspiration syndrome

MAS occurs when meconium is passed and aspirated during birth. Meconium is a thick and tenacious chemical irritant. When aspirated, it causes small and medium airway obstruction, chemical pneumonitis, and inactivation of surfactant. MAS is more common in children born after 40 weeks gestation.[83] Respiratory distress may range from mild to severe. MAS is the most common cause of mortality in term infants.[84]

Chest radiographs in MAS typically show hyperinflation with asymmetric irregular opacities due to combination of air-trapping, atelectasis, and chemical pneumonitis (**Fig. 11**). Pneumothorax is

relatively common, seen in 10% to 40% of cases.[51,83,85] Pleural effusion is seen in 10% to 20% of cases.[51,85] Occasionally, the only finding on chest radiograph is pneumothorax, with clear lungs.[51]

Patients with MAS are managed supportively to maintain oxygenation. Mechanical ventilation is optimized to reduce risk of pneumothorax and pneumomediastinum through use of low positive airway pressures and high-frequency oscillatory ventilation in select cases. Exogenous surfactant may be given via endotracheal tube to replace surfactant that has been chemically inactivated by meconium.[83,86] Extracorporeal membrane oxygenation may be required in severe cases to maintain oxygenation. Because patients with MAS are at higher risk for superimposed bacterial infection and their imaging findings are similar to neonatal pneumonia, patients with MAS are usually treated with antibiotics.[51]

Infection

Pulmonary infection and sepsis can be acquired via hematogenous transplacental spread in utero, during labor and delivery, or in the period soon after birth. Possible causes of neonatal pneumonia and sepsis include group A and B streptococcus, *Escherichia coli*, listeria, herpes simplex virus, and cytomegalovirus, among others. Signs and symptoms typically include respiratory distress and temperature instability.[87] Fever is not typical. Risk factors for neonatal pneumonia include maternal infection and prolonged rupture of membranes.

The imaging findings in neonatal pneumonia are variable. In a series by Haney and colleagues,[87]

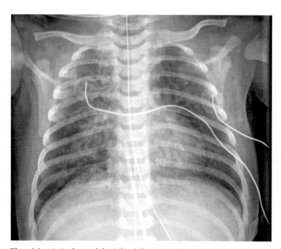

Fig. 11. A 1-day-old girl with meconium aspiration syndrome (MAS). Frontal chest radiograph demonstrates asymmetric bilateral irregular pulmonary opacities.

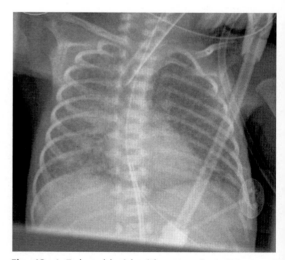

Fig. 12. A 7-day-old girl with group B streptococcus sepsis. Frontal chest radiograph shows bilateral diffuse hazy pulmonary opacities.

the most common pattern was bilateral alveolar opacities seen in 77% (**Fig. 12**). Findings were identical to RDS in 13% and identical to TTN in 17%.[87] Chest radiographs can be normal in up to 10%.[87] Because of the crossover in imaging findings with other entities, neonatal pneumonia may be difficult to differentiate from other causes of neonatal respiratory distress based on imaging findings alone. Blood or sputum culture are helpful when positive, though are often falsely negative. Therefore, affected patients are often treated presumptively with antibiotics.

SUMMARY

Respiratory distress has a variety of causes in the newborn. Conditions such as surfactant deficiency disorder and chronic lung disease of prematurity have been described since the beginning of pediatric radiology but advances in treatment have changed the patient population with these conditions and altered the imaging findings. A greater understanding of congenital lung malformations has changed the way clinicians approach imaging CPAM, pulmonary sequestration, and CLO. Newly characterized genetic causes of neonatal respiratory distress, including the congenital surfactant dysfunction disorders, have advanced appreciation of rare, previously unexplained cases of neonatal lung disease. An up-to-date knowledge of the imaging findings in the full range of neonatal lung diseases is essential for accurate diagnosis and optimal management.

REFERENCES

1. Soboleski D, Theriault C, Acker A, et al. Unnecessary irradiation to non-thoracic structures during pediatric chest radiography. Pediatr Radiol 2006;36(1):22–5.
2. Bader D, Datz H, Bartal G, et al. Unintentional exposure of neonates to conventional radiography in the Neonatal Intensive Care Units. J Perinatol 2007; 27(9):579–85.
3. Chavhan GB, Babyn PS, Cohen RA, et al. Multimodality imaging of the pediatric diaphragm: anatomy and pathologic. Radiographics 2010;30(7): 1797–817.
4. Laya BF, Lee EY. Congenital causes of upper airway obstruction in pediatric patients: updated imaging techniques and review of imaging findings. Semin Roentgenol 2012;47(2):147–58.
5. Coley BD. Chest sonography in children: current indications, techniques, and imaging findings. Radiol Clin North Am 2011;49(5):825–46.
6. Urvoas E, Pariente D, Fausser C, et al. Diaphragmatic paralysis in children: diagnosis by TM-mode ultrasound. Pediatr Radiol 1994;24(8):564–8.
7. Epelman M, Navarro OM, Daneman A, et al. M-mode sonography of diaphragmatic motion: description of technique and. Pediatr Radiol 2005; 35(7):661–7.
8. Taylor GA, Atalabi OM, Estroff JA. Imaging of congenital diaphragmatic hernias. Pediatr Radiol 2009;39(1):1–16.
9. Nason LK, Walker CM, McNeeley MF, et al. Imaging of the diaphragm: anatomy and function. Radiographics 2012;32(2):E51–70.
10. Copetti R, Cattarossi L. The 'double lung point': an ultrasound sign diagnostic of transient tachypnea of the newborn. Neonatology 2007;91(3):203–9.
11. Avni EF, Braude P, Pardou A, et al. Hyaline membrane disease in the newborn: diagnosis by ultrasound. Pediatr Radiol 1990;20(3):143–6.
12. Miglioretti DL, Johnson E, Williams A, et al. The use of computed tomography in pediatrics and the associated radiation exposure and estimated cancer risk. JAMA Pediatr 2013;167(8):700–7.
13. Brenner DJ. Estimating cancer risks from pediatric CT: going from the qualitative to the quantitative. Pediatr Radiol 2002;32(4):228–31 [discussion: 242–4].
14. Kim JE, Newman B. Evaluation of a radiation dose reduction strategy for pediatric chest CT. AJR Am J Roentgenol 2010;194(5):1188–93.
15. Goo HW. Individualized volume CT dose index determined by cross-sectional area and mean density of the body to achieve uniform image noise of contrast-enhanced pediatric chest CT obtained at variable kV levels and with combined tube current modulation. Pediatr Radiol 2011;41(7):839–47.
16. Wielputz M, Kauczor HU. MRI of the lung: state of the art. Diagn Interv Radiol 2012;18(4):344–53.
17. Liszewski MC, Hersman FW, Altes TA, et al. Magnetic resonance imaging of pediatric lung parenchyma, airways, vasculature, ventilation, and perfusion: state of the art. Radiol Clin North Am 2013;51(4):555–82.
18. Walkup LL, Tkach JA, Higano NS, et al. Quantitative Magnetic Resonance Imaging of Bronchopulmonary Dysplasia in the Neonatal Intensive Care Unit Environment. Am J Respir Crit Care Med 2015;192(10): 1215–22.
19. Adams EW, Harrison MC, Counsell SJ, et al. Increased lung water and tissue damage in bronchopulmonary dysplasia. J Pediatr 2004;145(4):503–7.
20. Flors L, Mugler JP 3rd, Paget-Brown A, et al. Hyperpolarized helium-3 diffusion-weighted magnetic resonance imaging detects abnormalities of lung structure in children with bronchopulmonary dysplasia. J Thorac Imaging 2017. [Epub ahead of print].
21. Walkup LL, Woods JC. Newer imaging techniques for bronchopulmonary dysplasia. Clin Perinatol 2015;42(4):871–87.
22. Okuyama H, Kubota A, Kawahara H, et al. Correlation between lung scintigraphy and long-term

outcome in survivors of congenital diaphragmatic hernia. Pediatr Pulmonol 2006;41(9):882–6.

23. Hayward MJ, Kharasch V, Sheils C, et al. Predicting inadequate long-term lung development in children with congenital diaphragmatic hernia: an analysis of longitudinal changes in ventilation and perfusion. J Pediatr Surg 2007;42(1):112–6.

24. Bjorkman KC, Kjellberg M, Bergstrom SE, et al. Postoperative regional distribution of pulmonary ventilation and perfusion in infants with congenital diaphragmatic hernia. J Pediatr Surg 2011;46(11): 2047–53.

25. Kjellberg M, Bjorkman K, Rohdin M, et al. Bronchopulmonary dysplasia: clinical grading in relation to ventilation/perfusion mismatch measured by single photon emission computed tomography. Pediatr Pulmonol 2013;48(12):1206–13.

26. Soler C, Figueras J, Roca I, et al. Pulmonary perfusion scintigraphy in the evaluation of the severity of bronchopulmonary dysplasia. Pediatr Radiol 1997; 27(1):32–5.

27. Grant FD, Treves ST. Nuclear medicine and molecular imaging of the pediatric chest: current practical imaging assessment. Radiol Clin North Am 2011; 49(5):1025–51.

28. Shinohara G, Morita K, Uno Y, et al. Scimitar syndrome in an infant with right lung hypoplasia, ventricular septal defect, and severe pulmonary hypertension. Gen Thorac Cardiovasc Surg 2010; 58(10):524–7.

29. Lee EY, Boiselle PM, Cleveland RH. Multidetector CT evaluation of congenital lung anomalies. Radiology 2008;247(3):632–48.

30. Newman B. Congenital bronchopulmonary foregut malformations: concepts and controversies. Pediatr Radiol 2006;36(8):773–91.

31. Riedlinger WF, Vargas SO, Jennings RW, et al. Bronchial atresia is common to extralobar sequestration, intralobar sequestration, congenital cystic adenomatoid malformation, and lobar emphysema. Pediatr Dev Pathol 2006;9(5):361–73.

32. Epelman M, Daltro P, Soto G, et al. Congenital lung anomalies. In: Coley BD, editor. Caffey's pediatric diagnostic imaging. 12th edition. Philadelphia: Elsevier; 2013. p. 550–66.

33. Lee EY, Dorkin H, Vargas SO. Congenital pulmonary malformations in pediatric patients: review and update on etiology, classification, and imaging findings. Radiol Clin North Am 2011;49(5):921–48.

34. Holder PD, Langston C. Intralobar pulmonary sequestration (a nonentity?). Pediatr Pulmonol 1986;2(3):147–53.

35. Laurin S, Hagerstrand I. Intralobar bronchopulmonary sequestration in the newborn–a congenital malformation. Pediatr Radiol 1999;29(3):174–8.

36. Stocker JT, Madewell JE, Drake RM. Congenital cystic adenomatoid malformation of the lung.

Classification and morphologic spectrum. Hum Pathol 1977;8(2):155–71.

37. Stocker J. The respiratory tract. In: Stocker JT, Dejner LP, editors. Pediatric pathology. 2nd edition. Philadelphia: Lippincott, Williams & Wilkins; 2001. p. 466–73.

38. Langston C. New concepts in the pathology of congenital lung malformations. Semin Pediatr Surg 2003;12(1):17–37.

39. Priest JR, Williams GM, Hill DA, et al. Pulmonary cysts in early childhood and the risk of malignancy. Pediatr Pulmonol 2009;44(1):14–30.

40. Griffin N, Devaraj A, Goldstraw P, et al. CT and histopathological correlation of congenital cystic pulmonary lesions: a common pathogenesis? Clin Radiol 2008;63(9):995–1005.

41. MacSweeney F, Papagiannopoulos K, Goldstraw P, et al. An assessment of the expanded classification of congenital cystic adenomatoid malformations and their relationship to malignant transformation. Am J Surg Pathol 2003;27(8):1139–46.

42. Hill DA, Dehner LP. A cautionary note about congenital cystic adenomatoid malformation (CCAM) type 4. Am J Surg Pathol 2004;28:554–5 [author reply: 555].

43. Stocker JT. Cystic lung disease in infants and children. Fetal Pediatr Pathol 2009;28(4):155–84.

44. Epelman M, Kreiger PA, Servaes S, et al. Current imaging of prenatally diagnosed congenital lung lesions. Semin Ultrasound CT MR 2010;31(2): 141–57.

45. Alamo L, Gudinchet F, Reinberg O, et al. Prenatal diagnosis of congenital lung malformations. Pediatr Radiol 2012;42(3):273–83.

46. Kao SW, Zuppan CW, Young LW. AIRP best cases in radiologic-pathologic correlation: type 2 congenital cystic adenomatoid malformation (type 2 congenital pulmonary airway malformation). Radiographics 2011;31(3):743–8.

47. Pryce DM. Lower accessory pulmonary artery with intralobar sequestration of lung; a report of seven cases. J Pathol Bacteriol 1946;58(3):457–67.

48. Savic B, Birtel FJ, Tholen W, et al. Lung sequestration: report of seven cases and review of 540 published cases. Thorax 1979;34(1):96–101.

49. Clements BS, Warner JO. Pulmonary sequestration and related congenital bronchopulmonary-vascular malformations: nomenclature and classification based on anatomical and embryological considerations. Thorax 1987;42(6):401–8.

50. Berrocal T, Madrid C, Novo S, et al. Congenital anomalies of the tracheobronchial tree, lung, and mediastinum: embryology, radiology, and pathology. Radiographics 2004;24(1):e17.

51. Cleveland RH. A radiologic update on medical diseases of the newborn chest. Pediatr Radiol 1995; 25(8):631–7.

52. Dinger J, Schwarze R, Rupprecht E. Radiological changes after therapeutic use of surfactant in infants with respiratory distress syndrome. Pediatr Radiol 1997;27(1):26–31.

53. Agrons GA, Courtney SE, Stocker JT, et al. From the archives of the AFIP: Lung disease in premature neonates: radiologic-pathologic correlation. Radiographics 2005;25(4):1047–73.

54. Boothroyd AE, Barson AJ. Pulmonary interstitial emphysema–a radiological and pathological correlation. Pediatr Radiol 1988;18(3):194–9.

55. Donnelly LF, Lucaya J, Ozelame V, et al. CT findings and temporal course of persistent pulmonary interstitial emphysema in neonates: a multiinstitutional study. AJR Am J Roentgenol 2003;180(4): 1129–33.

56. Donnelly LF, Frush DP. Localized radiolucent chest lesions in neonates: causes and differentiation. AJR Am J Roentgenol 1999;172(6):1651–8.

57. Jabra AA, Fishman EK, Shehata BM, et al. Localized persistent pulmonary interstitial emphysema: CT findings with radiographic-pathologic correlation. AJR Am J Roentgenol 1997;169(5):1381–4.

58. Swischuk LE, Shetty BP, John SD. The lungs in immature infants: how important is surfactant therapy in preventing chronic lung problems? Pediatr Radiol 1996;26(8):508–11.

59. Northway WH Jr, Rosan RC, Porter DY. Pulmonary disease following respirator therapy of hyaline-membrane disease. Bronchopulmonary dysplasia. N Engl J Med 1967;276(7):357–68.

60. Edwards DK, Jacob J, Gluck L. The immature lung: radiographic appearance, course, and complications. AJR Am J Roentgenol 1980;135(4): 659–66.

61. Jobe AH, Bancalari E. Bronchopulmonary dysplasia. Am J Respir Crit Care Med 2001;163(7):1723–9.

62. Ehrenkranz RA, Walsh MC, Vohr BR, et al. Validation of the National Institutes of Health consensus definition of bronchopulmonary dysplasia. Pediatrics 2005;116(6):1353–60.

63. Bancalari E, Wilson-Costello D, Iben SC. Management of infants with bronchopulmonary dysplasia in North America. Early Hum Dev 2005;81(2): 171–9.

64. Clouse BJ, Jadcherla SR, Slaughter JL. Systematic review of inhaled bronchodilator and corticosteroid therapies in infants with bronchopulmonary dysplasia: implications and future directions. PLoS One 2016;11(2):e0148188.

65. O'Shea TM, Kothadia JM, Klinepeter KL, et al. Randomized placebo-controlled trial of a 42-day tapering course of dexamethasone to reduce the duration of ventilator dependency in very low birth weight infants: outcome of study participants at 1-year adjusted age. Pediatrics 1999;104(1 Pt 1):15–21.

66. Yeh TF, Lin YJ, Huang CC, et al. Early dexamethasone therapy in preterm infants: a follow-up study. Pediatrics 1998;101(5):E7.

67. Watterberg KL. Policy statement–postnatal corticosteroids to prevent or treat bronchopulmonary dysplasia. Pediatrics 2010;126(4):800–8.

68. Hamvas A. Inherited surfactant protein-B deficiency and surfactant protein-C associated disease: clinical features and evaluation. Semin Perinatol 2006; 30(6):316–26.

69. Wilder MA. Surfactant protein B deficiency in infants with respiratory failure. J Perinat Neonatal Nurs 2004;18(1):61–7.

70. Whitsett JA. Genetic disorders of surfactant homeostasis. Paediatr Respir Rev 2006;7(Suppl 1):S240–2.

71. Yonker LM, Kinane TB. Pediatric interstitial lung disease: thyroid transcription factor-1 mutations and their phenotype potpourri. Chest 2013;144: 728–30.

72. Greenhill SR, Kotton DN. Pulmonary alveolar proteinosis: a bench-to-bedside story of granulocyte-macrophage colony-stimulating factor dysfunction. Chest 2009;136(2):571–7.

73. Lee EY. Interstitial lung disease in infants: new classification system, imaging technique, clinical presentation and imaging findings. Pediatr Radiol 2013;43(1):3–13 [quiz: 128–9].

74. Guillerman RP. Imaging of Childhood Interstitial Lung Disease. Pediatr Allergy Immunol Pulmonol 2010;23(1):43–68.

75. Guillerman RP, Brody AS. Contemporary perspectives on pediatric diffuse lung disease. Radiol Clin North Am 2011;49(5):847–68.

76. Mechri M, Epaud R, Emond S, et al. Surfactant protein C gene (SFTPC) mutation-associated lung disease: high-resolution computed tomography (HRCT) findings and its relation to histological analysis. Pediatr Pulmonol 2010;45(10):1021–9.

77. Olver RE, Ramsden CA, Strang LB, et al. The role of amiloride-blockable sodium transport in adrenaline-induced lung liquid reabsorption in the fetal lamb. J Physiol 1986;376:321–40.

78. Niisato N, Ito Y, Marunaka Y. cAMP stimulates Na(+) transport in rat fetal pneumocyte: involvement of a PTK- but not a PKA-dependent pathway. Am J Physiol 1999;277(4 Pt 1):L727–36.

79. Norlin A, Folkesson HG. Ca(2+)-dependent stimulation of alveolar fluid clearance in near-term fetal guinea pigs. Am J Physiol Lung Cell Mol Physiol 2002;282(4):L642–9.

80. O'Brodovich H, Hannam V, Seear M, et al. Amiloride impairs lung water clearance in newborn guinea pigs. J Appl Physiol (1985) 1990;68(4):1758–62.

81. Morrison JJ, Rennie JM, Milton PJ. Neonatal respiratory morbidity and mode of delivery at term: influence of timing of elective caesarean section. Br J Obstet Gynaecol 1995;102(2):101–6.

82. Guglani L, Lakshminrusimha S, Ryan RM. Transient tachypnea of the newborn. Pediatr Rev 2008; 29(11):e59–65.

83. Dargaville PA, Copnell B. The epidemiology of meconium aspiration syndrome: incidence, risk factors, therapies, and outcome. Pediatrics 2006; 117(5):1712–21.

84. Lee J, Romero R, Lee KA, et al. Meconium aspiration syndrome: a role for fetal systemic inflammation. Am J Obstet Gynecol 2016;214(3):366.e1-9.

85. Yeh TF, Harris V, Srinivasan G, et al. Roentgenographic findings in infants with meconium aspiration syndrome. JAMA 1979;242(1):60–3.

86. El Shahed AI, Dargaville PA, Ohlsson A, et al. Surfactant for meconium aspiration syndrome in term and late preterm infants. Cochrane Database Syst Rev 2014;(12):CD002054.

87. Haney PJ, Bohlman M, Sun CC. Radiographic findings in neonatal pneumonia. AJR Am J Roentgenol 1984;143(1):23–6.

Children with Cough and Fever
Up-to-date Imaging Evaluation and Management

Gary R. Schooler, MD[a],*, Joseph T. Davis, MD[a],
Victoria M. Parente, MD[b], Edward Y. Lee, MD, MPH[c]

KEYWORDS

• Cough • Fever • Lung infection • Pneumonia • Imaging management • Pediatric patients

KEY POINTS

• A broad spectrum of pulmonary infectious disorders may present in the pediatric population, ranging from the commonly encountered viral and bacterial pathogens to fungal and other atypical entities occurring in those patients who are immune compromised.
• Complications of pneumonia, including pleural effusion, empyema, necrotizing pneumonia, and abscess formation, often require ultrasonography and/or computed tomography for complete imaging evaluation.
• Recurrent chest infections, especially those occurring in the same anatomic region in the lung, should raise suspicion for underlying congenital pulmonary abnormality.
• Airway foreign bodies are common in the pediatric population and may present with cough and fever when the airway is obstructed or partially obstructed on a subacute or chronic basis.
• Follow-up chest radiographs are not routinely recommended in pediatric patients who are adequately treated and have recovered from lung infections.

INTRODUCTION

Cough and fever in the pediatric population are frequent but nonspecific symptoms at presentation. There are a wide range of underlying causes for these symptoms and clinicians are charged with determining what disorders may be present and how best to detect and treat each process. One of the more commonly encountered causes in children with fever and cough is pneumonia, an entity with a broad scope of infectious causes ranging from common viral and bacterial pathogens to atypical infectious agents. The incidence of pneumonia approaches 150 million cases per year worldwide and in children less than 5 years of age accounts for approximately 15% of deaths.[1,2]

Although community-acquired viral and bacterial pneumonia are encountered most frequently, clinicians and radiologists must remain cognizant of less common but equally important situations.

Disclosure: The authors have nothing to disclose.
[a] Department of Radiology, Duke University Medical Center, 1905 Children's Health Center, Box 3808–DUMC, Durham, NC 27710, USA; [b] Department of Pediatrics, Duke University Medical Center, Box 3127–DUMC, Durham, NC 27710, USA; [c] Department of Radiology, Boston Children's Hospital and Harvard Medical School, 300 Longwood Avenue, Boston, MA 02115, USA
* Corresponding author.
E-mail address: gary.schooler@duke.edu

Radiol Clin N Am 55 (2017) 645–655
http://dx.doi.org/10.1016/j.rcl.2017.02.007
0033-8389/17/© 2017 Elsevier Inc. All rights reserved.

Such situations include when the inflammatory or infectious condition is superimposed on immune dysfunction/suppression or congenital/acquired structural airway and pulmonary abnormalities. Underlying immunologic or structural abnormality may not be known at the time of presentation, and the radiologist may be the first to suggest that such a disorder is potentially present.

In most pediatric patients with cough and fever, imaging plays an important role in the initial diagnosis and management of infants and children with signs and symptoms indicating the presence of an infectious or inflammatory airway or pulmonary process. This article reviews a range of pathologic entities occurring in children with cough and fever in daily clinical practice. In addition, this article also discusses updated imaging algorithms, typical imaging findings, and practical recommendations for follow-up imaging.

IMAGING MODALITIES AND TECHNIQUES

The 3 most commonly used imaging modalities for evaluating infants and children who present with cough and fever are radiography, computed tomography (CT), and ultrasonography.

Radiography

Imaging pediatric patients presenting with cough and fever usually begins with radiography, an imaging modality that remains a mainstay in pediatric diagnostic imaging assessment. Although imaging evaluation may not be needed in pediatric patients with typical mild lower respiratory symptoms,[1,3] the cluster of classic clinical symptoms of pneumonia may be less accurate in infants and young children compared with adults, prompting the need for imaging if pneumonia is clinically suspected.[4]

The current standard practice for the imaging assessment of pneumonia includes obtaining frontal and lateral radiographs of the chest with the lungs at maximum inspiration. In efforts to reduce radiation exposure and cost, the necessity of the lateral radiograph in the evaluation process has been evaluated, revealing that the frontal radiograph alone has a slightly lower sensitivity than a combination of frontal and lateral radiographs and that pneumonia can be underdiagnosed in approximately 15% of patients.[5] However, in circumstances in which a radiologist can preview the frontal radiograph and a confluent lobar pneumonia can be confidently identified based on the frontal radiograph alone, the lateral radiograph may be safely omitted.[5] Such tailored practice has great potential for reducing the overall radiation dose, which is particularly important in the pediatric population.

Computed Tomography

CT is generally reserved for assessment of complications in the setting of chest infection or inflammation. In this clinical situation, intravenous contrast administration is typically needed. CT has shown enhanced diagnostic accuracy in assessing complications of lung infection such as necrosis, cavitation, abscess formation, and pleural complications, including complex pleural effusion and empyema.[6] In addition, CT may be beneficial in pediatric patients with atypical infections in the setting of immune compromise as well as those with underlying congenital lung malformations. Particular attention should be paid to using child-sized radiation dosing strategies as well as dose optimization techniques (including automatic exposure control and body size–specific dose modulation) to assist radiologists in ensuring adherence to ALARA (as low as reasonably achievable) principles.

Ultrasonography

For the past several decades, ultrasonography has been used for evaluation of pleural complications of pneumonia, predominantly evaluating for the presence and complexity of pleural fluid. More specifically, ultrasonography has been shown to be capable of detecting effusions as small as 3 to 5 mL,[7] which is typically achieved using a systematic approach that includes obtaining anterior, lateral, and posterior views of the chest using high-frequency linear and/or curved ultrasonography probes.

More recently, the use of ultrasonography to evaluate the lung parenchyma in the setting of infection has been explored. A meta-analysis performed by Pereda and colleagues[8] found that performing lung ultrasonography with a high-resolution linear transducer had a collective sensitivity of 96% and specificity of 93% for diagnosis of pneumonia in children less than 18 years of age. However, it is important to recognize that the infective consolidative process must reach the pleura to be detected by ultrasonography. In addition, differentiating between atelectasis and pneumonia may be difficult, because both may display sonographic air bronchograms (airless lung with gas or fluid filling the bronchi) resulting in some question of reliability and accuracy of ultrasonography in diagnosis of pneumonia.[9] Other investigators have suggested lung ultrasonography as a follow-up examination that may be useful in detection of ongoing infection and pulmonary and pleural complications.[9,10]

SPECTRUM OF UNDERLYING CAUSES OF CHILDREN WITH COUGH AND FEVER
Common Pediatric Chest Infections

Pneumonia, whether occurring as a result of viral, bacterial, or atypical pathogens, is a common infectious process in the pediatric patient population. It occurs in approximately 2.6% of children less than 17 years of age.[1] A familiarity with typical clinical manifestations and radiographic patterns of disease can help distinguish among pathologic entities and benefit radiologists and clinicians.

Viral infection
Of the many pathologic agents capable of causing infection in the pediatric chest, viral agents are the most common. A multicenter evaluation of children hospitalized for community-acquired pneumonia with radiographic evidence of pneumonia revealed detection of a viral pathogen in 73% of patients.[9] The more commonly encountered viral pathogens include respiratory syncytial virus (RSV), human rhinovirus, and human metapneumovirus.[1,11] Children with viral chest infection frequently present with an insidious onset of cough, upper and lower respiratory congestion, and fever. Differentiation between viral and bacterial pathogens clinically can be exceedingly difficult, particularly in the pediatric population. Although an abrupt and more severe onset of symptoms can suggest a bacterial pathogen, this is frequently inaccurate and imaging may aid clinicians in discerning the most likely cause.

Differentiation between viral and bacterial causes of lung infections on chest radiograph has long been, and continues to be, a source of consternation for radiologists. Classically, viral infections manifest as increased lung volumes with foci of air trapping and/or atelectasis. Multifocal or generalized perihilar/peribronchial opacities representing underlying bronchial wall thickening caused by inflammation favor a viral origin as well. The radiographic appearance of a viral lung infection is typified by RSV, which is commonly seen in children less than 2 years of age. This infection usually manifests as hyperexpanded lungs and thickening of the bronchial walls and pulmonary interstitium as a result of inflammation localized to and obstructing the airways, particularly those of small caliber[12] (**Fig. 1**). However, distinction between viral and bacterial pathogens remains difficult in many cases, especially those with patchy bilateral opacities, diffuse airspace consolidation, and lobar consolidation, which have been shown to occur in both viral and bacterial pneumonias.[13,14] Radiologists must also remain cognizant of the possibility of

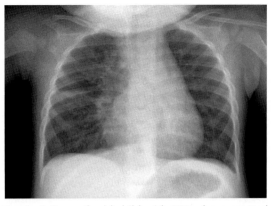

Fig. 1. A 9-month-old child with RSV who presented with cough and fever. Frontal chest radiograph shows mildly hyperexpanded lungs with streaky bilateral perihilar opacities and peribronchial cuffing. Right midlung subsegmental atelectasis is also noted. This constellation of findings and clinical history suggests a viral respiratory tract infection (bronchiolitic pattern).

superimposition of bacterial infection, which can lead to abrupt patient decompensation. Determining this based solely on imaging can be challenging but the rapid evolution or progression of consolidation, especially in pediatric patients who fail to show the expected clinical improvement or deteriorate clinically, should raise concern for this complication.

Bacterial infection
Bacterial lung infections, although considerably less frequent in children younger than 5 years of age, remain an important cause of morbidity and worldwide mortality.[1,2] Similar to viral pneumonia, a wide array of bacterial species can infect the pediatric lungs, the most common being *Streptococcus pneumoniae*. A large study of patients hospitalized with community-acquired pneumonia revealed a bacterial pathogen in 15% of patients.[11] Pediatric patients with bacterial pneumonia tend to present with more abrupt symptom onset, show more severe symptoms, and may have localized chest pain.[1]

Chest radiography in pediatric bacterial pneumonia can yield several patterns of disease, including lobar, diffuse, and segmental/subsegmental opacities, which can be in a peribronchovascular distribution. When diffuse or multifocal, it can be difficult to distinguish bacterial from viral infection. A unique pattern of airspace consolidation, the so-called round pneumonia, is occasionally seen in the pediatric patient population presenting with cough and fever. Most commonly seen in patients less than 8 years of age (mean age of 5 years), round pneumonia manifests as a spherical or rounded pulmonary mass, frequently with well-delineated borders and located in the posterior lower lobes[15] (Fig. 2). The rounded configuration is suspected to be a result of immature collateralization of distal airways secondary to underdevelopment of pores of Kohn and absence of canals of Lambert.[16] Round pneumonias typically resolve with appropriate antimicrobial treatment. Follow-up radiographs may be obtained to ensure interval resolution.

Complications of bacterial pneumonia, although infrequent, can arise. These complications include pleural effusion, pleural empyema, necrotizing pneumonia, and pulmonary abscess. The most frequent of these complications are pleural effusion and empyema, occurring in as many as 40% of hospitalized patients.[17,18] Although chest radiographs are not very specific for the nature of pleural fluid collections, they are often the first to suggest their presence. Occasionally, fluid collections become lenticular in shape or do not show the expected layering on supine/decubitus imaging, both findings suggestive of loculation. Ultrasonography can be used to further evaluate the fluid composition. Complex pleural effusions show echogenic debris, fibrinous strands, and septations within the fluid[19] (Fig. 3).

CT may be used for assessment of pleural fluid, and when performed with intravenous contrast can show pleural thickening, increased pleural enhancement, and loculation. However, CT is generally not able to visualize septations/stranding because their thickness is frequently less than the resolution threshold of CT. In a comparison of ultrasonography with CT for evaluation of parapneumonic effusion, Kurian and colleagues[20] concluded that CT did not provide any additional clinically useful information that was not seen on chest ultrasonography.

Similar to the pleural complications of pneumonia, the parenchymal complications are suboptimally evaluated on radiographs. Necrotizing pneumonia results from the thrombotic occlusion of alveolar capillaries associated with adjacent inflammation, resulting in ischemia and eventual necrosis of the affected lung parenchyma.[21] CT evaluation reveals nonenhancement of necrotic lung, frequently with gas-filled and fluid-filled cavities, distinguishable from a pulmonary abscess, which has a solitary cavity with thick, contrast-enhancing walls[21,22] (Fig. 4). The utility of ultrasonography in evaluation of pulmonary complications of pneumonia has been explored, and this showed that chest ultrasonography and chest CT are similar in diagnosing lung necrosis or abscess resulting from complicated pneumonia.[20] However, chest CT may be necessary when the chest ultrasonography is technically limited or discrepant with the clinical findings.

Atypical Pediatric Chest Infections

Mycoplasma infection

Mycoplasma pneumoniae is an important cause of community-acquired respiratory infection in school-aged children and younger children who attend day care centers. The symptoms of mycoplasma infection are usually nonspecific and viral-like with gradual onset of mild pharyngitis, low-grade fever, headache, myalgias, and eventually a dry, nagging cough. However, unlike viral respiratory infections, mycoplasma infections are treatable with appropriate antibiotic therapy. A

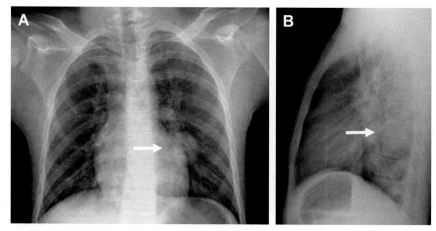

Fig. 2. A 3-year-old child with cough and fever. Frontal (*A*) and lateral (*B*) radiographs of the chest show a round masslike opacity (*arrow*) in the superior left lower lobe. Following appropriate antimicrobial therapy, the patient's symptoms resolved, confirming that this masslike lesion is a round pneumonia. In this clinical setting, immediate additional advanced or follow-up imaging is necessary.

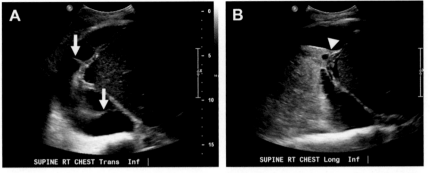

Fig. 3. A 7-year-old boy with bacterial pneumonia. Ultrasonography images in transverse (*A*) and longitudinal (*B*) orientation of the chest show complex pleural fluid with multiple internal fibrous septations (*arrows*). Note the consolidated lung (*arrowhead*) adhering to the diaphragm on the longitudinal image (*B*).

well-known feature of mycoplasma pulmonary infection is the discrepancy between the radiographic findings and the mild clinical presentation.[23]

The radiographic patterns in *M pneumoniae* infection are variable. However, most commonly seen is a reticulonodular pattern, correlating with histopathologic findings of peribronchitis, with a lower lobe predominance (**Fig. 5**). Diffuse interstitial and parahilar peribronchial opacities are also common patterns of *M pneumoniae* infection. In one study, 33% of patients with *M pneumoniae* infection had consolidations that were either homogeneous areas of ground-glass opacification or patchy inhomogeneous increased opacity.[23] Pleural effusions and hilar adenopathy are uncommon.

Fungal infection

Pulmonary fungal infection in the pediatric population is most commonly caused by histoplasmosis and aspergillosis. Histoplasmosis is a systemic mycosis caused by *Histoplasma capsulatum*, an organism that is a natural soil contaminant and is endemic in the Ohio River valley. In pediatric patients affected with *H capsulatum*, cough and fever are two of the most common presenting symptoms. Pulmonary infection can result in diffuse reticulonodular opacities, small diffuse pulmonary nodules, and mediastinal lymph node enlargement. Typically, pulmonary nodules heal leaving granulomata that calcify. Involved lymph nodes frequently calcify as well.[24,25]

Aspergillus infection can be caused by infection with several *Aspergillus* species. The fungus is ubiquitous and asymptomatic colonization is common. Infection is a result of type and amount of exposure, the virulence of the organism present, and most importantly the immune competency of the pediatric patient. The spectrum of infectious

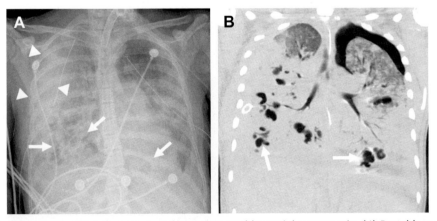

Fig. 4. A 12-year-old girl with influenza A and superimposed bacterial pneumonia. (*A*) Portable supine frontal radiograph of the chest shows hazy bilateral pulmonary opacities with areas of denser consolidation in the lower lobes and larger geographic parenchymal lucencies (*arrows*) in the right greater than left lower lobes. Also note the large right pleural effusion (*arrowheads*). (*B*) Coronal reformatted lung window CT image shows the presence of large gas-filled spaces (*arrows*) to better detail, caused by pulmonary necrosis.

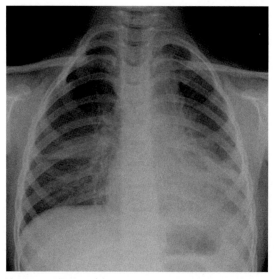

Fig. 5. A 6-year-old girl with mycoplasma infection who presented with fatigue, headache, fever, and cough. Frontal chest radiograph shows reticulonodular opacities in the right lower lobe and airspace disease characterized by ground-glass opacity and consolidation in the right midlung zone, medial left upper lobe, and left lower lobe.

manifestations is broad, ranging from allergic pulmonary reaction to systemic involvement from invasive pulmonary infection. The allergic form of infection (allergic bronchopulmonary aspergillosis) affects children with asthma and cystic fibrosis, resulting in proximal and segmental bronchiectasis with mucous plugging and scattered consolidations as a result of a hypersensitivity reaction to the fungus. Formation of an aspergilloma is an uncommon finding in children, but may be seen within a cavity from prior pulmonary infection or in congenital bronchopulmonary malformations.[24] Angioinvasive disease is most commonly seen in immune-compromised pediatric patients and is discussed in further detail later.

Tuberculosis infection

Compared with the aforementioned causes of chest infection, tuberculosis (TB) is uncommon in the pediatric patient population living in developed countries. However, there has been a resurgence of the disease worldwide and children represent one of the highest-risk groups, especially those younger than 5 years of age. A recent epidemiologic study performed on pediatric patients diagnosed with TB found that the TB rate for young children (<5 years of age) who are born in the United States but have at least 1 foreign-born parent to be more than 6 times that of US-born children with US-born parents.[26,27]

Primary TB, the most common form in children, is distinct from the postprimary TB seen in the adult population. Approximately 50% of affected patients are symptomatic, most commonly presenting with cough and fever.[27] Chest radiographs most frequently show hilar and mediastinal lymph node enlargement in 70% to 90% of patients, which may be predominantly right-sided, and airspace consolidation that can be indistinguishable from bacterial pneumonia. On CT, lymph nodes characteristically show low-attenuation centers caused by underlying caseous necrosis[24,27,28] (Fig. 6).

Recurrent Chest Infections

Immunodeficiency

Pediatric immunodeficiency may be the result of 1 or several primary deficiencies in the components of the immune system, including humoral, cellular, phagocytic, or complement systems. Dysfunction of each of these systems renders pediatric patients susceptible to particular sets of diseases. Humoral deficiencies (impaired antibody production) account for 70% of all primary immunodeficiency disorders and result in increased susceptibility to pyogenic bacteria such as *Haemophilus influenzae*, *S pneumoniae*, and

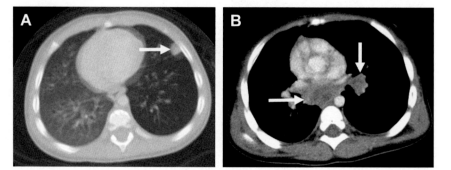

Fig. 6. Pediatric patient with primary tuberculosis who presented with cough and fever. Axial CT images show a soft tissue density perifissural left upper lobe nodule (*arrow in A*) with necrotic subcarinal and left hilar lymphadenopathy (*arrows in B*).

staphylococci. Recurrent pneumonia is one of the most common clinical manifestations. Dysfunction may also be present in the phagocytes (neutrophils, monocytes, and macrophages), resulting in recurrent pyogenic and fungal infections. Of the phagocytic deficiencies, chronic granulomatous disease is the most common, usually manifesting as recurrent pulmonary infection, with fungal infections encountered most frequently[29] (Fig. 7).

Acquired immune dysfunction, especially in the setting of chemotherapy and bone marrow transplant, is an important cause of recurrent pediatric chest infections. Infections usually initially manifest clinically as a fever, and are a major cause of morbidity and mortality early in pediatric cancer treatment.[30] Pulmonary aspergillosis is one of the frequently encountered infections in this patient population. Chest radiographs often reveal variable findings, ranging from scattered, randomly distributed pulmonary nodules to segmental and multilobar consolidation. In these patients, evaluation with chest CT is often warranted to help guide treatment. CT can show the multiplicity of nodules as well as cavitation of nodules, areas of consolidation, and chest wall involvement.[31]

Congenital lung malformations

Structural abnormalities of the pediatric lung parenchyma can result in recurrent pneumonia, which manifests clinically as recurrent cough and fever. The Infectious Disease Society of America (IDSA) guidelines for the management of community-acquired pneumonia in children recommend repeating chest radiographs 4 to 6 weeks after the diagnosis of recurrent pneumonia that involves the same lobe or in patients with lobar collapse at initial chest radiograph.[3] The reason for this recommendation is that these findings may raise suspicion of an anatomic anomaly, chest mass, or foreign body.[3]

On imaging studies, what may previously have been disguised as a round pneumonia may represent an infected pulmonary sequestration, congenital pulmonary airway malformation (CPAM), or bronchogenic cyst[32] (Fig. 8). Outside the neonatal period, infection is the most common presenting symptom for both CPAM and pulmonary sequestration.[33,34] When an underlying congenital lung malformation is suspected, contrast-enhanced CT of the chest with angiographic technique should be performed to evaluate the pulmonary parenchyma and for any aberrant vascular supply to the lung lesion (Fig. 9). Imaging findings include focal parenchymal opacities/consolidations, particularly in the lower lobes, and frequently with cysts of variable sizes that may contain gas and fluid.

Airway Foreign Body

Foreign body aspiration in the pediatric population is the most common cause of mortality caused by unintentional injury in children less than 1 year of age, resulting in approximately 3500 deaths per year in children of all ages.[35] Aspiration is substantially more common in children less than 3 years of age. The most commonly aspirated foreign bodies are food items, specifically peanuts, accounting for up to 50% of aspirated objects.[35] Many aspirations are unwitnessed and therefore present with variable signs and symptoms indicating airway obstruction ranging from partial to complete. Those pediatric patients with partial airway obstruction may have a much less acute presentation, with wheezing, recurrent coughing, and fever.

When a clinical history suggestive of foreign body aspiration is elicited, imaging of the airway should be performed. In general, anteroposterior and lateral radiographs of the neck and chest are indicated. When food material is aspirated, it is almost always radiolucent. Therefore, radiologists must rely on secondary signs to diagnose and localize the level of airway obstruction. The most common location for an aspirated foreign body

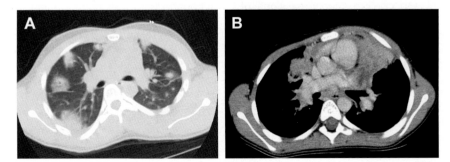

Fig. 7. Child with underlying chronic granulomatous disease and aspergillus fungal infection. Axial CT images show multiple bilateral nodular densities with surrounding ground glass opacity (*A*) and mediastinal adenopathy (*B*).

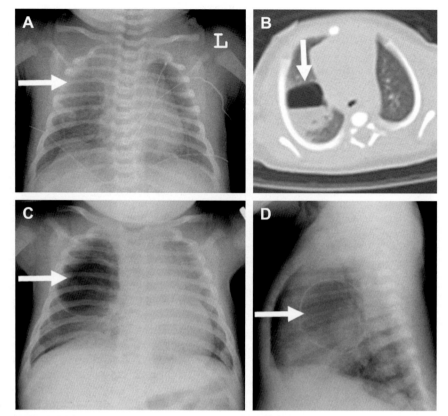

Fig. 8. A 3-month-old child with CPAM who presented with recurrent cough and fever. Frontal radiograph (*A*) shows a vague right upper lobe opacity (*arrow*). Subsequent axial lung window CT image (*B*) shows a cystic lesion with an internal air-fluid level (*arrow*) in the right upper lobe. This appearance suggests an infected, previously undiagnosed CPAM. Patient was treated with antibiotics, after which 3-week follow-up frontal and lateral radiographs (*C*, *D*) show interval resolution of fluid within the lesion with increased size/aeration of the CPAM (*arrows*), which was subsequently surgically resected.

to lodge is the lower airway, specifically the right lung (60%), followed by the left lung (23%), and least commonly the trachea (13%).[36]

Frontal radiographs are frequently normal or unremarkable, but can show unilateral pulmonary hyperexpansion indicating a partial main stem bronchial obstruction caused by a foreign body (**Fig. 10**). Often additional assessment is necessary to detect and confirm secondary signs of obstruction. Bilateral decubitus chest radiographs can be performed for evaluation of the lack of expected pulmonary deflation of the downside/affected lung with obstructed airway. Alternatively, radiologists can use fluoroscopy to observe the chest and lungs of patients being evaluated for the presence of symmetric inflation and deflation of the lungs. When airway obstruction is encountered, the affected lung shows a higher static volume and reduced volume changes during inspiration and expiration. Based on the author's experience, small children often begin to cry with fluoroscopic examination, which results in

increased respiration accentuating the findings discussed earlier.

In the subacute phase of aspiration, clinicians may not identify signs of airway obstruction but find sequelae of volume loss and postobstructive infection manifesting as lobar, segmental, or subsegmental consolidation. With aspiration of a radiopaque foreign body, these findings remain, although direct radiographic identification of the aspirate body is frequently possible. Bronchoscopy is currently the reference standard for evaluation and subsequent retrieval of aspirated foreign bodies, even if radiographs are negative in pediatric patients with high clinical suspicion of having aspirated foreign bodies and persistent symptoms.[36]

Follow-up Imaging

Follow-up chest radiographs are not routinely recommended in children who are adequately treated and have recovered from lung infections.

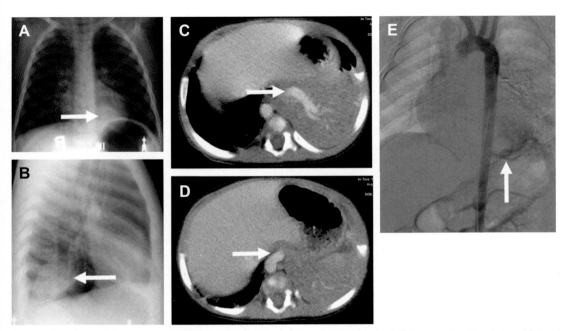

Fig. 9. Infant boy with recurrent infection of pulmonary sequestration in the left lower lobe. Frontal and lateral radiographs (*A*, *B*) show a left lower lobe/retrocardiac opacity (*arrows*). Given concern for possible congenital pulmonary lesion predisposing to recurrent infection, thoracic CT angiography (*C, D*) was performed, which shows consolidative density within the left lower lobe with an aberrant systemic arterial supply (*arrows*) arising from the aorta. This finding was confirmed with catheter-directed angiography (*E, arrow*). These findings are consistent with a left lower lobe sequestration.

Follow-up imaging is indicated in complicated pneumonias in pediatric patients receiving adequate antibiotic coverage for 48 to 72 hours with poor clinical improvement or worsening symptoms.[1,3] In addition, follow-up imaging should be considered in recurrent pneumonias that involve the same lobe in order to exclude a suspected underlying congenital anomaly, chest mass, or aspirated foreign body.[1,3] In pediatric patients who required cross-sectional imaging with ultrasonography or CT to further delineate complications of pneumonia, repeat imaging may be necessary in order to ensure satisfactory resolution of previously documented abnormalities or assess the sequelae of permanent damage.

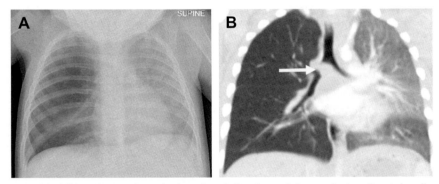

Fig. 10. A 1-year-old child with cough and wheezing following unobserved play. Frontal radiograph of the chest (*A*) shows hyperexpansion of the right lung without radiopaque foreign body. Appearance and history suggest air trapping secondary to an aspirated radiolucent foreign body. Subsequently obtained coronal reformatted lung window CT (*B*) image shows the hyperexpanded right lung as well as a soft tissue density (*arrow*) obstructing the right mainstem bronchus. This object was found to be an aspirated nut on bronchoscopy.

SUMMARY

Children presenting with cough and fever may have one of various airway or lung abnormalities. Infectious agents range from the most common viruses to which children are exposed each winter to ubiquitous fungal organisms found in the environment. A clear knowledge of common as well as less common but clinically important pathogens affecting children and how they manifest on imaging can help radiologists and clinicians arrive at an accurate diagnosis in a timely manner, pursue the proper imaging strategy, and deliver optimal pediatric patient management.

REFERENCES

1. Gereige RS, Laufer PM. Pneumonia. Pediatr Rev 2013;34:438–55.
2. McCulloh RJ, Patel K. Recent developments in pediatric community-acquired pneumonia. Curr Infect Dis Rep 2016;8:14.
3. Bradley JS, Byington CL, Shah SS, et al. The management of community-acquired pneumonia in infants and children older than 3 months of age: clinical practice guidelines by the Pediatric Infectious Disease Society and the Infectious Disease Society of America. Clin Infect Dis 2011;53:e25–76.
4. Grossman LK. Clinical, laboratory, and radiological information in the diagnosis of pneumonia in children. Ann Emerg Med 1988;17:43–6.
5. Rigsby CK, Strife JL, Johnson ND, et al. Is the frontal radiograph alone sufficient to evaluate for pneumonia in children? Pediatr Radiol 2004;34:379–83.
6. Kendrick APT, Ling H, Subramaniam R, et al. The value of early CT in complicated childhood pneumonia. Pediatr Radiol 2002;32:16–21.
7. Mong A, Epelman M, Darge K. Ultrasound of the pediatric chest. Pediatr Radiol 2012;42:1287–97.
8. Pereda MA, Chavez MA, Hooper-Miele CC, et al. Lung ultrasound of the diagnosis of pneumonia in children: a meta-analysis. Pediatrics 2015;135:714–22.
9. Toma P, Owens CM. Chest ultrasound in children: critical appraisal. Pediatr Radiol 2013;43:1427–34.
10. Caiulo VA, Gargani L, Caiulo S, et al. Lung ultrasound characteristics of community-acquired pneumonia in hospitalized children. Pediatr Pulmonol 2013;48:280–7.
11. Jain S, Williams DJ, Arnold SR, et al. Community-acquired pneumonia requiring hospitalization among U.S. children. N Engl J Med 2015;372:835–45.
12. Griscom NT. Pneumonia in children and some of its variants. Radiology 1988;167:297–302.
13. Virkki R, Juven T, Rikalainen H, et al. Differentiation of bacterial and viral pneumonia in children. Thorax 2002;57:438–41.
14. Guo W, Wang J, Sheng M, et al. Radiological findings in 210 paediatric patients with viral pneumonia: a retrospective case study. Br J Radiol 2012;85:1385–9.
15. Kim Y, Donnelly L. Round pneumonia: imaging findings in a large series of children. Pediatr Radiol 2007;37:1235–40.
16. Kirks D. Practical pediatric imaging: diagnostic radiology of infants and children. 3rd edition. Philadelphia: Lippincott-Raven; 1998. p. 639–42.
17. Tan TQ, Mason EO, Wald ER, et al. Clinical characteristics of children with complicated pneumonia caused by Streptococcus pneumoniae. Pediatrics 2002;110:1–6.
18. Grisaru-Soen G, Eisenstadt M, Paret G, et al. Pediatric parapneumonic empyema: risk factors, clinical characteristics, microbiology, and management. Pediatr Emerg Care 2013;29:425–9.
19. Calder A, Owens CM. Imaging of parapneumonic pleural effusions and empyema in children. Pediatr Radiol 2009;39:527–37.
20. Kurian J, Levin TL, Han BK, et al. Comparison of ultrasound and CT in the evaluation of pneumonia complicated by parapneumonic effusion in children. AJR Am J Roentgenol 2009;193:1648–54.
21. Donnelly LF, Klosterman LA. Cavitary necrosis complicating pneumonia in children: sequential findings on chest radiography. AJR Am J Roentgenol 1998;171:253–6.
22. Hodin M, Hanquinet S, Cotting J, et al. Imaging of cavitary necrosis in complicated childhood pneumonia. Eur Radiol 2002;12:391–6.
23. John SD, Ramanathan J, Swischuk LE. Spectrum of clinical and radiographic findings in pediatric mycoplasma pneumonia. Radiographics 2001;21:121–31.
24. Daltro P, Santos EN, Gaspretto TD, et al. Pulmonary infections. Pediatr Radiol 2011;41:S69–82.
25. Butler JP, Heller R, Wright PF. Histoplasmosis during childhood. South Med J 1994;87:476–80.
26. Pang J, Teeter LD, Katz DJ, et al. Epidemiology of tuberculosis in young children in the United States. Pediatrics 2014;133:e494–504.
27. Kim WS, Choi J, Cheon J, et al. Pulmonary tuberculosis in infants: radiographic and CT findings. AJR Am J Roentgenol 2006;187:1024–33.
28. Leung AN, Muller NL, Pineda PR, et al. Primary tuberculosis in childhood: radiographic manifestations. Radiology 1992;182:87–91.
29. Yin EZ, Frush DP, Donnelly LF, et al. Primary immunodeficiency disorders in pediatric patients: clinical features and imaging findings. AJR Am J Roentgenol 2001;176:1541–52.
30. Chavhan GB, Babyn PS, Nathan PC, et al. Imaging of acute and subacute toxicities of cancer therapy in children. Pediatr Radiol 2016;46:9–20.

31. Thomas KE, Owens CM, Veys PA, et al. The radiological spectrum of invasive aspergillosis in children: a 10-year review. Pediatr Radiol 2003;33: 453–60.

32. Restrepo R, Palani R, Matapathi UM, et al. Imaging of round pneumonia and mimics in children. Pediatr Radiol 2010;40:1931–40.

33. Parikh DH, Rsiah SV. Congenital lung lesions: postnatal management and outcome. Semin Pediatr Surg 2015;24:160–7.

34. Laberge JM, Bratu I, Flageole H. The management of asymptomatic congenital lung malformations. Paediatr Respir Rev 2004;5(suppl A):S305–15.

35. Pugmire BS, Lim R, Avery L. Review of ingested and aspirated foreign bodies in children and their clinical significance for radiologists. Radiographics 2015; 35:1528–38.

36. Darras KE, Roston AT, Yewchuk LK. Imaging acute airway obstruction in infants and children. Radiographics 2015;35:2064–79.

Thoracic Neoplasms in Children

Contemporary Perspectives and Imaging Assessment

Matthew A. Zapala, MD, PhD[a],*, Victor M. Ho-Fung, MD[b],
Edward Y. Lee, MD, MPH[c]

KEYWORDS

- Primary lung neoplasm • Primary airway neoplasm • Mediastinal neoplasm • Chest wall neoplasm
- Pediatric patients

KEY POINTS

- Pediatric thoracic neoplasms are rare and often present with nonspecific symptoms leading to a delay in diagnosis. Imaging evaluation is often first in identifying the unforeseen problem.
- A thorough understanding of the multiple imaging modalities and protocols available to assess pediatric thoracic neoplasms provides the optimal radiologic evaluation necessary for accurate diagnosis and proper surgical/treatment planning.
- Up-to-date knowledge of the typical imaging appearance of pediatric thoracic neoplasms narrows differential diagnoses for optimal clinical management and treatment.

INTRODUCTION

Radiology plays an increasingly critical role in the evaluation and characterization of thoracic neoplasms in the pediatric population.[1] In recent years, dramatic advances in imaging techniques from various currently available modalities, including digital radiography, ultrasound, multidetector computed tomography (MDCT), and MR imaging, have substantially increased the diagnostic capabilities of radiology and placed radiology at the forefront of clinical decision making.[2–6] Although primary thoracic neoplasms in children are rare, they are clinically challenging to diagnose because they are often asymptomatic.[7] In addition, when affected children do present with symptoms, they are often nonspecific, such as cough, prompting imaging as the initial work-up. Imaging of pediatric patients with thoracic neoplasms offers unique challenges distinct from adult patients. This article reviews the current radiologic work-up for pediatric thoracic neoplasms and provides imaging algorithms with the latest techniques and the characteristic imaging appearance of various thoracic neoplasms unique to the pediatric population.

IMAGING ALGORITHM

Initial imaging work-up in children with clinically suspected underlying thoracic neoplasm often begins with chest radiographs. Chest radiographs are

Disclosure Statement: All authors certify that there is no actual or potential conflict of interest in relation to this article.

[a] Department of Radiology and Biomedical Imaging, Benioff Children's Hospital, University of California, San Francisco, 1975 Fourth Street, San Francisco, CA 94158, USA; [b] Department of Radiology, The Children's Hospital of Philadelphia, 3401 Civic Center Boulevard, Philadelphia, PA 19104, USA; [c] Department of Radiology, Boston Children's Hospital, Harvard Medical School, 300 Longwood Avenue, Boston, MA 02115, USA
* Corresponding author.
E-mail address: Matthew.Zapala@ucsf.edu

Radiol Clin N Am 55 (2017) 657–676
http://dx.doi.org/10.1016/j.rcl.2017.02.008

an excellent first-line modality in providing the radiologist with an overview of the chest and can often identify sizable parenchymal lesions, pleural-based masses, mediastinal masses, and chest wall or bony-based neoplasms.[7] Although most thoracic neoplasms in children eventually require additional cross-sectional imaging for confirmation and further characterization,[6] chest radiographs remain a vital screening component in the initial work-up of pediatric thoracic neoplasms.

Ultrasound also plays an increasingly important role as a first-line screening modality in the assessment of palpable thoracic chest wall masses.[8] Some of these palpable chest wall masses are accurately diagnosed with ultrasound alone, such as vascular malformations.[9] However, chest wall masses without classic imaging features of vascular malformation need to go on to further characterization by CT or MR imaging. Typically, soft tissue chest wall masses that lack bony involvement can best be assessed by contrast-enhanced MR imaging.

MDCT remains the main workhorse in terms of image evaluation of thoracic neoplasms in the pediatric patient population.[6] After initial assessment by chest radiographs, MDCT is the imaging modality of choice given its superior ability to confirm and characterize airway, parenchymal, and pleural-based thoracic neoplastic masses.[10] However, it is important to recognize that, in comparison with chest radiographs, such increased ability to assess the lung parenchyma, pleura, and airways comes with a price of increased radiation dose to the patient. As such, every effort should be made to obtain the MDCT using the ALARA (as low as reasonably achievable) principle with the lowest possible radiation dose to obtain diagnostic quality images for the pertinent indication.[11]

Although MDCT remains the modality of choice for most pediatric thoracic neoplasms, MR imaging still can play an important role in the assessment of chest- and mediastinal-based neoplastic masses.[12] MR imaging is particularly useful in assessing for fat within lesions or for assessing atypical vascular malformations. MR imaging may be most useful in further characterizing isolated chest wall soft tissue masses with nonspecific imaging findings on ultrasound.[13] Although MR imaging lacks ionizing radiation, the increased scan time needed to acquire images may necessitate that pediatric patients be sedated. As such, it is critical that only the appropriate MR imaging sequences be performed to address the underlying specific diagnostic question. Imaging protocols for ultrasound, MDCT, and MR imaging are further discussed in the following sections.

IMAGING TECHNIQUES AND PROTOCOLS
Ultrasound

Sonographic technique for chest masses is usually reserved for palpable chest masses.[14] For ultrasound to be useful, the thoracic mass needs to be superficial and can usually be imaged with a high-frequency linear transducer (9–15 MHz) to increase image resolution.[15] Lesions may require a standoff pad to visualize appropriately. In addition to gray-scale images, color flow images documenting arterial and/or venous waveforms are critical in the sonographic assessment of chest wall masses. Ultrasound can also be useful for accurately identifying thymus versus other mediastinal masses given the typical sonographic appearance of the thymus in infants and young children. In contrast to superficial masses, a sector probe using a subxiphoid approach is often helpful to assess the mediastinum.[8] The advantages of ultrasound are the lack of ionizing radiation and the ability to image nonsedated pediatric patients in a dynamic and reproducible way.

Multidetector Computed Tomography

MDCT evaluation of neoplastic thoracic masses requires that the pediatric patient remain still and follow instruction. Although sedation can usually be avoided in older patients who can follow instruction, it is usually required for pediatric patients age 5 and younger.[16] MDCT scanning parameters should be adjusted and optimized to the ALARA principle to minimize the overall radiation exposure. This can usually be achieved by varying the kilovoltage peak (kVp) and tube current milliampere (mA) according to the patient's weight and age. Recommended weight- and age-based MDCT protocols are provided online at the Image Gently campaign from the Alliance for Radiation Safety in Pediatric Imaging.

When assessing purely airway-based or lung parenchymal–based lesions, intravenous (IV) contrast may not be necessary. However, when assessing mediastinal masses, lymphadenopathy, and involvement of major vasculature, IV contrast is beneficial. Often, initial evaluations of thoracic neoplastic masses in pediatric patients are evaluated with IV contrast. The recommended dose of contrast is usually 1.5 to 2 mL per kg body weight not to exceed 150 mL of total IV contrast. IV contrast is administered either by hand or mechanically depending on the catheter size and location.[17]

MR Imaging

MR imaging protocols should be indication-based with the field of view and coil selection tailored to answer the specific clinical question, particularly in the pediatric population.

Mediastinal or large chest wall masses may best be assessed with dedicated chest/cardiac coils.[18] Smaller chest wall masses can best be evaluated with surface coils. Electrocardiac gating and respiratory ordered phase encoding is used to reduce motion artifact. Pediatric chest MR imaging is challenging because of the long acquisition times and because children usually have difficulty with long breath holds or the concept of quite breathing.[19] In pediatric patients that have difficulty following breath-holding instructions, one can take advantage of sequences that do not require breath holding, such as axial T2 PROPELLER/BLADE sequences, performed with the patient free breathing. Respiratory gating can also be used with external respiratory devices, such as pneumobelts.[20] MR imaging evaluations of chest wall masses typically include a T2 fat-saturated or short T1 inversion recovery sequence, often in the axial and coronal plane. T2 single-shot fast spin echo sequences are used given their quick acquisition times, high sensitivity, and high signal-to-noise ratio for fluid. Additional T1 fat-saturated postcontrast images are also usually obtained.

Although MR imaging is not typically used to evaluate the lung parenchyma, certain larger lung masses are assessed with MR imaging. In fact, a recent study compared the efficacy of fast imaging sequences for thoracic MR imaging with MDCT findings and showed that MR imaging could reliably detect pulmonary nodules or masses greater than 3 mm in size in children.[21] MR imaging sequences that evaluate the lung parenchyma include variations of two-dimensional (2D) and three-dimensional (3D) short and ultrashort gradient recall echo sequences, which overcome the short T2* of lung parenchyma and minimize signal loss created by air-tissue interfaces.[22] Spoiled gradient echo sequences have been used in several clinical studies and were rated the best sequence for nodule detection.[23] Postcontrast images are usually required often with 3D gradient recalled echo T1 fat-saturated postcontrast sequences. Gadolinium contrast agents used in pediatric patients include the nonlinear macrocyclic contrast agents, such as gadobutrol or gadoterate meglumine.

PET/Computed Tomography and PET/MR Imaging

Currently, PET/CT has proven value in pediatric oncologic imaging and is specifically used in the staging of pediatric lymphoma and some patients with sarcomas.[24,25] Because PET/CT can assess metabolic activity, it has increased sensitivity and specificity for metastatic disease and disease recurrence.[26] For thoracic chest wall masses and mediastinal masses, it is useful in the initial work-up to assess metabolic activity and assess additional areas of disease that may be more amenable to biopsy. It is also useful in follow-up examinations to assess for metastatic disease and disease recurrence for chest wall sarcomas and thoracic lymphoma. The most widespread and basic CT acquisition is a free breathing low-dose protocol used for anatomic and attenuation correction purposes. Diagnostic CT with IV contrast can also be performed if required.

More recently, PET/MR imaging has become available and is used in similar circumstances as PET/CT. Although PET/MR imaging has advantages over PET/CT given the lack of ionizing radiation for pediatric patients, it lacks some of the contrast resolution, specifically in the chest, to be used routinely. However, PET/MR imaging has shown utility in imaging neoplasms in the chest, specifically lymphoma, soft tissue sarcomas, primary bone tumors, and neuroblastoma.[27] PET/MR imaging also requires an attenuation correction sequence and for the body a 2D or 3D isotropic Dixon sequence is typically used. Additional sequences can be performed but are time consuming. Whole-body sequences should be tailored to the specific clinical indication cognizant of overall scan time for pediatric patients.

SPECTRUM OF THORACIC NEOPLASTIC DISORDERS

Pediatric thoracic neoplasms are uncommon and can have a varied appearance across multiple imaging modalities. However, the radiologist with knowledge of specific imaging features and anatomic location can provide appropriate differential diagnoses expediting optimal clinical and surgical management. This article focuses on pediatric thoracic neoplastic disorders affecting lungs, airways, mediastinum, and chest wall.

Primary Neoplasms of the Lung

Malignant primary neoplasms of the lung
Although primary lung parenchymal neoplasms in the pediatric population are uncommon, most are malignant.[28] Common malignant lung masses in the adult population, such as small cell carcinoma, adenocarcinoma, and squamous cell carcinoma, are exceedingly rare in the pediatric population. The most common malignant pediatric primary lung parenchymal neoplasm is pleuropulmonary blastoma (PPB).[29]

Pleuropulmonary blastoma PPB is a primary lung neoplasm found only in the pediatric population with a median age of diagnosis of 3 years.[30] Affected pediatric patients may be asymptomatic or present with varying degrees of respiratory distress with fever, cough, or chest pain. PPB can also initially present with pneumothorax.[31] PPB comes from the dysembryonic/dysontogenetic neoplasm family, which includes common pediatric malignancies, such as neuroblastoma, retinoblastoma, Wilms tumor, and hepatoblastoma.[32] This family of tumors is related in that they all have histologic features of the developing organ or tissue from which they develop into. PPBs arise from lung parenchyma, or infrequently the parietal pleura. PPB is genetically determined in approximately 70% of cases and is associated with an inherited tumor predisposition syndrome.[32] These cases are associated with germline mutations of the DICER1 gene, which encodes an enzyme required for the production of mature microRNAs. MicroRNAs are critical regulators of gene expression in normal organ development. Radiographic screening of infants and young children with the DICER1 mutation for PPB has been advocated.[33]

PPBs are classified into three types based on their underlying pathologic features. Type I PPBs are purely cystic masses without a detectable solid component and typically present in younger patients with a median age of 10 months (**Fig. 1**). The cysts in type I PPBs are lined with benign respiratory epithelium covering primitive malignant cells. Type II PPBs have solid and cystic areas. Type III PPBs are completely solid and typically affect slightly older children with a median age of approximately 4 years.[31] Because the age range varies between the various types of PPBs, it is hypothesized that PPBs evolve from type I cystic lesion to type II mixed lesions to finally type III completely solid lesions through a continued overgrowth of mesenchymal primitive malignant cells.

Given that PPBs can range from completely cystic to completely solid, they can have a varied imaging appearance. Radiographically, PPBs present as a peripherally located lung-based mass with or without cysts more often in the right hemithorax.[31] In older children with type III lesions, the entire hemithorax can be opacified with shift of the cardiomediastinal contents. Initial radiographic appearance of PPB is confusing and invariably leads to additional cross-sectional imaging with

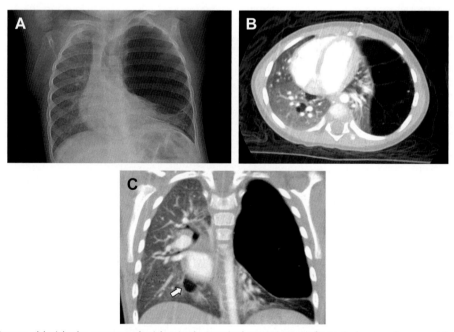

Fig. 1. A 2-year-old girl who presented with cough. Surgical resection confirmed pleuropulmonary blastoma and patient was found to have the DICER1 mutation. (A) Frontal chest radiograph shows a large cystic lesion with mass effect on the adjacent mediastinum located in the left hemithorax. (B) Axial lung window CT image demonstrates a large cystic lesion in the left lung with several internal septations. (C) Coronal reformatted lung window CT image shows a large cystic lesion in the left lung. Additional smaller cystic lesion (*arrow*) is also seen in the right lower lobe concerning for pleuropulmonary blastoma.

MDCT being the imaging study of choice. Type I PPB is cystic with the cysts sometimes causing mass effect or leading to lobar expansion on CT (see **Fig. 1**). There can be intralesion cystic hemorrhage causing gas liquid levels. Type II lesions are mixed with some solid component. Type I and II can have pneumothorax in addition to pleural effusions. Given the cystic appearance of type I and type II PPBs, they can be confused with benign congenital pulmonary airway malformations. However, congenital pulmonary airway malformations are present in utero and are often detected on prenatal ultrasound. The presence of cystic or mixed cystic-solid lesions, especially if they involve multiple lobes, should raise suspicion for PPB in a young child, particularly if not present on prenatal imaging.[34] Type III PPBs have a CT imaging appearance of a solid lesion with mixed enhancement.[35] Although CT is the imaging modality of choice, there have been limited published reports of the MR imaging appearance of the solid portion of PPB, which has been shown to demonstrate mixed heterogeneous enhancement on postcontrast imaging.[36] Hemorrhagic cysts with intrinsic T1 hyperintensity also may be present. On PET imaging, the solid components of PPB demonstrate peripheral heterogeneous fluorodeoxyglucose (FDG) avidity.[36]

PPBs are treated with complete surgical resection. Neoadjuvant chemotherapy may be necessary to decrease tumor bulk before resection, especially if the solid tumor is extensive or adjacent to vital structures. Type I lesions demonstrate overall better survival than type II and III lesions.[37]

Kaposi sarcoma Kaposi sarcoma (KS) is a vascular tumor associated with the human herpes virus 8.[38] KS is seen in pediatric patients with human immunodeficiency virus and is the most common AIDS-defining malignancy in children. KS typically affects the skin; however, 10% of cases of mucocutaneous KS have concomitant pulmonary involvement.[39] Pediatric patients with pulmonary KS typically present with cough, dyspnea, and enlarged lymph nodes.[40] Histologically, KS is a low-grade tumor of proliferating endothelial spindle cells.[41] In KS, human herpes virus 8 reprograms host blood endothelial cells to more resemble lymphatic endothelium resulting in abnormal vessels lined by thinned endothelial cells.[42]

The radiographic appearance of KS demonstrates bilateral opacities typically in the perihilar and basal regions with hilar lymphadenopathy and large bilateral pleural effusions (**Fig. 2**A).[43] The radiographic appearance of nodules in pulmonary KS has been characterized as flame-shaped or spiculated and often numbers more than 10. Septal thickening may be present because of lymphatic obstruction or tumor invasion. Although the imaging feature of KS can resemble pulmonary infection, in a patient with known mucocutaneous KS and abnormal chest radiographs, pulmonary involvement should be suspected.[43] CT is the imaging modality of choice and an accurate diagnosis is made based on the CT findings in approximately 90% of cases.[44] CT findings mirror the radiographic findings with bronchial wall thickening, septal thickening, hilar lymphadenopathy, and ill-defined nodules in a perihilar distribution (**Fig. 2**B).[43] Some of the nodules may have a halo of ground glass indicating hemorrhage. MR imaging is helpful to assess thoracic wall involvement but is limited in terms of pulmonary involvement. PET imaging has somewhat limited utility with pulmonary KS and has more utility in identifying malignant KS skin lesions and nodal involvement.[45]

Pulmonary KS is considered a more advanced form of KS and has a poorer prognosis. The treatment of choice is chemotherapy with concurrent

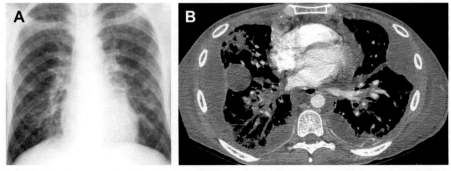

Fig. 2. AIDS related pulmonary Kaposi sarcoma. (*A*) Frontal radiograph in a 24-year-old man with AIDS shows multiple bilateral pulmonary nodules. (*B*) Axial soft tissue CT image in a different 25 year-old man with AIDS demonstrates multiple pulmonary nodules with bilateral pleural effusions, septal thickening, and hilar lymphadenopathy.

antiretroviral human immunodeficiency virus treatment that can have a large impact on survival rates. However, treatment may cause an immune reactivation inflammatory response, which may need to be titrated with chemotherapy to ameliorate and reverse the disease progression.[46]

Adenocarcinoma Pulmonary adenocarcinomas are malignant epithelial neoplasms much more common in the adult population.[47] However, adenocarcinomas have been linked with congenital pulmonary airway malformations in children. Also, a rare subtype of adenocarcinoma called fetal adenocarcinoma of the lung presents in pediatric patients and histologically resembles epithelium of the fetal lung.[48] Affected pediatric patients present with postobstructive pneumonias if the masses are located centrally and otherwise may be asymptomatic in peripheral masses that are found incidentally. Adenocarcinomas demonstrate glandular differentiation with mucin production histologically.

Imaging features of pediatric adenocarcinomas have been confined to the nonradiology case reports given their rarity. Pulmonary adenocarcinomas in the pediatric population have been described to have a similar varied appearance as in the adult population ranging from solitary pulmonary nodule to consolidative opacity.[49,50] CT findings have also been described in similar fashion ranging from ground glass opacities to more solid nodular opacities. There are no standard treatment protocols in pediatric patients for lung adenocarcinomas. Surgical resection is the treatment but metastases are usually present and prognosis remains poor.

Benign primary neoplasms of the lung

Most solid lung masses seen in children are caused by benign inflammatory, infectious, or reactive process, such as round pneumonia. If the mass is identified as a primary neoplasm of the lung, only 1% to 5% are benign.[28] The three most common benign primary neoplasms of the lung that occur in the pediatric population are pulmonary hamartoma, inflammatory myofibroblastic tumor, and pulmonary sclerosing hemangioma.

Pulmonary hamartoma Pulmonary hamartomas are benign primary neoplasm of the lung found in all age groups.[51] They are more common in elderly adults with a peak age of incidence in the sixth decade of life, but they do also sometimes occur in pediatric patients.[52] Affected patients are usually asymptomatic and masses are typically identified incidentally. Hamartomas are composed of variable amounts of mature disorganized tissue that is normally found in the lung and bronchi, such as cartilage, fat, and connective tissue.[53]

On imaging studies, hamartomas are typically well-circumscribed masses located peripherally. The classic chest radiograph appearance seen in adults, which can also be seen in children, is a smooth or lobulated peripheral mass with the classic popcorn calcifications (**Fig. 3**). CT is the imaging study of choice to identify intralesion fat and calcifications that can be diagnostic. The presence of calcifications in hamartomas varies from 5% to 50% and fat is seen in up to 60% of lesions.[54] The presence of fat in a nongrowing well-circumscribed pulmonary mass is diagnostic of pulmonary hamartoma.[55] Hamartomas do demonstrate FDG uptake on PET studies and are not recommended if the classic findings of fat are present because they can lead to potential confusion.[54] MR imaging is useful to demonstrate fat signal with heterogeneous T1 and T2 signal and heterogeneous enhancement.[56]

In asymptomatic patients, pulmonary hamartomas found incidentally with classic imaging findings can be safely left alone. However, pulmonary hamartomas that cause endobronchial obstruction can be surgically removed and lesions with atypical features biopsied for further assessment. Although fine-needle aspirates have been shown to be diagnostic, prior reports have commented on the difficulty of obtaining biopsy material from hard and partially calcified pulmonary hamartomas.[57] Therefore, in some cases surgical wedge resection may be needed for definitive diagnosis.

Inflammatory myofibroblastic tumor Inflammatory myofibroblastic tumors of the lung are rare benign pulmonary tumors composed of spindle cell fibroblast and myofibroblast proliferation with a mixture of plasma cells, lymphocytes, and histiocytes.[58] However, they are the most common benign pulmonary neoplasm in children with approximately 25% of all cases occurring in the pediatric population.[59] Most of the neoplasms arise from the lung parenchyma but approximately 12% can arise from the bronchi.[60] Most affected pediatric patients are asymptomatic; when patients do present, symptoms are variable with cough, fever, shortness of breath, and hemoptysis.[61]

On chest radiographs, inflammatory myofibroblastic tumors typically appear as well-defined solitary pulmonary masses with peripheral and lower lobe predominance sometimes in combination with atelectasis and pleural effusion. In 5% of cases, masses are multiple. Calcifications can occur and are actually more common among pediatric patients.[62] CT can better demonstrate these

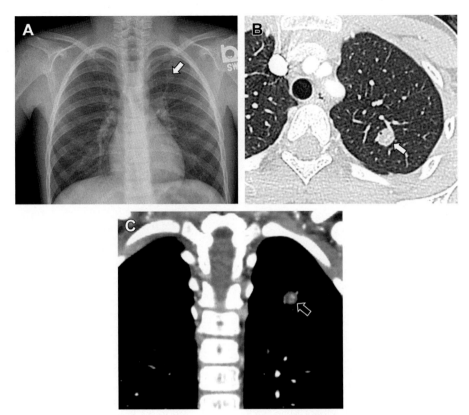

Fig. 3. An 8-year-old girl who presented with dry cough and an incidentally detected pulmonary hamartoma. (*A*) Frontal chest radiograph shows a well-defined pulmonary nodule (*arrow*) located in the left upper lobe. (*B*) Axial lung window CT image demonstrates a well-defined pulmonary nodule (*arrow*) located in the left upper lobe corresponding well with the findings seen on frontal chest radiograph in *A*. (*C*) Coronal soft tissue window CT image shows a well-defined pulmonary nodule (*arrow*) with the classic popcorn-type calcifications in the left upper lobe.

calcifications that have been described as amorphous, fine fleck-like, or dystrophic (**Fig. 4**A).[63] The inflammatory components of these tumors can demonstrate increased FDG avidity on PET imaging (**Fig. 4**B).[64] Inflammatory myofibroblastic tumors typically have low to intermediate T1 signal and high T2 signal with one case report describing delayed homogenous enhancement on MR imaging (**Fig. 4**C, D).[65]

The current treatment of inflammatory myofibroblastic tumor is surgical. Diagnosis based on biopsy is difficult given that the inflammatory cells and fibrosis present in this tumor can be present at the periphery of multiple other neoplasms. However, frozen sections from surgical specimens can usually provide the diagnosis. Prognosis in patients with complete resection is excellent with a low risk for recurrence.[66]

Pulmonary sclerosing hemangioma Pulmonary sclerosing hemangioma is a rare benign pulmonary tumor that was originally thought to be vascular in origin but has since been shown to originate from primary lung epithelium based on immunohistochemical and molecular analyses.[67] Histologically, the tumor is composed of sclerotic and ectatic vascular spaces considered to be secondary changes in an epithelial neoplasm.[68] Although the tumor commonly affects middle-age adults, case reports have demonstrated the tumor in adolescent patients.[69] Most affected patients are asymptomatic; however, they can also present with hemoptysis, cough, and chest pain.[70]

On chest radiographs, pulmonary sclerosing hemangiomas typically appear as a well-defined solitary pulmonary mass with peripheral predominance usually less than 3 cm in size. CT demonstrates a well-defined smooth round or oval enhancing pulmonary mass usually adjacent to the pleural surface at the periphery.[71] On MR imaging, pulmonary sclerosing hemangiomas are typically hyperintense on T1 and T2 sequences with marked enhancement.[72] Pulmonary sclerosing hemangiomas also typically demonstrate increased FDG avidity on PET imaging.[73,74]

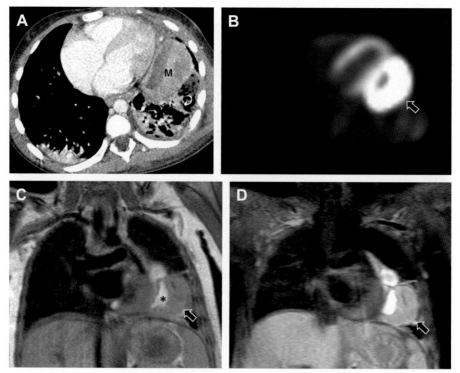

Fig. 4. A 7-year-old boy who presented with chest pain and decreased ability to use his left arm. The results of surgical biopsy of the left lung mass confirmed the diagnosis of inflammatory myofibroblastic tumor. (*A*) Axial soft tissue window CT image shows a mass (M) in the lingula adjacent to the left ventricle with a pleural effusion and chest tube. (*B*) Axial PET image demonstrates intense peripheral FDG avidity of the mass (*arrow*) with central necrosis. (*C*) Coronal T1-weighted MR image shows a mass (*arrow*) composed of soft tissue component showing intermediate signal intensity and central internal hemorrhagic necrosis (*asterisk*). (*D*) Postcontrast T1-weighted MR image with fat saturation demonstrates enhancement of the soft tissue component (*arrow*).

Surgical resection is needed for diagnosis and treatment. Prognosis is excellent with a rare chance of recurrence that does not affect long-term prognosis.[75]

Primary Neoplasms of the Airway

In pediatric patients, most primary neoplasms of the airway are benign. Pediatric benign neoplasms of the airway tend to be located in the proximal portion of the central airways, whereas malignant neoplasms of the airway tend to be located in the distal trachea or bronchi.[76]

Malignant primary neoplasms of the airway
Carcinoid tumor Carcinoid tumors are types of low-grade slow-growing neuroendocrine tumors derived from amine precursor uptake and decarboxylation cells.[77] Carcinoid tumors are typically endobronchial lesions that arise in the large airways. They cause obstructive-type symptoms, such as postobstructive pneumonia or wheezing.[78] A smaller percentage of carcinoid tumors also originate from the lung parenchyma.[79]

Because carcinoids are neuroendocrine tumors, they can secrete serotonin and kalikrein and can cause carcinoid syndrome characterized by flushing and diarrhea as the most common symptoms.

On chest radiographs, postobstructive pneumonia or atelectasis is often seen that does not resolve with treatment in affected pediatric patients. Less commonly, a perihilar mass may be seen or lung hyperinflation from partial airway obstruction. CT demonstrates a well-defined lobulated soft tissue endobronchial mass with marked enhancement (**Fig. 5**).[80] Calcifications are seen in approximately 30% of cases.[81] MR imaging is useful for distinguishing carcinoid tumor from adjacent vessels given that bronchial carcinoids demonstrate marked increased T2 signal.[81] Carcinoid tumors do not typically demonstrate FDG uptake on PET imaging; however, they have somatostatin receptors and are positive on octreotide scans.[82]

Complete surgical resection is typically the treatment of choice with lobectomy.[83] Carcinoid tumors have a better prognosis than other

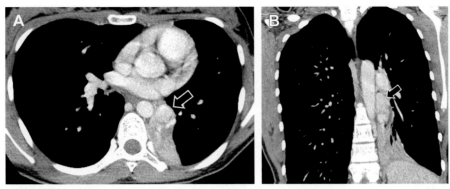

Fig. 5. A 14-year-old girl who presented with left lower lobe consolidation on chest radiograph. Endobronchial lesion located in the left lower lobe bronchus was found to be a typical carcinoid on surgical pathology. (A) Axial enhanced CT image shows an enhancing endobronchial lesion (*arrow*) obstructing a left lower lobe bronchus resulting in postobstructive atelectasis and pneumonia. (B) Coronal enhanced CT image better demonstrates the longitudinal extent of an enhancing endobronchial lesion (*arrow*). Also noted are postobstructive atelectasis and pneumonia.

pulmonary neoplasms with 10-year survival rates of 77% to 90% in the absence of lymph node metastases. When nodal metastases are present, the 10-year survival rate drops to 22% to 80%.[83]

Mucoepidermoid carcinoma Mucoepidermoid carcinomas in pediatric patients are typically low-grade slow-growing tumors originating from a combination of mucin-secreting cells, squamous cells, and intermediate-type cells.[84] Like carcinoid tumors, they are endobronchial lesions that arise in the large airways and typically present with postobstructive pneumonia or wheezing.[85]

On chest radiographs, a central mass or endoluminal nodule is seen with postobstructive pneumonia or atelectasis. CT can demonstrate calcifications seen in 50% of cases.[86] A well-defined lobulated soft tissue endobronchial mass with moderate to marked enhancement is seen similar to carcinoid.[87] MR imaging is not particularly helpful in the imaging assessment of mucoepidermoid carcinomas. High-grade mucoepidermoid carcinomas demonstrate FDG update; however, the lower grade mucoepidermoid carcinomas typically do not.[88] It is challenging to differentiate mucoepidermoid carcinomas from carcinoid tumors based on imaging alone. Regardless, the treatment of both lesions is typically the same with surgical resection.

Benign primary neoplasms of the airway
Subglottic hemangioma Subglottic hemangiomas are infantile hemangiomas that usually present in infancy (mean age, 3–4 months) with stridor.[89] Subglottic hemangiomas undergo a proliferative phase during which they cause symptoms and then involute over time. Subglottic hemangiomas

can also involve the supraglottic region, trachea, or main stem bronchi. Infants with subglottic hemangiomas often have cutaneous hemangiomas. Histopathologically, subglottic hemangiomas are infantile benign vascular neoplasms composed of rapidly proliferating vascular endothelial cells with specific high immunoreactivity to the GLUT1 protein.[90]

Infants with stridor are typically first evaluated with soft tissue neck radiographs and chest radiographs. Subglottic hemangiomas are suggested on frontal or lateral radiographs with asymmetric narrowing of the subglottic trachea (**Fig. 6**A). Congenital subglottic stenosis and croup typically cause symmetric narrowing of the subglottic trachea. However, rarely circumferential subglottic hemangiomas can cause symmetric narrowing of the subglottic airway.[91] CT with contrast is the imaging study of choice usually demonstrating a lesion with early intense and homogeneous contrast enhancement (**Fig. 6**B). The early intense enhancement of hemangiomas can differentiate them from other causes of airway narrowing, such as congenital or iatrogenic tracheal stenosis, or other masses, such as lymphatic malformations or laryngeal papillomas.[92] MR imaging for subglottic hemangiomas demonstrate heterogeneous T1 signal, high T2 signal, and rapid enhancement.[93] PET imaging is not routinely used for subglottic hemangiomas but studies focused on hemangiomas of the extremities have demonstrated low FDG avidity with standardized uptake values ranging from 0.7 to 1.67.[94]

The diagnosis is confirmed with bronchoscopy and management is initially medical with systemic and intralesional steroids and recently propranolol to temporize the lesion until it naturally involutes.

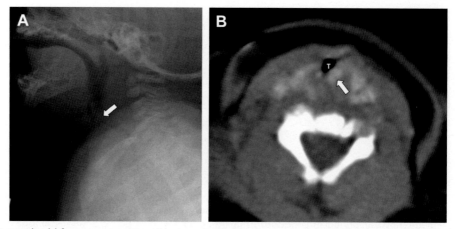

Fig. 6. A 2-month-old former premature girl presented to the emergency department with stridor and was found to have a subglottic hemangioma. (A) Lateral soft tissue neck radiograph shows soft tissue fullness in the posterior subglottic airway (arrow). (B) Axial enhanced soft tissue CT image demonstrates a homogenous enhancing mass (arrow) with mass effect on the trachea (T).

Surgical and laser excision is reserved for lesions that are symptomatic and do not respond to medical treatment.[95] Additional options are tracheostomy with removal after lesion involution.[96]

Recurrent respiratory papillomatosis Recurrent respiratory papillomatosis is the recurrent growth of warts in the airways caused by the human papillomavirus transmitted via infected mothers to their infants during vaginal birth. It is the most common neoplasm of the large airway in the pediatric population.[97] The warty lesions demonstrate papillary fronds covered by stratified squamous epithelium. Affected pediatric patients typically present with hoarseness between 2 and 4 years of age. However, symptoms may vary depending on the location and degree of airway obstruction.[98] Recurrent respiratory papillomatosis most commonly affects the larynx but can affect the lower trachea and bronchi and rarely the lung parenchyma.

Chest radiographs demonstrate nodular involvement of the larynx and subglottic region (**Fig. 7**A). Postobstructive atelectasis/pneumonia may be present with endobronchial lesions. CT demonstrates numerous nodular lesions within the airway, many of which show cavitation (**Fig. 7**B). Virtual bronchoscopy can provide additional noninvasive assessment with 3D MDCT.[99] MR imaging is not typically useful in the imaging assessment of respiratory papillomatosis but may show intraluminal airway lesions. For PET imaging, increased FDG avidity has been seen in lesions with malignant transformation.[100] However, other case reports have demonstrated heterogeneous FDG avidity of lesions suggesting variability in the metabolic behavior of these lesions.[101]

Treatment is typically reserved for symptomatic lesions to relieve airway obstruction. Surgical debulking is the mainstay of treatment usually

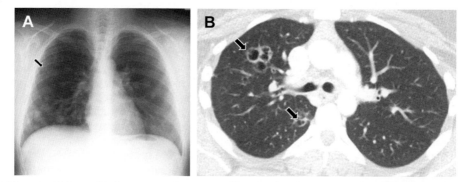

Fig. 7. A 16-year-old boy with known respiratory papillomatosis who presented with hemoptysis. (A) Frontal chest radiograph shows multiple pulmonary nodules in both lungs. Some of these pulmonary nodules have central cavitation (arrow). (B) Axial lung window CT image demonstrates cavitary pulmonary nodules (arrows).

with microdebridement or angiolytic laser.[102] This may be followed by an injection of cidofovir into the resection site in patients with moderate-to-severe disease.[103] Tracheostomy may be needed if significant airway obstruction occurs.

Mediastinal Masses

Mediastinal masses are the most common thoracic neoplasms in the pediatric population with the most common location being the anterior mediastinum. The three most common pediatric mediastinal neoplasms are lymphoma, neuroblastoma, and teratoma.

Malignant mediastinal masses

Lymphoma Lymphoma is the most common cause of pediatric mediastinal masses and accounts for approximately 13% of all childhood cancers.[104] Non-Hodgkin lymphoma is more common; however, Hodgkin lymphoma more commonly affects the anterior mediastinum.[105] Affected pediatric patients typically present with painless adenopathy or may present with cough, shortness of breath, or chest pain. Additional constitutional symptoms, such as fever, weight loss, and night sweats, may be present.

Chest radiographs demonstrate a mediastinal soft tissue mass with obscuration of the retrosternal clear space and widening of the mediastinum.[106] Chest CT exhibits an anterior mediastinal soft tissue attenuating mass with lobulated smooth borders.[107] Cystic low-attenuating areas can be present within the mass representing underlying hemorrhage, necrosis, or cystic degeneration. Unilateral pleural effusions are common and pericardial effusions are seen less frequently.[108] Beyond mediastinal involvement, pediatric patients have been known to have pulmonary involvement of lymphoma with three distinct patterns of lung abnormalities.[109] The most common is the presence of pulmonary nodules with irregular borders. Another pattern is increased interstitial thickening from venous or lymphatic obstruction from hilar nodes or interstitial tumor.[110] The last pattern is segmental consolidation that can mimic pneumonia.[111]

MR imaging is more accurate than CT in assessing thoracic wall invasion from lymphoma and MR imaging has also been useful in evaluating the response to therapy in lymphoma.[112] PET/CT is more sensitive than other imaging modalities and is useful in staging patients with lymphoma and for monitoring recurrence.[113,114] Recently, studies have demonstrated that PET/MR imaging shows comparable sensitivity to PET/CT with significantly reduced radiation exposure for pediatric lymphoma.[115]

Neuroblastoma Neuroblastoma is in a group of tumors, including ganglioneuroblastoma and ganglioneuroma, which come from primordial neural crest cells, the precursors of the sympathetic nervous system.[116] When these tumors occur in the chest, they typically occur along the paraspinal area in the location of the sympathetic ganglia.[117] However, neuroblastoma has also been described in the anterior mediastinum.[118] Most affected children present between 1 and 5 years and symptoms vary based on the location of the neuroblastoma. Thoracic neuroblastoma has a higher incidence of causing opsoclonus-myoclonus, a known symptom of neuroblastoma, which is usually associated with a better prognosis.[119] Thoracic neuroblastoma can also cause dyspnea or be discovered as a mass incidentally on chest radiographs.[118]

Chest radiographs demonstrate a paravertebral mass in the posterior mediastinum with splaying of the posterior ribs and possible erosion of the vertebral pedicles (**Fig. 8A, B**).[120] Calcification in the mass is sometimes present. Further cross-sectional imaging is needed to properly stage thoracic neuroblastoma (**Fig. 8C**). MR imaging has been considered superior to CT for staging given its superior assessment of marrow involvement and intraspinal extension.[120] Neuroblastoma is typically heterogeneous in signal with variable enhancement. Nuclear scintigraphy studies with ^{123}I-MIBG are useful for assessment of primary and metastatic disease and for disease follow-up. However, only about 70% of neuroblastomas are MIBG avid.[121] PET/CT can also be used in neuroblastoma, which is FDG avid. PET has been shown to have higher accuracy than MIBG studies in selected populations and has been shown to provide prognostic information[121]

Benign mediastinal masses

Teratoma/germ cell tumors Germ cell tumors arise from pluripotent stem cells that fail to migrate from the ectoderm to the gonad and are found throughout the body.[122] The most common extragonadal location for germ cell tumors is the mediastinum.[123] The most common extragonadal germ cell tumors are mediastinal teratomas, which make up to 25% of pediatric anterior mediastinal masses. Teratomas are classified histologically as mature (well differentiated) or immature (poorly differentiated) with variable levels of neoplastic potential, although most mediastinal teratomas identified in utero or within the first year of life are immature.[124] Most mature and immature teratomas are benign with a low incidence of malignant transformation. Mediastinal teratomas are

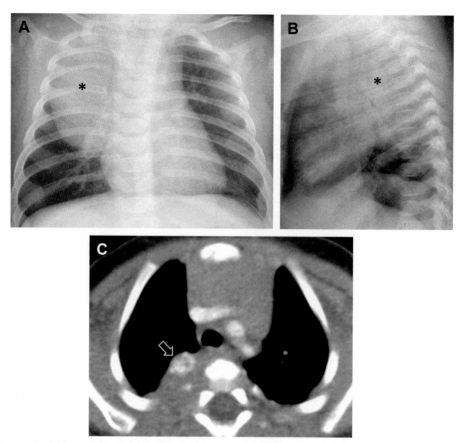

Fig. 8. A 4-month-old boy with respiratory distress initially presumed to have pneumonia but subsequently found to have a posterior mediastinal neuroblastoma. (*A*) Frontal radiograph shows a large opacity (*asterisk*) located in the right upper to mid hemithorax. (*B*) Lateral radiograph demonstrates a mass (*asterisk*) located in the posterior mediastinum. (*C*) Axial enhanced CT image from a different patient (2-month-old girl) shows an enhancing posterior mediastinal mass (*arrow*) with calcification. Surgical pathology confirmed the diagnosis of neuroblastoma.

often asymptomatic but may present because of mass effect or rupture.[125]

Chest radiographs demonstrate an anterior mediastinal mass sometimes with calcifications.[126] Although most teratomas are located in the anterior mediastinum, a smaller fraction is found in the posterior or middle mediastinum. CT is the examination study of choice demonstrating varying degrees of soft tissue, fat, calcification, and fluid/cystic densities, with teeth or bone seen in up to 8% of cases (**Fig. 9**).[127] Immature teratomas are usually completely solid. Cystic teratomas may rupture and show a higher prevalence of inhomogeneity.[128,129] MR imaging appearance of teratomas demonstrates variable components of fat, fluid, soft tissue, and calcification. A fat-saturation technique can be used to identify fat distinct from hemorrhage or sebum.[130] Given the typical benign nature of mediastinal teratomas, PET imaging is often not warranted. PET imaging

has been useful in mediastinal seminomas to identify residual viable tumor.[131]

Chest Wall Masses

Chest wall masses can arise from any tissue within the thoracic wall. Although chest radiographs are the initial study of choice, ultrasound has proved invaluable in the initial assessment for palpable lesions.[15] CT and MR imaging can further define the extent of a pediatric chest wall mass and narrow the differential diagnosis.[132]

Malignant chest wall masses

Rhabdomyosarcoma Rhabdomyosarcomas are high-grade mesenchymal tumors of skeletal muscle that often present as rapidly growing painful chest masses.[133] It is one of the most common malignant soft tissue neoplasms that occur in the pediatric population. Radiographs may show a soft tissue mass but ultrasound can identify a

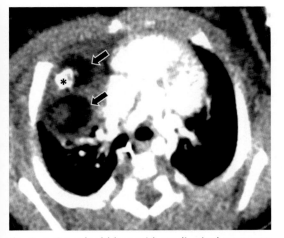

Fig. 9. A 2-week-old boy with mediastinal mass seen on prenatal imaging. Axial enhanced CT image shows a large anterior mediastinal mass composed of soft tissue, fat (*arrows*), and calcific (*asterisk*) components compatible with a mediastinal teratoma.

predominantly hypoechoic mass with internal vascularity (**Fig. 10**A, B).[134] CT and MR imaging are useful to identify the extent of the mass and metastatic involvement (**Fig. 10**C). On MR imaging, rhabdomyosarcoma typically shows intermediate T1 signal, isointense to hyperintense T2 signal with marked contrast enhancement.[135] PET is useful for staging rhabdomyosarcomas and to assess initial response to chemotherapy.[136]

Ewing sarcoma of the chest wall Ewing sarcoma of the chest wall is a primary bone tumor from the small round blue cell tumor family that can arise from the osseous or soft tissue components of the chest wall.[137] The Ewing sarcoma family of tumors shares a common cytogenetic rearrangement resulting in the formation of a fusion gene.[138] These tumors often present as rapidly growing painful chest masses. Radiographs typically demonstrate an extrapleural mass that may or may not cause rib destruction with aggressive

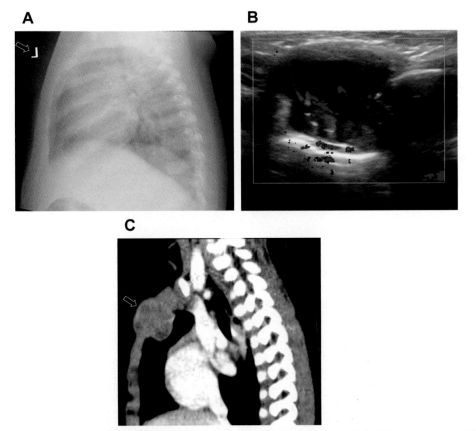

Fig. 10. A 4-year-old boy with palpable right chest mass found to have chest wall rhabdomyosarcoma. (*A*) Lateral chest radiograph shows soft tissue prominence of the anterior upper chest (*arrow*). (*B*) Focused ultrasound with color Doppler demonstrates a predominantly hypoechoic mass with internal vascularity. (*C*) Sagittal soft tissue window CT image shows a heterogeneous enhancing mass (*arrow*) splaying the ribs with mass effect on the pleural space.

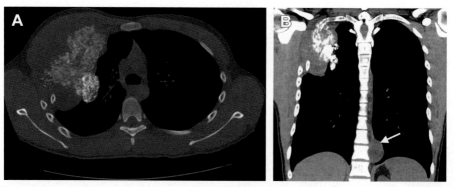

Fig. 11. A 20-year-old man who presented with right side chest pain and a growing mass for the past 2 years. Axial (*A*) bone widow and coronal (*B*) soft tissue window CT images show a large and destructive mass arising for the right second rib with substantial new bone formation compatible with osteosarcoma with paraspinal soft tissue metastasis (*arrow*).

periosteal reaction, typically lamellated.[139] Ultrasound demonstrates a soft tissue mass with internal vascularity and may be useful to guide biopsy; however, bony involvement is difficult to discern.[140] CT demonstrates a heterogeneous mass with or without cystic degeneration and bony involvement; however, calcifications are rare. MR imaging also demonstrates heterogeneous hyperintense T1 and T2 signal along with heterogeneous enhancement given areas of necrosis.[141] PET has high sensitivity and specificity for staging and restaging of Ewing sarcoma.[142]

Osteosarcoma Osteosarcoma is a high-grade primary bone tumor that typically arises in the long bones but can occur in the chest wall with pain as the primary presenting symptom.[143] Chest radiographs show a destructive osseous lesion with areas of ossification. CT is superior to MR imaging and radiographs in assessing the extent of cortical osseous involvement from osteosarcoma (**Fig. 11**).[15] CT is also the best modality to assess for pulmonary metastatic involvement. However, MR imaging is superior to assess for marrow involvement with soft tissue components typically

demonstrating hyperintense T1 and T2 signal with marked enhancement.[144] Foci of low signal on all sequences correspond to areas of ossification and/or calcification. Osteosarcomas are strongly PET avid with heterogeneous uptake and PET is useful for staging and follow-up.[145]

Benign chest wall masses
Hemangioma Hemangiomas are benign vascular tumors composed of vascular endothelial cells.[146] Hemangiomas are classified as congenital or infantile. Infantile hemangiomas are the most common vascular tumor of infancy and are differentiated from congenital hemangiomas by the expression of GLUT-1.[147] They typically appear during the first week of life with a proliferative phase during the first 3 to 6 months of life and then an involution phase by 12 months of age with complete regression by age 5 to 10 years.[148] Infantile hemangiomas are typically diagnosed on physical examination but imaging can confirm the diagnosis. Ultrasound demonstrates a heterogeneous hyperechoic mass with multiple vessels that demonstrate arterial and venous waveforms (**Fig. 12**). The hyperechoic soft tissue components

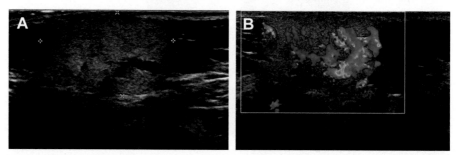

Fig. 12. A 2-year-old with an enlarging bluish lesion in the right upper chest wall. (*A*) Focused gray-scale ultrasound image demonstrates a well-defined hyperechoic mass. (*B*) Focused ultrasound with color Doppler demonstrates internal vascularity with the waveforms (not shown) showing arterial and venous flow compatible with a hemangioma.

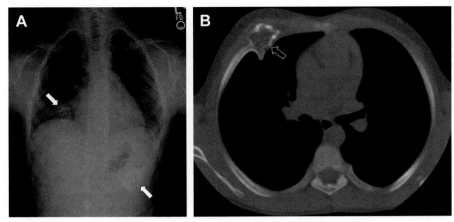

Fig. 13. An 11-year-old with known multiple hereditary exostoses presenting with lower chest discomfort. (*A*) Frontal chest radiograph demonstrates bony exostoses originating from the anterior ribs bilaterally (*arrows*). (*B*) Axial bone window CT demonstrates an exostosis (*arrow*) extending anteriorly from the anterior rib with continuity with the medullary cavity.

distinguish hemangiomas from arterial venous malformations, which contain no soft tissue components.[9] CT demonstrates a well-defined mass in the superficial soft tissues with marked enhancement. MR imaging shows a T2 hyperintense enhancing mass with multiple flow voids.[149] As the infantile hemangioma involutes its signal characteristics across the imaging spectrum become more heterogeneous.[149] PET imaging has not shown much utility in the assessment of infantile hemangiomas.[94]

Osteochondroma Osteochondromas are benign bony tumors that develop as an outgrowth of the physeal cartilage, which herniates through the periosteal bone collar.[150] In the chest, osteochondromas frequently affect the costochondral junctions, but can also affect the ribs, scapula, sternum, and clavicles. Osteochondromas can present as palpable masses that sometimes cause pain if they are related to bursa formation.[151]

Radiographs demonstrate a sessile or pedunculated osseous protuberance in continuity with the medullary bone (**Fig. 13**A). CT is superior in demonstrating that the cortex of the osteochondroma is in continuity with the medullary cavity (**Fig. 13**B). CT can also sometimes demonstrate the cartilage cap. MR imaging best visualizes the cartilage cap, which demonstrate T2 hyperintense signal. In adults, thickening of the cartilage cap greater than 2 cm is suspicious for malignant transformation to chondrosarcoma, although it may be unreliable in growing pediatric patients.[152] Malignant transformation in children is rare and is usually associated with multiple hereditary exostoses.[153] Unfortunately, identifying imaging features of malignant transformation in pediatric patients

has been challenging. Case reports have described cortical invasion with loss of distinct regular margins and cortical erosion of the stalk.[154] PET imaging has not been informative in the work-up of malignant transformation.[154,155]

SUMMARY

Pediatric primary thoracic neoplasms are rare. However, given the nonspecific symptoms of these neoplasms, imaging evaluation is often required for identifying underlying abnormalities and provides a reasonable differential to help guide subsequent clinical management. Radiologists with up-to-date knowledge of the imaging work-up, imaging protocols, and imaging appearance of these pediatric thoracic neoplasms can greatly expedite initial diagnosis and follow-up assessment leading to optimal pediatric patient management.

REFERENCES

1. Nelson BA, Lee EY, Ranganath SH, et al. Oncological diseases. In: Cleveland RH, editor. Imaging in pediatric pulmonology. New York: Springer-Verlag; 2012. p. 265–98.
2. Burris NS, Johnson KM, Larson PE, et al. Detection of small pulmonary nodules with ultrashort echo time sequences in oncology patients by using a PET/MR system. Radiology 2016;278:239–46.
3. Thacker PG, Mahani MG, Heider A, et al. Imaging evaluation of mediastinal masses in children and adults: practical diagnostic approach based on a new classification system. J Thorac Imaging 2015;30:247–67.
4. Szucs-Farkas Z, Patak MA, Yuksel-Hatz S, et al. Improved detection of pulmonary nodules on

energy-subtracted chest radiographs with a commercial computer-aided diagnosis software: comparison with human observers. Eur Radiol 2010; 20:1289–96.

5. Coley BD. Chest sonography in children: current indications, techniques, and imaging findings. Radiol Clin North Am 2011;49:825–46.

6. Amini B, Huang SY, Tsai J, et al. Primary lung and large airway neoplasms in children: current imaging evaluation with multidetector computed tomography. Radiol Clin North Am 2013;51:637–57.

7. Dichop MK, Kuruvilla S. Primary and metastatic lung tumors in the pediatric population. Arch Pathol Lab Med 2008;132:1079–103.

8. Mong A, Epelman M, Darge K. Ultrasound of the pediatric chest. Pediatr Radiol 2012;42:1287–97.

9. Paltiel HJ, Burrows PE, Kozakewich HP, et al. Soft-tissue vascular anomalies: utility of ultrasound for diagnosis. Radiology 2000;214(3):747–54.

10. Honda O, Johkoh T, Yamamoto S, et al. Comparison of quality of multiplanar reconstructions and direct coronal multidetector CT scans of the lung. AJR Am J Roentgenol 2002;179(4):875–9.

11. Frush DP. Overview of CT technologies for children. Pediatr Radiol 2014;44(Suppl 3):422–6.

12. Baez JC, Ciet P, Mulkern R, et al. Pediatric chest MR imaging: lung and airways. Magn Reson Imaging Clin N Am 2015;23(2):337–49.

13. Carter BW, Gladish GW. MR imaging of chest wall tumors. Magn Reson Imaging Clin N Am 2015; 23(2):197–215.

14. Trinavarat P, Riccabona M. Potential of ultrasound in the pediatric chest. Eur J Radiol 2014;83: 1507–18.

15. Baez JC, Lee EY, Restrepo R, et al. Chest wall lesions in children. AJR Am J Roentgenol 2013; 200(5):W402–19.

16. Macias CG, Chumpitazi CE. Sedation and anesthesia for CT: emerging issues for providing high-quality care. Pediatr Radiol 2011;41(Suppl 2): 517–22.

17. Schooler GR, Zurakowski D, Lee EY. Evaluation of contrast injection site effectiveness: thoracic CT angiography in children with hand injection of IV contrast material. AJR Am J Roentgenol 2015; 204(2):423–7.

18. Ackman JB. MR imaging of mediastinal masses. Magn Reson Imaging Clin N Am 2015;23(2): 141–64.

19. Ciet P, Tiddens HA, Wielopolski PA, et al. Magnetic resonance imaging in children: common problems and possible solutions for lung and airways imaging. Pediatr Radiol 2015;45(13):1901–15.

20. Scott AD, Keegan J, Firmin DN. Motion in cardiovascular MR imaging. Radiology 2009;250:331–51.

21. Gorkem SB, Coskun A, Yikilmaz A, et al. Evaluation of pediatric thoracic disorders: comparison of unenhanced fast-imaging-sequence 1.5T MRI and contrast-enhanced MDCT. AJR 2013;200(6): 1352–7.

22. Wild JM, Marshall H, Bock M, et al. MRI of the lung (1/3): methods. Insights Imaging 2012;3(4):345–53.

23. Fink C, Puderbach M, Biederer J, et al. Lung MRI at 1.5 and 3 Tesla: observer preference study and lesion contrast using five different pulse sequences. Invest Radiol 2007;42:377–83.

24. Hudson MM, Krasin MJ, Kaste SC. PET imaging in pediatric Hodgkin's lymphoma. Pediatr Radiol 2004;34(3):190–8.

25. Uslu L, Donig J, Link M, et al. Value of 18F-FDG PET and PET/CT for evaluation of pediatric malignancies. J Nucl Med 2015;56(2):274–86.

26. Sioka C. The utility of FDG PET in diagnosis and follow-up of lymphoma in childhood. Eur J Pediatr 2013;172(6):733–8.

27. Purz S, Sabri O, Viehweger A, et al. Potential pediatric applications of PET/MR. J Nucl Med 2014; 55(Suppl 2):32S–9S.

28. Tischer W, Reddemann H, Herzog P, et al. Experience in surgical treatment of pulmonary and bronchial tumours in childhood. Prog Pediatr Surg 1987;21:118–35.

29. Dishop MK, Kuruvilla S. Primary and metastatic lung tumors in the pediatric population: a review and 25-year experience at a large children's hospital. Arch Pathol Lab Med 2008;132(7):1079–103.

30. Priest JR, McDermott MB, Bhatia S, et al. Pleuropulmonary blastoma: a clinicopathologic study of 50 cases. Cancer 1997;80(1):147–61.

31. Naffaa LN, Donnelly LF. Imaging findings in pleuropulmonary blastoma. Pediatr Radiol 2005;35(4): 387–91.

32. Schultz KA, Pacheco MC, Yang J, et al. Ovarian sex cord-stromal tumors, pleuropulmonary blastoma and DICER1 mutations: a report from the International Pleuropulmonary Blastoma Registry. Gynecol Oncol 2011;122(2):246–50.

33. Sabapathy DG, Guillerman RP, Orth RC, et al. Radiographic screening of infants and young children with genetic predisposition for rare malignancies: DICER1 mutations and pleuropulmonary blastoma. AJR Am J Roentgenol 2015;204(4): W475–82.

34. Griffin N, Devaraj A, Goldstraw P, et al. CT and histopathological correlation of congenital cystic pulmonary lesions: a common pathogenesis? Clin Radiol 2008;63(9):995–1005.

35. Orazi C, Inserra A, Schingo PM, et al. Pleuropulmonary blastoma, a distinctive neoplasm of childhood: report of three cases. Pediatr Radiol 2007; 37(4):337–44.

36. Geiger J, Walter K, Uhl M, et al. Imaging findings in a 3-year-old girl with type III pleuropulmonary blastoma. In Vivo 2007;21(6):1119–22.

37. Venkatramani R, Malogolowkin MH, Wang L, et al. Pleuropulmonary blastoma: a single-institution experience. J Pediatr Hematol Oncol 2012;34(5): e182–5.

38. Chang Y, Cesarman E, Pessin MS, et al. Identification of herpesvirus-like DNA sequences in AIDS-associated Kaposi's sarcoma. Science 1994; 266(5192):1865–9.

39. Antman K, Chang Y. Kaposi's sarcoma. N Engl J Med 2000;342(14):1027–38.

40. Stefan DC, Stones DK, Wainwright L, et al. Kaposi sarcoma in South African children. Pediatr Blood Cancer 2011;56(3):392–6.

41. Radu O, Pantanowitz L. Kaposi Sarcoma. Arch Pathol Lab Med 2013;137(2):289–94.

42. Hong YK, Foreman K, Shin JW, et al. Lymphatic reprogramming of blood vascular endothelium by Kaposi sarcoma-associated herpesvirus. Nat Genet 2004;36(7):683–5.

43. Theron S, Andronikou S, Du Plessis J, et al. Pulmonary Kaposi sarcoma in six children. Pediatr Radiol 2007;37(12):1224–9.

44. Khalil AM, Carette MF, Cadranel JL. Intrathoracic Kaposi's sarcoma. CT findings. Chest 1995; 108(6):1622–6.

45. Davison JM, Subramaniam RM, Surasi DS, et al. FDG PET/CT in patients with HIV. AJR Am J Roentgenol 2011;197(2):284–94.

46. De Bruin GP, Stefan DC. Children with Kaposi sarcoma in two South African hospitals: clinical presentation, management and outcome. J Trop Med 2013;2013:213490.

47. Lai DR, Clark I, Shalkow J, et al. Primary epithelial lung malignancies in the pediatric population. Pediatr Blood Cancer 2005;45(5):683–6.

48. Kodama T, Shimosato Y, Watanabe S, et al. Six cases of well-differentiated adenocarcinoma simulating fetal lung tubules in pseudoglandular stage. Comparison with pulmonary blastoma. Am J Surg Pathol 1984;8(10):735–44.

49. Park JA, Park HJ, Lee JS, et al. Adenocarcinoma of lung in never smoked children. Lung Cancer 2008; 61(2):266–9.

50. Kayton ML, He M, Zakowski MF, et al. Primary lung adenocarcinomas in children and adolescents treated for pediatric malignancies. J Thorac Oncol 2010;5(11):1764–71.

51. Thomas JW, Staerkel GA, Whitman GJ. Pulmonary hamartoma. AJR Am J Roentgenol 1999;172(6): 1643.

52. Bateson EM, Abbott EK. Mixed tumors of the lung, or hamarto-chondromas. A review of the radiological appearances of cases published in the literature and a report of fifteen new cases. Clin Radiol 1960;11:232–47.

53. Gjevre JA, Myers JL, Prakash UB. Pulmonary hamartomas. Mayo Clin Proc 1996;71(1):14–20.

54. Klein JS, Braff S. Imaging evaluation of the solitary pulmonary nodule. Clin Chest Med 2008; 29(1):15–38.

55. Ledor K, Fish B, Chaise L, et al. CT diagnosis of pulmonary hamartomas. J Comput Tomogr 1981; 5(4):343–4.

56. Alexopoulou E, Economopoulos N, Priftis KN, et al. MR imaging findings of an atypical pulmonary hamartoma in a 12-year-old child. Pediatr Radiol 2008;38(10):1134–7.

57. Sinner WN. Fine-needle biopsy of hamartomas of the lung. AJR Am J Roentgenol 1982;138(1):65–9.

58. Gleason BC, Hornick JL. Inflammatory myofibroblastic tumors: where are we now? J Clin Pathol 2008;61(4):428–37.

59. Hedlund GL, Navoy JF, Galliani CA, et al. Aggressive manifestations of inflammatory pulmonary pseudotumor in children. Pediatr Radiol 1999; 29(2):112–6.

60. Matsubara O, Tan-Liu NS, Kenney RM, et al. Inflammatory pseudotumors of the lung: progression from organizing pneumonia to fibrous histiocytoma or to plasma cell granuloma in 32 cases. Hum Pathol 1988;19(7):807–14.

61. Patankar T, Prasad S, Shenoy A, et al. Pulmonary inflammatory pseudotumour in children. Australas Radiol 2000;44:318–20.

62. Agrons GA, Rosado-de-Christenson ML, Kirejczyk WM, et al. Pulmonary inflammatory pseudotumor: radiologic features. Radiology 1998; 206(2):511–8.

63. Kim TS, Han J, Kim GY, et al. Pulmonary inflammatory pseudotumor (inflammatory myofibroblastic tumor): CT features with pathologic correlation. J Comput Assist Tomogr 2005;29(5):633–9.

64. Huellner MW, Schwizer B, Burger I, et al. Inflammatory pseudotumor of the lung with high FDG uptake. Clin Nucl Med 2010;35(9):722–3.

65. Takayama Y, Yabuuchi H, Matsuo Y, et al. Computed tomographic and magnetic resonance features of inflammatory myofibroblastic tumor of the lung in children. Radiat Med 2008;26(10):613–7.

66. Copin MC, Gosselin BH, Ribet ME. Plasma cell granuloma of the lung: difficulties in diagnosis and prognosis. Ann Thorac Surg 1996;61(5): 1477–82.

67. Keylock JB, Galvin JR, Franks TJ. Sclerosing hemangioma of the lung. Arch Pathol Lab Med 2009; 133(5):820–5.

68. Kuo KT, Hsu WH, Wu YC, et al. Sclerosing hemangioma of the lung: an analysis of 44 cases. J Chin Med Assoc 2003;66(1):33–8.

69. Liebow AA, Hubbell DS. Sclerosing hemangioma (histiocytoma, xanthoma) of the lung. Cancer 1956;9(1):53–75.

70. Devouassoux-Shisheboran M, Hayashi T, Linnoila RI, et al. A clinicopathologic study of 100 cases of

pulmonary sclerosing hemangioma with immunohistochemical studies: TTF-1 is expressed in both round
and surface cells, suggesting an origin from primitive
respiratory epithelium. Am J Surg Pathol 2000;24(7):
906–16.

71. Im JG, Kim WH, Han MC, et al. Sclerosing hemangiomas of the lung and interlobar fissures: CT findings. J Comput Assist Tomogr 1994;18(1):34–8.

72. Fujiyoshi F, Ichinari N, Fukukura Y, et al. Sclerosing
hemangioma of the lung: MR findings and correlation with pathological features. J Comput Assist Tomogr 1998;22(6):1006–8.

73. Patrini D, Shukla R, Lawrence D, et al. Sclerosing
hemangioma of the lung showing strong FDG avidity on PET scan: case report and review of the current literature. Respir Med Case Rep 2015;17:20–3.

74. Lee E, Park CM, Kang KW, et al. 18F-FDG PET/CT
features of pulmonary sclerosing hemangioma.
Acta Radiol 2012;54(1):24–9.

75. Wei S, Tian J, Song X, et al. Recurrence of pulmonary sclerosing hemangioma. Thorac Cardiovasc
Surg 2008;56(2):120–2.

76. Roby BB, Drehner D, Sidman JD. Pediatric tracheal
and endobronchial tumors: an institutional experience. Arch Otolaryngol Head Neck Surg 2011;
137(9):925–9.

77. Reznek RH. CT/MRI of neuroendocrine tumours.
Cancer Imaging 2006;6:S163–77.

78. Yu DC, Grabowski MJ, Kozakewich HP, et al. Primary lung tumors in children and adolescents: a
90-year experience. J Pediatr Surg 2010;45(6):
1090–5.

79. Fisseler-Eckhoff A, Demes M. Neuroendocrine tumors of the lung. Cancer 2012;4(3):777–98.

80. Chong S, Lee KS, Chung MJ, et al. Neuroendocrine tumors of the lung: clinical, pathologic,
and imaging findings. Radiographics 2006;26(1):
41–57.

81. Doppman JL, Pass HI, Nieman LK, et al. Detection
of ACTH-producing bronchial carcinoid tumors:
MR imaging vs CT. AJR Am J Roentgenol 1991;
156(1):39–43.

82. Yellin A, Zwas ST, Rozenman J, et al. Experience
with somatostatin receptor scintigraphy in the management of pulmonary carcinoid tumors. Isr Med
Assoc J 2005;7(11):712–6.

83. Rea F, Rizzardi G, Zuin A, et al. Outcome and surgical strategy in bronchial carcinoid tumors: single
institution experience with 252 patients. Eur J Cardiothorac Surg 2007;31(2):186–91.

84. Torres AM, Ryckman FC. Childhood tracheobronchial mucoepidermoid carcinoma: a case report
and review of the literature. J Pediatr Surg 1988;
23(4):367–70.

85. Desai DP, Holinger LD, Gonzalez-Crussi F. Tracheal
neoplasms in children. Ann Otol Rhinol Laryngol
1998;107(9 Pt 1):790–6.

86. Kim TS, Lee KS, Han J, et al. Mucoepidermoid carcinoma of the tracheobronchial tree: radiographic
and CT findings in 12 patients. Radiology 1999;
212(3):643–8.

87. Wang YQ, Mo YX, Li S, et al. Low-grade and high-
grade mucoepidermoid carcinoma of the lung: CT
findings and clinical features of 17 cases. AJR Am
J Roentgenol 2015;205(6):1160–6.

88. Lee EY, Vargas SO, Sawicki GS, et al. Mucoepidermoid carcinoma of bronchus in a pediatric patient:
(18)F-FDG PET findings. Pediatr Radiol 2007;
37(12):1278–82.

89. Shikhani AH, Jones MM, Marsh BR, et al. Infantile
subglottic hemangiomas. An update. Ann Otol Rhinol Laryngol 1986;95(4 Pt 1):336–47.

90. Badi AN, Kerschner JE, North PE, et al. Histopathologic and immunophenotypic profile of subglottic
hemangioma: multicenter study. Int J Pediatr Otorhinolaryngol 2009;73(9):1187–91.

91. Koplewitz BZ, Springer C, Slasky BS, et al. CT of
hemangiomas of the upper airways in children.
AJR Am J Roentgenol 2005;184(2):663–70.

92. Cooper M, Slovis TL, Madgy DN, et al. Congenital
subglottic hemangioma: frequency of symmetric
subglottic narrowing on frontal radiographs of the
neck. AJR Am J Roentgenol 1992;159(6):1269–71.

93. Bhat V, Salins PC, Bhat V. Imaging spectrum of
hemangioma and vascular malformations of the
head and neck in children and adolescents.
J Clin Imaging Sci 2014;4:31.

94. Hatayama K, Watanabe H, Ahmed AR, et al. Evaluation of hemangioma by positron emission tomography: role in a multimodality approach. J Comput
Assist Tomogr 2003;27(1):70–7.

95. Wu L, Wu X, Xu X, et al. Propranolol treatment of
subglottic hemangiomas: a review of the literature.
Int J Clin Exp Med 2015;8(11):19886–90.

96. Bajaj Y, Hartley BE, Wyatt ME, et al. Subglottic
haemangioma in children: experience with open
surgical excision. J Laryngol Otol 2006;120(12):
1033–7.

97. Niyibizi J, Rodier C, Wassef M, et al. Risk factors for
the development and severity of juvenile-onset
recurrent respiratory papillomatosis: a systematic
review. Int J Pediatr Otorhinolaryngol 2014;78:
186–97.

98. Zacharisen MC, Conley SF. Recurrent respiratory
papillomatosis in children: masquerader of common respiratory diseases. Pediatrics 2006;118(5):
1925–31.

99. Frauenfelder T, Marincek B, Wildermuth S. Pulmonary spread of recurrent respiratory papillomatosis
with malignant transformation: CT-findings and
airflow simulation. Eur J Radiol 2005;56:11–6.

100. Pipavath SN, Manchanda V, Lewis DH, et al. 18F
FDG-PET/CT findings in recurrent respiratory papillomatosis. Ann Nucl Med 2008;22(5):433–6.

101. Yu JP, Barajas RF Jr, Olorunsola D, et al. Heterogeneous 18F-FDG uptake in recurrent respiratory papillomatosis. Clin Nucl Med 2013; 38(5):387–9.

102. Myer CM 3rd, Willging JP, McMurray S, et al. Use of a laryngeal micro resector system. Laryngoscope 1999;109:1165–6.

103. McMurray JS, Connor N, Ford CN. Cidofovir efficacy in recurrent respiratory papillomatosis: a randomized, double-blind, placebo-controlled study. Ann Otol Rhinol Laryngol 2008;117(7):477–83.

104. McCarville MB. Malignant pulmonary and mediastinal tumors in children: differential diagnoses. Cancer Imaging 2010;10:S35–41.

105. Duwe BV, Sterman DH, Musani AI. Tumors of the mediastinum. Chest 2005;128(4):2893–909.

106. Toma P, Granata C, Rossi A, et al. Multimodality imaging of Hodgkin disease and non-Hodgkin lymphomas in children. Radiographics 2007;27(5): 1335–54.

107. Turner CA, Tung K. CT appearances of amyloid lymphadenopathy in a patient with non-Hodgkin's lymphoma. Br J Radiol 2007;80(958):e250–2.

108. Rostock RA, Siegelman SS, Lenhard RE, et al. Thoracic CT scanning for mediastinal Hodgkin's disease: results and therapeutic implications. Int J Radiat Oncol Biol Phys 1983;9:1451–6.

109. White KS. Thoracic imaging of pediatric lymphomas. J Thorac Imaging 2001;16:224–37.

110. Au V, Leung AN. Radiologic manifestations of lymphoma in the thorax. AJR Am J Roentgenol 1997; 168:93–8.

111. Urasinski T, Kamienska E, Gawlikowska-Sroka A, et al. Pediatric pulmonary Hodgkin lymphoma: analysis of 10 years data from a single center. Eur J Med Res 2010;15(Suppl 2):206–10.

112. Wyttenbach R, Vock P, Tschäppeler H. Cross-sectional imaging with CT and/or MRI of pediatric chest tumors. Eur Radiol 1998;8(6):1040–6.

113. Hutchings M, Barrington S. PET/CT for therapy response assessment in lymphoma. J Nucl Med 2009;50(Suppl 1):S21–30.

114. Lu P. Staging and classification of lymphoma. Semin Nucl Med 2005;35:160–4.

115. Sher AC, Seghers V, Paldino MJ, et al. Assessment of sequential PET/MRI in comparison with PET/CT of pediatric lymphoma: a prospective study. AJR Am J Roentgenol 2016;206(3):623–31.

116. Papaioannou G, McHugh K. Neuroblastoma in childhood: review and radiological findings. Cancer Imaging 2005;5:116–27.

117. Lonergan GJ, Schwab CM, Suarez ES, et al. Neuroblastoma, ganglioneuroblastoma, and ganglioneuroma: radiologic–pathologic correlation. Radiographics 2002;22:911–34.

118. Hiorns MP, Owens CM. Radiology of neuroblastoma in children. Eur Radiol 2001;11:2071–81.

119. Kushner BH. Neuroblastoma: a disease requiring a multitude of imaging studies. J Nucl Med 2004;45: 1172–88.

120. McCarville MB. Imaging neuroblastoma: what the radiologist needs to know. Cancer Imaging 2011; 11:S44–7.

121. Dhull VS, Sharma P, Patel C, et al. Diagnostic value of 18F-FDG PET/CT in paediatric neuroblastoma: comparison with 131I-MIBG scintigraphy. Nucl Med Commun 2015;36(10):1007–13.

122. Albany C, Einhorn LH. Extragonadal germ cell tumors: clinical presentation and management. Curr Opin Oncol 2013;25(3):261–5.

123. Ueno T, Tanaka YO, Nagata M, et al. Spectrum of germ cell tumors: from head to toe. Radiographics 2004;24(2):387–404.

124. Juanpere S, Cañete N, Ortuño P, et al. A diagnostic approach to the mediastinal masses. Insights Imaging 2013;4(1):29–52.

125. Moeller KH, Rosado-de-Christenson ML, Templeton PA. Mediastinal mature teratoma: imaging features. AJR Am J Roentgenol 1997;169(4): 985–90.

126. Jeung MY, Gasser B, Gangi A, et al. Imaging of cystic masses of the mediastinum. Radiographics 2002;22(Spec No):S79–93.

127. Takahashi K, Al-Janabi NJ. Computed tomography and magnetic resonance imaging of mediastinal tumors. J Magn Reson Imaging 2010;32:1325–39.

128. Choi SJ, Lee JS, Song KS, et al. Mediastinal teratoma: CT differentiation of ruptured and unruptured tumors. AJR Am J Roentgenol 1998;171(3):591–4.

129. Escalon JG, Arkin J, Chaump M, et al. Ruptured anterior mediastinal teratoma with radiologic, pathologic, and bronchoscopic correlation. Clin Imaging 2015;39(4):689–91.

130. Peterson CM, Buckley C, Holley S, et al. Teratomas: a multimodality review. Curr Probl Diagn Radiol 2012;41(6):210–9.

131. Koizumi T, Katou A, Ikegawa K, et al. Comparative analysis of PET findings and clinical outcome in patients with primary mediastinal seminoma. Thorac Cancer 2013;4(3):241–8.

132. Nam SJ, Kim S, Lim BJ, et al. Imaging of primary chest wall tumors with radiologic-pathologic correlation. Radiographics 2011;31(3):749–70.

133. Saenz NC, Ghavimi F, Gerald W, et al. Chest wall rhabdomyosarcoma. Cancer 1997;80(8):1513–7.

134. Gladish GW, Sabloff BM, Munden RF, et al. Primary thoracic sarcomas. Radiographics 2002;22(3): 621–37.

135. McCarville MB. What MRI can tell us about neurogenic tumors and rhabdomyosarcoma. Pediatr Radiol 2016;46(6):881–90.

136. Eugene T, Corradini N, Carlier T, et al. 18F-FDG-PET/CT in initial staging and assessment of early response to chemotherapy of pediatric

rhabdomyosarcomas. Nucl Med Commun 2012; 33(10):1089–95.

137. Saenz NC, Hass DJ, Meyers P, et al. Pediatric chest wall Ewing's sarcoma. J Pediatr Surg 2000; 35(4):550–5.

138. Burchill SA. Ewing's sarcoma: diagnostic, prognostic, and therapeutic implications of molecular abnormalities. J Clin Pathol 2003;56(2):96–102.

139. Tateishi U, Gladish GW, Kusumoto M, et al. Chest wall tumors: radiologic findings and pathologic correlation: part 2. Malignant tumors. Radiographics 2003;23(6):1491–508.

140. Foran P, Colleran G, Madewell J, et al. Imaging of thoracic sarcomas of the chest wall, pleura, and lung. Semin Ultrasound CT MR 2011;32(5):365–76.

141. O'Sullivan P, O'Dwyer H, Flint J, et al. Malignant chest wall neoplasms of bone and cartilage: a pictorial review of CT and MR findings. Br J Radiol 2007;80(956):678–84.

142. Al-Ibraheem A, Buck AK, Benz MR, et al. (18) F-fluorodeoxyglucose positron emission tomography/ computed tomography for the detection of recurrent bone and soft tissue sarcoma. Cancer 2013; 119(6):1227–34.

143. Wong KS, Hung IJ, Wang CR, et al. Thoracic wall lesions in children. Pediatr Pulmonol 2004;37(3): 257–63.

144. Carter BW, Benveniste MF, Betancourt SL, et al. Imaging evaluation of malignant chest wall neoplasms. Radiographics 2016;36(5):1285–306.

145. Amini B, Jessop AC, Ganeshan DM, et al. Contemporary imaging of soft tissue sarcomas. J Surg Oncol 2015;111(5):496–503.

146. North PE, Mihm MC Jr. Histopathological diagnosis of infantile hemangiomas and vascular malformations. Facial Plast Surg Clin North Am 2001;9(4):505–24.

147. Leon-Villapalos J, Wolfe K, Kangesu L. GLUT-1: an extra diagnostic tool to differentiate between haemangiomas and vascular malformations. Br J Plast Surg 2005;58:348–52.

148. Chang LC, Haggstrom AN, Drolet BA, et al, Hemangioma Investigator Group. Growth characteristics of infantile hemangiomas: implications for management. Pediatrics 2008;122(2):360–7.

149. Lowe LH, Marchant TC, Rivard DC, et al. Vascular malformations: classification and terminology the radiologist needs to know. Semin Roentgenol 2012;47:106–17.

150. Giudici MA, Moser RP Jr, Kransdorf MJ. Cartilaginous bone tumors. Radiol Clin North Am 1993; 31(2):237–59.

151. Murphey MD, Choi JJ, Kransdorf MJ, et al. Imaging of osteochondroma: variants and complications with radiologic-pathologic correlation. Radiographics 2000;20(5):1407–34.

152. Bernard SA, Murphey MD, Flemming DJ, et al. Improved differentiation of benign osteochondromas from secondary chondrosarcomas with standardized measurement of cartilage cap at CT and MR imaging. Radiology 2010;255(3):857–65.

153. Czajka CM, DiCaprio MR. What is the proportion of patients with multiple hereditary exostoses who undergo malignant degeneration? Clin Orthop Relat Res 2015;473(7):2355–61.

154. Schmale GA, Hawkins DS, Rutledge J, et al. Malignant progression in two children with multiple osteochondromas. Sarcoma 2010;2010:417105.

155. Feldman F, Van Heertum R, Saxena C, et al. 18FDG-PET applications for cartilage neoplasms. Skeletal Radiol 2005;34(7):367–74.

Pediatric Thoracic Anatomic Variants
What Radiologists Need to Know

Abbey J. Winant, MD, MFA[a],*, Joo Cho, MD[a],
Tahiya Salem Alyafei, MD[b], Edward Y. Lee, MD, MPH[a]

KEYWORDS

• Thoracic anatomic variants • Thymus • Accessory fissures • Tracheobronchial variants

KEY POINTS

• Anatomic variants are commonly encountered in the pediatric thorax, including the mediastinum, tracheobronchial tree, pulmonary parenchyma, and chest wall.
• Accurate differentiation of normal pediatric thymic variants from pathologic masses is important to prevent unnecessary intervention and delayed diagnosis. Normal pediatric thymus can be quite large with biconvex margins throughout early childhood. Ectopic thymus and cervical thymus are normal variants that can be confirmed with ultrasound or cross-sectional imaging.
• Tracheobronchial variants are more common on the right, and may be asymptomatic or may predispose to recurrent pulmonary infections.
• Accessory fissures, the most common pulmonary developmental variant, are asymptomatic, but important for disease localization and operative planning.
• Thoracic cage anatomic variants, including prominent anterior convexity, bifid ribs, and fused ribs, may be isolated and sporadic, or may be associated with malformation syndromes.

INTRODUCTION

Anatomic variants are common incidental findings in pediatric chest imaging and can be mistaken for true underlying pathology, sometimes resulting in unnecessary additional imaging evaluation or invasive procedures. Clear understanding of the underlying cause and imaging characteristics of thoracic variants is important for accurate diagnosis and avoidance of unnecessary intervention. This article provides an up-to-date review of the imaging findings of anatomic variations in the pediatric thorax, including the mediastinum, tracheobronchial tree, pulmonary parenchyma, and chest wall, to increase knowledge of these variants among practicing radiologists and help with timely, accurate diagnosis.

MEDIASTINAL VARIANTS
Age-Dependent Changes in Thymus

There is wide variability in the normal radiologic appearance of the pediatric thymus. The thymus is a bilobed, lymphatic organ important for cellular immunity, especially T-cell lymphopoesis. The thymus demonstrates unique age-dependent morphologic changes over time. Achieving its maximum weight relative to body weight in the perinatal period, the pediatric thymus can be quite large relative to the thorax with convex margins until approximately age 5 (**Figs. 1–3**).[1–3] Differentiating normal age-appropriate thymus from an anterior mediastinal mass is critical for preventing unnecessary intervention and delay in diagnosis.

[a] Department of Radiology, Boston Children's Hospital, Harvard Medical School, 300 Longwood Avenue, Boston, MA 02115, USA; [b] Clinical Imaging Department, Hamad General Hospital, Hamad Medical Corporation, PO Box 3050, Doha, Qatar
* Corresponding author.
E-mail address: Abbey.Winant@childrens.harvard.edu

Radiol Clin N Am 55 (2017) 677–691
http://dx.doi.org/10.1016/j.rcl.2017.02.002
0033-8389/17/Published by Elsevier Inc.

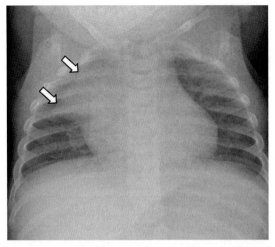

Fig. 1. A 3-week-old boy with normal thymus. Frontal chest radiograph demonstrates "thymic sail sign" (*arrows*), with a triangular extension of thymus over the right lung.

On chest radiographs, two signs, the thymic sail sign and the thymic wave sign, may help confirm normal thymus.[4,5] First, the thymic sail sign denotes a triangular extension of thymic tissue, extending laterally from the mediastinum, commonly projecting over the right upper lobe (see **Fig. 1**).[4,5] The thymic sail sign is a common normal radiographic appearance of the thymus in infants and should not be mistaken for an upper lobe mass or pneumonia.[4] The thymic wave sign describes a subtle undulation in thymic contour caused by the impression on the overlying ribs

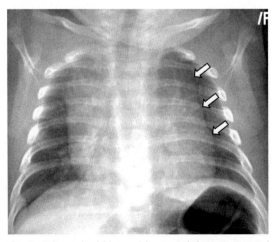

Fig. 2. A 4-week-old boy with normal thymus. Frontal chest radiograph shows "thymic wave sign" (*arrows*) with undulating thymic contour along the left heart border, caused by impression of the overlying ribs on pliable thymic parenchyma.

on its soft parenchyma (see **Fig. 2**).[4] The thymic wave sign confirms the presence of normal pliable thymic tissue.[4,5]

On cross-sectional imaging studies, such as computed tomography (CT) or MR imaging, normal pediatric thymus often appears as generous anterior mediastinal soft tissue, draping over the superior aspect of the heart, with a quadrilateral morphology in the coronal plane (see **Fig. 3C**; **Figs. 4** and **5**).[2,6] Although the contour of normal pediatric thymus may be convex, significant lobulations or irregular margins are abnormal.[2,6] Normal thymus is soft, and should not displace or compress adjacent airways or vessels.[2,7] On CT, normal thymic tissue demonstrates homogeneous soft tissue attenuation, without calcifications or focal fat.[6] On MR imaging, thymus is homogenously T2 hyperintense, and isointense to slightly hyperintense to muscle on T1-weighted MR imaging.[2,7] After intravenous contrast administration, normal thymus demonstrates mild uniform enhancement on CT and MR imaging.[8]

Normal thymus regresses with age, near completely involuting with biconcave margins by late adolescence (**Fig. 6**).

Ectopic Thymus

Ectopic thymic tissue can be discovered anywhere along the path of normal thymic development, including the cervical region and the middle and posterior mediastinum, and may present a diagnostic dilemma (**Fig. 7**).[8,9] During gestation, the two lobes of the thymus arise from the third pharyngeal pouch and descend inferomedially to fuse in the superior anterior mediastinum.[1,9] Furthermore, cervical extension of pediatric thymus, in which the thymic tissue extends superiorly through the thoracic inlet, often attaching to the inferior aspect of the thyroid gland, is a common variant in children (**Fig. 8**).[10] Ectopic thymic tissue in the mediastinum and cervical regions can be mistaken for mass or adenopathy, and accurate recognition is important to prevent unnecessary intervention.[2,8,10]

Ultrasound is a helpful problem-solving tool for ectopic thymus in infants and young children with an appropriate sonographic window, especially in the anterior cervical region. Ectopic thymus often has an angulated morphology and drapes over adjacent structures, such as vessels and airways, without displacing or invading them.[2,7] Ultrasound of ectopic or cervical thymus typically demonstrates a characteristic thymic dot-dash echotexture, with alternating hyperechoic linear striations and punctate echogenic foci, corresponding to septa and vessels (see

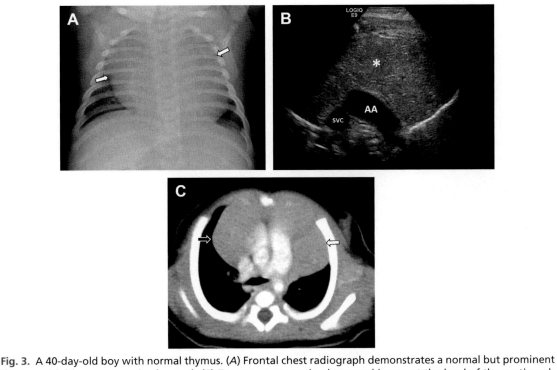

Fig. 3. A 40-day-old boy with normal thymus. (A) Frontal chest radiograph demonstrates a normal but prominent thymus with biconvex margins (arrows). (B) Transverse grayscale ultrasound image at the level of the aortic arch demonstrates homogeneous, predominantly hypoechoic soft tissue in the anterior mediastinum (asterisk) with alternating linear striations and punctate echogenic foci, compatible with normal thymus. Despite its large size and convex margins, this normal infant thymus does not exert any mass effect on the underlying vascular structures. (C) Axial contrast-enhanced computed tomography image shows normal age-appropriate thymus (arrows) in the anterior mediastinum with biconvex margins and homogenous attenuation, without compression or invasion of adjacent structures. AA, aortic arch; SVC, superior vena cava.

Fig. 3B).[11] Mediastinal ectopic thymus, which is less accessible by ultrasound, may be visualized on cross-sectional imaging as soft tissue islands in the middle or posterior mediastinum, in the retrocaval region or interposed between vessels, including the superior vena cava, brachiocephalic vessels, or aorta.[2,8] Ectopic thymic tissue demonstrates the same imaging characteristics as normally located thymus. On CT, similar to normal thymus, ectopic or cervical thymic tissue

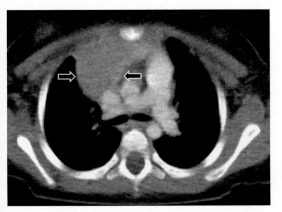

Fig. 4. An 18-month-old girl with normal thymus. Axial contrast-enhanced CT image demonstrates homogeneously enhancing anterior mediastinal soft tissue (arrows) with biconvex margins consistent with normal age-appropriate thymus.

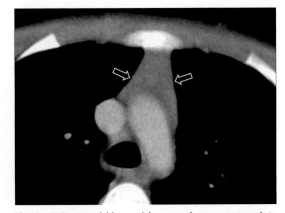

Fig. 5. A 6-year-old boy with normal, age-appropriate thymus. Axial contrast-enhanced CT image shows homogeneously enhancing anterior mediastinal soft tissue (arrows) consistent with normal age-appropriate thymus.

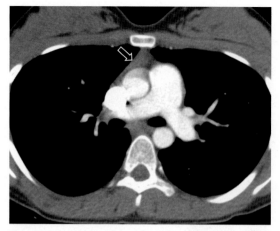

Fig. 6. An 18-year-old girl with normal involuting thymus. Axial contrast-enhanced CT image demonstrates homogeneous triangular anterior mediastinal soft tissue (*arrow*) with biconcave margins, consistent with involuting thymus.

demonstrates homogenous soft tissue attenuation, without focal fat or calcification, and does not exert mass effect on adjacent structures, such as vessels and airways (**Fig. 9**).[8] On MR imaging, ectopic thymus may demonstrate continuity with the normal thymus, especially on multiplanar reformats, and identical signal intensity (homogeneously T2 hyperintense, T1 isointense to hyperintense to muscle) and enhancement patterns.[2,7,8] Both normal and ectopic thymic tissue demonstrate mild homogenous enhancement on CT and MR imaging.[8]

Cervical extension of pediatric thymus, in which thymic tissue extends superiorly through the thoracic inlet, is a common variant in children.[12] Furthermore, intermittent superior movement of normal thymus into the cervical region is

often a physiologic consequence of increased intrathoracic pressure, for example, during forced exhalation and/or Valsalva maneuver.[12,13] Suprasternal herniation of normal pediatric thymus has been described to cause intermittent, asymptomatic, subclinical posterior buckling of the cervicothoracic trachea and often rightward tracheal deviation, without tracheal luminal narrowing or respiratory distress.[12,13] Diagnosis of superior extension of thymus is made by location, continuity with mediastinal thymic tissue, and the previously described characteristic imaging features.[12]

Ectopic thymus is a benign normal variant that typically regresses with age and requires no further evaluation or intervention.

TRACHEOBRONCHIAL VARIANTS

Congenital variations in tracheobronchial anatomy are common and important to recognize. Thought to be the result of abnormal lung budding during development, most tracheobronchial anomalies occur on the right.[14,15] Anomalous bronchi are classified as either displaced or supernumerary.[14] Displaced bronchi arise at a lower level than normal in the bronchial tree.[14] Conversely, supernumerary anomalous bronchi supply a segment of lung that is also ventilated by a coexisting normal bronchus.[14] Although variant large airway branching may be often an incidental finding, some tracheobronchial anomalies can predispose to the development of respiratory problems.

Tracheal Bronchus

Classic tracheal bronchus, also known as "bronchus suis" or "pig bronchus," is a displaced upper lobe bronchus that arises directly from the trachea, superior to the carina (**Fig. 10**).[16] Far more

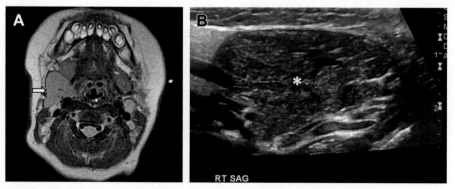

Fig. 7. A 4-month-old girl with palpable right neck mass. (*A*) Axial T2-weighted MR image shows asymmetric, well-circumscribed, triangular soft tissue (*arrow*) with homogeneously T2-hyperintense signal relative to adjacent muscle, interposed between the right submandibular gland and the right carotid sheath, compatible with ectopic thymus. (*B*) Sagittal gray-scale high-frequency ultrasound image demonstrates a predominantly hypoechoic mass (*asterisk*) with the characteristic dot-dash echotexture, consistent with ectopic thymus.

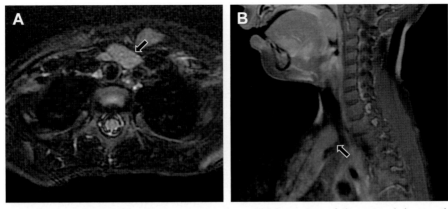

Fig. 8. A 4-year-old boy with incidentally demonstrated cervical extension of the normal thymus. (*A*) Axial T2-weighted MR image shows homogeneously mildly T2-hyperintense, anterior mediastinal soft tissue (*arrow*), draping anteriorly over the trachea, without mass effect or invasion of adjacent structures. (*B*) Sagittal T2-weighted MR image with fat saturation shows T2-hyperintense anterior mediastinal soft tissue (*arrow*), extending superiorly above the thoracic inlet, consistent with cervical extension of thymus.

common on the right, tracheal bronchus can occur on either side or bilaterally. Occurring in up to 5% of the population, tracheal bronchus is the most common tracheobronchial variant.[14] Although classically only referring to displaced upper lobe bronchus arising from the trachea, recent literature has suggested that the term tracheal bronchus encompass any upper lobe bronchus, displaced or supernumerary, originating from the trachea, mainstem bronchi, or any segmental airway.[17] Vascularization is typically normal for the pulmonary parenchyma ventilated by the anomalous tracheal bronchus.[17] Although most frequently an asymptomatic incidental finding, tracheal bronchus can cause recurrent upper lobe atelectasis and/or pneumonia.[16] Management depends patient symptoms; however, surgical resection of tracheal bronchus may be considered in symptomatic pediatric patients.

Esophageal Bronchus

Esophageal bronchus is a rare anomaly, in which a bronchus arises directly from the esophagus. There is a higher incidence of esophageal bronchus in patients with esophageal atresia, tracheoesophageal fistula, and VACTERL (vertebral defects, anal atresia, cardiac defects, tracheoesophageal fistula, renal anomalies, and limb anomalies).[18] The esophageal bronchus may supply an entire lung (eg, esophageal lung), a lobe, or pulmonary segment, most commonly the right lower lobe medial basal segment (**Fig. 11**).[16] As expected, pediatric patients with esophageal bronchus may present early in life with respiratory distress during feeding and recurrent pulmonary infections.[18]

Esophageal bronchus may present with unilateral complete hemithorax opacification, especially in patients with predisposing conditions

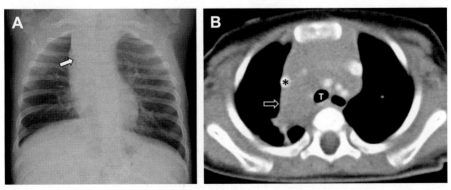

Fig. 9. A 10-month-old boy with abnormal chest radiograph. (*A*) Frontal chest radiograph demonstrates prominent thymus with biconvex margins, and a suggestion of double density (*arrow*) along the right paratracheal strip, suspicious for mediastinal mass. (*B*) Contrast-enhanced axial CT image demonstrates posterior extension of the normal thymus (*arrow*) between the superior vena cava (*asterisk*) and the great vessels, without mass effect on vessels or trachea (T).

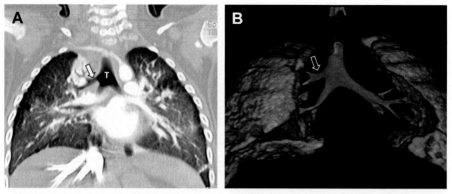

Fig. 10. A 9-month-old girl with tracheal bronchus (bronchus suis). (*A*) Coronal lung window CT image demonstrates a tracheal bronchus (*arrow*), arising from the right aspect of the distal trachea (T) and supplying a segment of the right upper lobe. (*B*) Three-dimensional volume-rendered CT image demonstrates the tracheal bronchus (*arrow*) arising from the distal trachea.

(esophageal atresia, tracheoesophageal fistula, VACTERL).[18] Esophagram demonstrates the direct communication between the esophagus and the pulmonary parenchyma via the anomalous esophageal bronchus.[16] CT demonstrates atelectasis and/or consolidation in the affected lung segment.[18] CT may also reveal additional tracheal or vascular anomalies, such as hypoplastic trachea and hypoplastic right pulmonary artery.[18]

Treatment of esophageal bronchus is surgical: traditionally, resection of the esophageal bronchus and its ventilated pulmonary segments. Recently, however, bronchial reconstruction has been described and may salvage pulmonary parenchyma.[16,18] Early diagnosis of esophageal bronchus may prevent lung-damaging complications, including aspiration and infection, allowing for lung-sparing tracheobronchial reconstructive surgery.[18]

Accessory Cardiac Bronchus

Accessory cardiac bronchus (ACB) is a rare tracheobronchial anomaly, in which a supernumerary bronchus arises from the medial aspect of the bronchus intermedius or right mainstem

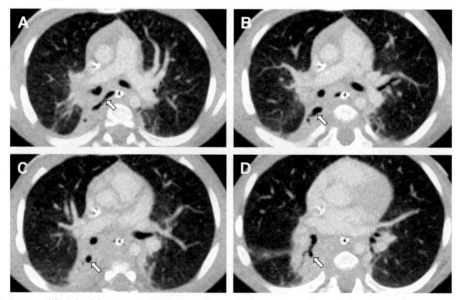

Fig. 11. A 2-year-old girl with recurrent pneumonia secondary to esophageal bronchus. Sequential axial lung window CT images (*A–D*) demonstrate esophageal bronchus (*arrow*), arising from the right aspect of the mid-distal thoracic esophagus and communicating with the right lower lobe, which is partially consolidated and scarred.

bronchus and advances inferomedially toward the heart (**Fig. 12**).[17,19] Slightly more common in males, with a reported incidence of 0.07% to 0.5%, ACB is the only true supernumerary anomalous bronchus.[17,19,20] Histologically, the ACB airway wall is normal. Most ACBs are asymptomatic; however ACBs can present with recurrent infection and hemoptysis.[20,21]

ACBs are typically undetectable on chest radiographs and are usually discovered on CT.[22] Most ACBs arise from the bronchus intermedius (86%–100%), opposite to the origin of the right upper lobe bronchus.[22,23] ACBs are variable in morphology and length (typically ranging between 0.5 cm and 5.0 cm).[20] ACBs have been classified into three types; however, most are blind-ending type 1 (diverticulum stump type, 50%–71%), which do not actually ventilate any pulmonary parenchyma.[19,22,23] Less commonly, ACBs are type 2 (cystic type, 25%–50%), ending in cystic degeneration of rudimentary bronchiolar tissue, and type 3 (ventilated type, 25%–29%), culminating in a ventilated lobulus, usually in the azygoesophageal recess, often demarcated from the right lower lobe by an accessory fissure.[19,22,23]

No treatment is required for most ACBs, which are asymptomatic. However, if recurrent infection is attributed to poor drainage from ACB, surgical resection may be considered.[20]

Bridging Bronchus

Bridging bronchus (BB) is a very rare tracheobronchial anomaly, in which a displaced bronchus crosses the midline of the mediastinum to ventilate contralateral pulmonary parenchyma (**Fig. 13**).[19]

Strongly associated with left pulmonary artery sling, BB is also associated with partial anomalous pulmonary venous return, bilobed right lung, and cardiac anomalies, among others.[24–27] BB may be asymptomatic, or may present with recurrent wheeze and/or respiratory distress.[28]

Radiologically, BB denotes a displaced bronchus intermedius, arising from the medial aspect of the left mainstem bronchus and crossing the midline to ventilate portions of the right lung.[19] Two types of BB have been described, based on the anatomy of the trachea and right mainstem bronchus. In the first type of BB, the right mainstem bronchus is absent or hypoplastic, often a small blind-ending diverticulum. Often associated with tracheal stenosis and right lung hypoplasia, this first pattern of BB is unique because the BB ventilates the entire right lung.[19] In the second type of BB, the right mainstem bronchus and trachea are normal in structure, and the right mainstem bronchus ventilates the right upper lobe (and sometimes the right middle lobe), with the BB ventilating the right lower lobe (and sometimes the right middle lobe).[19] Parenchyma ventilated by the BB may be poorly aerated, often demonstrating atelectasis and/or cystic changes, especially when there is coexisting tracheal stenosis and/or left pulmonary artery sling.[19,24] In the second subtype of BB, the normal right mainstem bronchus may hyperinflate the right upper lobe (and right middle lobe), which can be mistaken for congenital lobar emphysema, leading to inadvertent right upper lobe resection.[19]

On CT and bronchoscopy, the first subtype of BB may be confused with a tracheal bronchus,

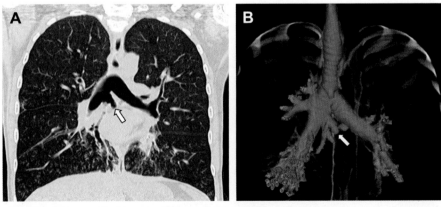

Fig. 12. An 11-year-old boy with Mounier-Kuhn syndrome and incidentally discovered accessory cardiac bronchus. Coronal lung window (*A*) and coronal three-dimensional airway reconstruction (*B*) CT images demonstrate an accessory cardiac bronchus (*arrow*) arising from the left inferior aspect of the bronchus intermedius. Tracheobronchomegaly and bronchial diverticuli, in keeping with patient's known history of Mounier-Kuhn, are also noted.

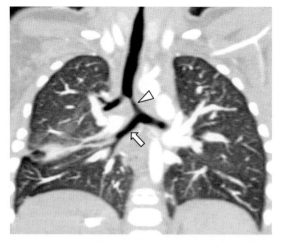

Fig. 13. An 11-month-old boy with bridging bronchus who presented with respiratory distress. Coronal lung window CT image demonstrates a bridging bronchus (*arrow*) arising from the inferior aspect of the left mainstem bronchus, crossing the midline to ventilate the right lower lobe. Associated high-grade stenosis of the left mainstem bronchus (*arrowhead*) is also present.

with the hypoplastic right mainstem bronchus mistaken for a tracheal bronchus and the pseudo-carina (formed by the bifurcation of the left mainstem bronchus and BB) mistaken for the true carina.[19,29] The location of the apparent carina helps to differentiate BB from tracheal bronchus: the normal carina is located at approximately the T4-T5 level and midline, whereas the pseudo-carina of BB is typically located at approximately T5-T7 level and left of midline.[19] In addition, the BB typically follows a more horizontal course than the normal right mainstem bronchus and bronchus intermedius.[19] Three-dimensional

reconstructions of the tracheobronchial tree can aide in diagnosis.

Treatment of BB depends on patient symptoms. Asymptomatic pediatric patients may be treated conservatively. Tracheobronchial reconstruction may be considered in symptomatic pediatric patients.

LUNG PARENCHYMAL VARIANTS
Accessory Fissures

Accessory fissures are the most common pulmonary developmental variant.[30] Although the expected major and minor fissures are identified on nearly 100% of chest CTs, accessory fissures are identified on up to 40% of CTs and present in up to 50% pathologic specimens.[31–34] Usually occurring at the boundaries between bronchopulmonary segments, accessory fissures are clefts, lined by two closely apposed layers of visceral pleura, that can be either partial or complete, depending on the depth of extension toward the hilum (**Fig. 14**).[34] The segment of lung separated by an accessory fissure is often denoted an accessory lobe.[30,34] Note that accessory fissures do not denote the presence of additional lung tissue: only the fissure is supernumerary.[30] Furthermore, the bronchial and vascular anatomy is normal.[30] Pediatric patients with accessory fissures are typically asymptomatic; however, accurate depiction of fissural anatomy on CT is important for precise localization of disease (eg, pleural tumors along an accessory fissure may be mistaken for intraparenchymal masses) and for preoperative planning.[32]

On chest radiographs, an accessory fissure often appears as a thin white line, which may be mistaken for a scar, atelectasis, bulla wall, or pleural line made apparent by pneumothorax.[30]

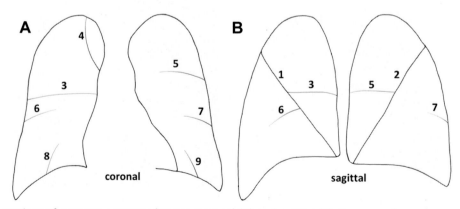

Fig. 14. Locations of common accessory fissures. Coronal (*A*) and sagittal (*B*) diagrams of common accessory fissures. 1 = right major fissure, 2 = left major fissure, 3 = right minor fissure, 4 = azygous fissure, 5 = left minor (horizontal) fissure, 6 = right superior accessory fissure, 7 = left superior accessory fissure, 8 = right inferior accessory fissure, 9 = left inferior accessory fissure.

On CT, pneumonias may be bound by an accessory fissure, which may either contain or exclude airspace exudates from the separated segment.[30] The most common accessory fissures are the inferior accessory fissure (5%–21%), superior accessory fissure (1%–6%), and left minor (horizontal) fissure (8%–18%).[32–35] Nearly any segmental boundary can be accentuated by an accessory fissure, and additional unnamed accessory fissures occur with less frequency, including between the right middle lobe medial and lateral segments, and between the lower lobe anterior and lateral basal segments bilaterally.

Accessory fissures are incidental normal variants requiring no further management.

Inferior Accessory Fissure

The inferior accessory fissure, also known as Twining's line, is seen in 5% to 21% of patients.[30,33,34] The inferior accessory fissure divides the medial basal bronchopulmonary segment from the remainder of the lower lobe, and is at least five times more common on the right (**Figs. 15** and **16**).[34] The separated medial basal segment is often referred to as the inferior accessory, cardiac, retrocardiac, or infracardiac lobe.[34] When complete, the inferior accessory fissure extends from the major fissure to the pulmonary ligament. On frontal radiographs, inferior accessory fissure often appears as a diaphragmatic peak.[30] On CT, inferior accessory fissure is a partial or complete thin curvilinear arc extending from the major fissure toward the inferior pulmonary ligament, near the esophagus.[30,34] The inferior accessory fissure is often thicker anteriorly, where the cleft is often deeper on anatomic specimens.[30]

Superior Accessory Fissure

More common on the right, and seen in up to 6% of patients, the superior accessory fissure, is horizontal in configuration and demarcates the lower lobe superior segment from the lower lobe basal segments (**Figs. 17** and 18).[32,34] The excluded lower lobe superior segment has been called the posterior or dorsal lobe.[30,34] On lateral radiographs and sagittal CT, superior accessory fissure resembles the minor fissure, but is slightly more inferior in position and directed posteriorly.[30] The superior accessory fissure extends posteriorly from the major fissure toward the patient's back, often with a slight superior angulation, whereas the normal right minor fissure extends anteriorly from the right major fissure.[30] If the superior accessory fissure lies at the same level as the minor fissure, then the right major fissure, minor fissure, and superior accessory fissure form an X configuration on lateral radiographs and sagittal CT.[30]

Left Minor Fissure

Analogous to the right minor fissure, the left minor fissure separates the lingula from the remainder of the left upper lobe, specifically separating the left upper lobe anterior segment from the lingular superior segment (**Fig. 19**).[35] Of note, the normal superior and inferior segmental anatomy of lingula is preserved.[30,32–34] Radiographically, the left minor fissure is frequently dome-shaped (convex superior), and usually more superior in location than the right minor fissure.[35] In addition, the left minor fissure is infrequently horizontal; rather, it is often obliquely oriented, with its lateral margin more superior than the medial margin.[35]

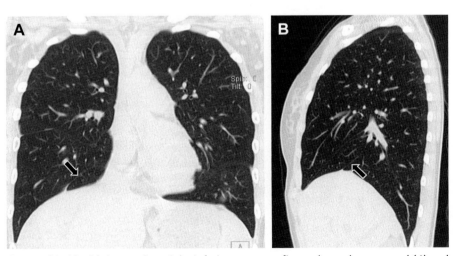

Fig. 15. A 13-year-old girl with incomplete right inferior accessory fissure (*arrow*) on coronal (*A*) and sagittal (*B*) lung window CT images.

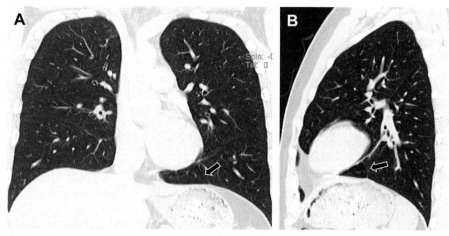

Fig. 16. A 19-year-old woman with incomplete left inferior accessory fissure (*arrow*) on coronal (*A*) and sagittal (*B*) lung window CT images.

Horseshoe Lung

Horseshoe lung is a rare congenital variant in which an isthmus of pulmonary parenchyma extends across the midline, posterior to the pericardium, to connect the bilateral lung bases (**Fig. 20**).[36] Nearly all documented cases of horseshoe lung have been associated with unilateral pulmonary hypoplasia, and most occurred in the context of scimitar syndrome (right lung hypoplasia, partial anomalous pulmonary venous return).[37] Horseshoe lung is also frequently associated with additional abnormalities, including lobation, bronchial, pleural, diaphragmatic, and cardiac anomalies.[36–39] Horseshoe lung may be an asymptomatic incidental finding, or may present with recurrent pulmonary infections.[40]

Horseshoe lung is not easily identified on radiographs alone. On frontal radiographs, horseshoe lung has been associated with a faint linear or curvilinear white line at the medial left lung base, denoting the left lateral pleural margin of the pulmonary isthmus as it extends beyond the left aspect of the spine.[36] In a pediatric patient with predisposing condition (eg, scimitar syndrome, unilateral pulmonary hypoplasia), a linear density at the medial left lung base can suggest the coexistence of horseshoe lung.

CT demonstrates a narrow band of pulmonary parenchyma that extends from the often hypoplastic right lung to the left lung base, crossing the midline posterior to the pericardium and anterior to the spine, esophagus, and aorta.[36] This

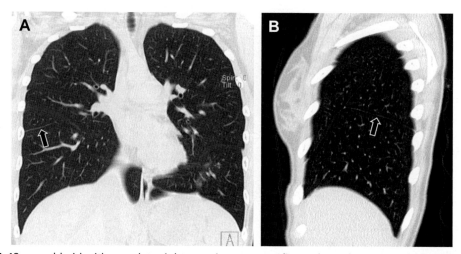

Fig. 17. A 13-year-old girl with complete right superior accessory fissure (*arrow*) on coronal (*A*) and sagittal (*B*) lung window CT images.

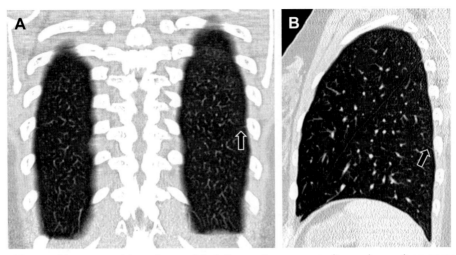

Fig. 18. An 18-year-old woman with an incomplete left superior accessory fissure (*arrows*) on coronal (*A*) and sagittal (*B*) lung window CT images.

horseshoe lung isthmus may be fused to the left lower lobe parenchyma, with or without intervening pleura or fissure.[36] Frequently, the isthmus has its own pleural sheath, which is often incomplete and may allow some communication between the right and left pleura.[38] The isthmus typically receives arterial supply from the right pulmonary artery and bronchi from the right bronchial tree, resulting in right-sided vessels and bronchi also crossing the midline.[38] Pulmonary parenchyma from the horseshoe lung isthmus is histologically normal.[36]

Treatment of horseshoe lung depends on symptoms. Surgical resection of the isthmus may be considered in pediatric patients with recurrent pulmonary infections.[36]

CHEST WALL VARIANTS

Although anatomic variations in thoracic cage anatomy are often seen in the setting of additional malformations, most chest wall variants are sporadic, isolated findings.[41,42] Chest wall variants may occasionally result in an asymmetric or palpable abnormality discovered by parent or physician on close physical examination. Radiologists should be familiar with congenital variations in thoracic cage anatomy to avoid unnecessary evaluation and intervention.

Prominent Anterior Chest Wall Convexity

Incidental variations in anterior chest wall osteochondral anatomy occur in approximately 33% of

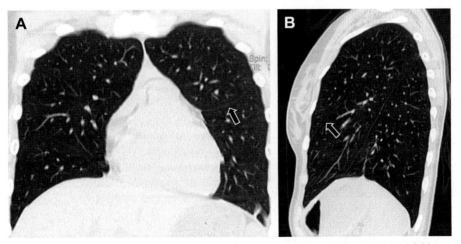

Fig. 19. A 13-year-old girl with complete left minor fissure (*arrow*) on coronal (*A*) and sagittal (*B*) lung window CT images.

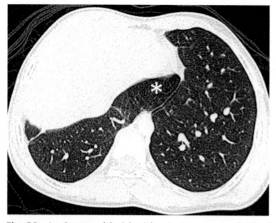

Fig. 20. An 8-year-old girl with scimitar syndrome and horseshoe lung. Axial lung window CT image reveals a band of lung parenchyma (*asterisk*) extending from the hypoplastic right lung to the left lung base, crossing the midline, posterior to the heart and anterior to the spine and aorta.

children.[43] The most frequently occurring incidental anterior chest wall variants include tilted sternum (45%), prominent convexity of anterior rib or costal cartilage (29%), and asymmetrically prominent costal cartilage (31%) (**Fig. 21**).[43] There is no significant association between the occurrence of anterior chest wall variants and patient age or sex.[43] In a large study of children presenting with an asymptomatic palpable anterior chest wall abnormality, prominent anterior rib convexity or costal cartilage was the most frequent cause.[44]

These variants are commonly incidentally noted on chest CT examinations performed for other reasons. Tilted sternum is present when the sternum is oriented oblique to the horizontal axis of the body, resulting in a unilateral anterior convexity.[43] Prominent anterior rib or cartilage convexity is

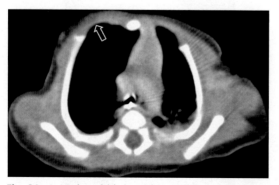

Fig. 21. A 15-day-old boy with prominent right anterior costal cartilage convexity (*arrow*). Axial contrast-enhanced CT image shows asymmetrically prominent apex anterior convexity (*arrow*) of the right anterior costal cartilage.

defined as a rib or costal cartilage with an apex anterior convexity with angulation greater than the adjacent ipsilateral and/or contralateral ribs.[43] Asymmetrically prominent costal cartilage is denoted by a costal cartilage whose anteroposterior diameter is more than 3 mm greater than the contralateral costal cartilage at the same level.[43]

No further management is indicated for prominent anterior chest wall convexity. Indeed, benign history and physical examination, especially the absence of pain or growth of a palpable pediatric chest wall abnormality, have a high negative predictive value for excluding sinister etiologies, such as infection or malignancy, even in the absence of imaging.[44] Painless asymptomatic prominent anterior chest wall convexities are common findings that should be considered normal, warranting no further work-up.[43]

Bifid Rib

Bifid rib is a congenital deformity in which a portion of a rib or costal cartilage is bifurcated, most commonly the anteromedial portion, resulting in a cleaved or forked appearance (**Fig. 22**).[41,45] Bifid rib is uncommon with an estimated prevalence of 0.15% to 0.6% and a slight female predilection.[41,46,47] Bifid rib most commonly occurs in the upper right-sided ribs, especially the right fourth rib.[41,45,48] Most frequently an isolated anomaly, bifid ribs also have been associated with congenital scoliosis and multisystem malformations. For example, bifid ribs were discovered in up to 26% of patients with nevoid basal cell carcinoma syndrome (Gorlin syndrome) in one series, most commonly affecting the third, fourth, and fifth ribs.[49,50] In addition, bifid ribs were identified in 24% of patients with congenital scoliosis, and have been associated with Kindler syndrome.[51,52]

Chest radiographs and CT demonstrate duplication and bifurcation of the bifid rib, most common the anteromedial aspect, often with metaphyseal flaring and/or downward extension of the rib.[48] Typically, each (duplicated) branch of the bifid rib has its own costal cartilage; however, the duplicated costal cartilages reunite before their articulation with the sternum.[48] Rarely, the duplication involves only the nonossified costal cartilage, which cannot be visualized on plain radiographs.[41,48] In the absence of additional malformations, bifid rib most likely represents an isolated, sporadic anomaly, requiring no further evaluation or treatment.[48]

Rib Fusion

Rib fusion is a structural rib anomaly with multiple etiologies. Fused ribs may be an incidental

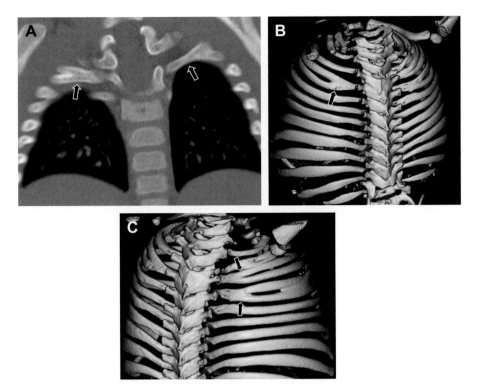

Fig. 22. A 23-month-old boy with thoracolumbar myelomeningocele and congenital kyphosis. (*A*) Coronal bone window CT image shows bilateral third bifid ribs (*arrows*), with cleaved appearance posteriorly. (*B*) Three-dimensional reconstruction bone CT image demonstrates left third bifid rib (*arrow*). (*C*) Three-dimensional reconstruction bone CT image shows right third and fourth bifid ribs (*arrows*).

anatomic variant; however, they are also frequently seen in association with vertebral segmentation anomalies and multisystem malformation syndromes, among other causes.[41] Indeed, fused ribs are identified in up to 30% of patients with congenital scoliosis (**Fig. 23**).[51] Rib fusion was the most common rib anomaly (72%) discovered in a series of patients with multiple congenital

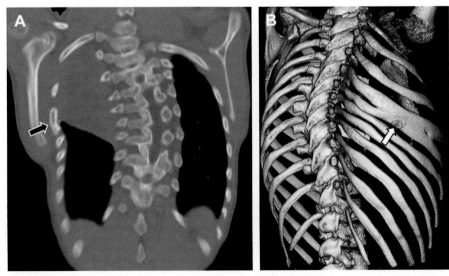

Fig. 23. A 13-year-old girl with VATER syndrome and scoliosis with fused right fourth and fifth ribs. (*A*) Coronal bone window CT image shows fusion (*arrow*) of the lateral portions of the right fourth and fifth ribs. (*B*) Three-dimensional reconstruction bone CT image redemonstrates osseous fusion (*arrow*) of the posterolateral portions of the right fourth and fifth ribs.

anomalies and has also been associated with nevoid basal cell carcinoma syndrome (Gorlin syndrome, 16%).[42,49] Furthermore, rib fusion may also result from surgery (thoracotomy), trauma, or infection, and may result in scoliosis and/or restriction of chest wall expansion.[53]

Radiologically, rib fusion is characterized by the osseous bridging of two adjacent ribs, most frequently involving the first and second ribs when it is an isolated and incidental finding.[41] Rib fusion may involve any segment of the rib (posterior, lateral, or anterior) and may be partial or complete.[47] The presence of fused ribs may be incidental; however, it should raise suspicion for additional anomalies.

SUMMARY

Anatomic variation is a common finding in pediatric chest imaging. Anatomic variants are encountered throughout the structures of the pediatric thorax, including the mediastinum, tracheobronchial tree, pulmonary parenchyma, and thoracic cage. Clear knowledge of the underlying cause, optimum imaging modality for assessment, and imaging characteristics of pediatric thoracic variants is important for accurate and timely diagnosis, and avoidance of unnecessary intervention.

REFERENCES

1. Nishino M, Ashiku SK, Kocher ON, et al. The thymus: a comprehensive review. Radiographics 2006;26(2): 335–48.
2. Siegel MJ, Glazer HS, Wiener JI, et al. Normal and abnormal thymus in childhood: MR imaging. Radiology 1989;172(2):367–71.
3. Jacobs MT, Frush DP, Donnelly LF. The right place at the wrong time: historical perspective of the relation of the thymus gland and pediatric radiology. Radiology 1999;210(1):11–6.
4. Alves ND, Sousa M. Images in pediatrics: the thymic sail sign and thymic wave sign. Eur J Pediatr 2013; 172(1):133.
5. Mulvey RB. The thymic "wave" sign. Radiology 1963;81:834–8.
6. St Amour TE, Siegel MJ, Glazer HS, et al. CT appearances of the normal and abnormal thymus in childhood. J Comput Assist Tomogr 1987;11(4):645–50.
7. Zielke AM, Swischuk LE, Hernandez JA. Ectopic cervical thymic tissue: can imaging obviate biopsy and surgical removal? Pediatr Radiol 2007;37(11):1174–7.
8. Slovis TL, Meza M, Kuhn JP. Aberrant thymus: MR assessment. Pediatr Radiol 1992;22(7):490–2.
9. Nasseri F, Eftekhari F. Clinical and radiologic review of the normal and abnormal thymus: pearls and pitfalls. Radiographics 2010;30(2):413–28.
10. Costa NS, Laor T, Donnelly LF. Superior cervical extension of the thymus: a normal finding that should not be mistaken for a mass. Radiology 2010;256(1): 238–42.
11. Han BK, Yoon HK, Suh YL. Thymic ultrasound. II. Diagnosis of aberrant cervical thymus. Pediatr Radiol 2001;31(7):480–7.
12. Wong KT, Lee DL, Chan MS, et al. Unusual anterior neck mass visible only during Valsalva's maneuver in a child. AJR Am J Roentgenol 2005;185(5): 1355–7.
13. Mandell GA, Bellah RD, Boulden ME, et al. Cervical trachea: dynamics in response to herniation of the normal thymus. Radiology 1993;186(2):383–6.
14. Wu JW, White CS, Meyer CA, et al. Variant bronchial anatomy: CT appearance and classification. AJR Am J Roentgenol 1999;172(3):741–4.
15. Atwell SW. Major anomalies of the tracheobronchial tree: with a list of the minor anomalies. Dis Chest 1967;52(5):611–5.
16. Lee EY, Restrepo R, Dillman JR, et al. Imaging evaluation of pediatric trachea and bronchi: systematic review and updates. Semin Roentgenol 2012;47(2): 182–96.
17. Ghaye B, Szapiro D, Fanchamps JM, et al. Congenital bronchial abnormalities revisited. Radiographics 2001;21(1):105–19.
18. Colleran GC, Ryan CE, Lee EY, et al. Computed tomography and upper gastrointestinal series findings of esophageal bronchi in infants. Pediatr Radiol 2017;47(2):154–60.
19. Desir A, Ghaye B. Congenital abnormalities of intrathoracic airways. Radiol Clin North Am 2009;47(2): 203–25.
20. McGuinness G, Naidich DP, Garay SM, et al. Accessory cardiac bronchus: CT features and clinical significance. Radiology 1993;189(2):563–6.
21. Keane MP, Meaney JF, Kazerooni EA, et al. Accessory cardiac bronchus presenting with haemoptysis. Thorax 1997;52(5):490–1.
22. Unlu EN, Yilmaz Aydin L, Bakirci S, et al. Prevalence of the accessory cardiac bronchus on multidetector computed tomography: evaluation and proposed classification. J Thorac Imaging 2016;31(5):312–7.
23. Ghaye B, Kos X, Dondelinger RF. Accessory cardiac bronchus: 3D CT demonstration in nine cases. Eur Radiol 1999;9(1):45–8.
24. Starshak RJ, Sty JR, Woods G, et al. Bridging bronchus: a rare airway anomaly. Radiology 1981;140(1): 95–6.
25. Medina-Escobedo G, Lopez-Corella E. Sling left pulmonary artery, bridging bronchus, and associated anomalies. Am J Med Genet 1992;44(3):303–6.
26. Bertucci GM, Dickman PS, Lachman RS, et al. Bridging bronchus and posterior left pulmonary artery: a unique association. Pediatr Pathol 1987; 7(5–6):637–43.

27. Berdon WE, Muensterer OJ, Zong YM, et al. The triad of bridging bronchus malformation associated with left pulmonary artery sling and narrowing of the airway: the legacy of wells and landing. Pediatr Radiol 2012;42(2):215–9.

28. Schnabel A, Glutig K, Vogelberg C. Bridging bronchus: a rare cause of recurrent wheezy bronchitis. BMC Pediatr 2012;12:110.

29. Gainor D, Kinzinger M, Carl J, et al. Bridging bronchus: importance of recognition on airway endoscopy. Int J Pediatr Otorhinolaryngol 2015;79(7):1145–7.

30. Godwin JD, Tarver RD. Accessory fissures of the lung. AJR Am J Roentgenol 1985;144(1):39–47.

31. Frija J, Schmit P, Katz M, et al. Computed tomography of the pulmonary fissures: normal anatomy. J Comput Assist Tomogr 1982;6(6):1069–74.

32. Cronin P, Gross BH, Kelly AM, et al. Normal and accessory fissures of the lung: evaluation with contiguous volumetric thin-section multidetector CT. Eur J Radiol 2010;75(2):e1–8.

33. Ariyurek OM, Gulsun M, Demirkazik FB. Accessory fissures of the lung: evaluation by high-resolution computed tomography. Eur Radiol 2001;11(12):2449–53.

34. Yildiz A, Golpinar F, Calikoglu M, et al. HRCT evaluation of the accessory fissures of the lung. Eur J Radiol 2004;49(3):245–9.

35. Austin JH. The left minor fissure. Radiology 1986;161(2):433–6.

36. Frank JL, Poole CA, Rosas G. Horseshoe lung: clinical, pathologic, and radiologic features and a new plain film finding. AJR Am J Roentgenol 1986;146(2):217–26.

37. Figa FH, Yoo SJ, Burrows PE, et al. Horseshoe lung: a case report with unusual bronchial and pleural anomalies and a proposed new classification. Pediatr Radiol 1993;23(1):44–7.

38. Dupuis C, Remy J, Remy-Jardin M, et al. The "horseshoe" lung: six new cases. Pediatr Pulmonol 1994;17(2):124–30.

39. Kamijoh M, Itoh M, Kijimoto C, et al. Horseshoe lung with bilateral vascular anomalies: a rare variant of hypogenetic lung syndrome (scimitar syndrome). Pediatr Int 2002;44(4):443–5.

40. Cipriano P, Sweeney LJ, Hutchins GM, et al. Horseshoe lung in an infant with recurrent pulmonary infections. Am J Dis Child 1975;129(11):1343–5.

41. Guttentag AR, Salwen JK. Keep your eyes on the ribs: the spectrum of normal variants and diseases that involve the ribs. Radiographics 1999;19(5):1125–42.

42. Wattanasirichaigoon D, Prasad C, Schneider G, et al. Rib defects in patterns of multiple malformations: a retrospective review and phenotypic analysis of 47 cases. Am J Med Genet A 2003;122A(1):63–9.

43. Donnelly LF, Frush DP, Foss JN, et al. Anterior chest wall: frequency of anatomic variations in children. Radiology 1999;212(3):837–40.

44. Donnelly LF, Taylor CN, Emery KH, et al. Asymptomatic, palpable, anterior chest wall lesions in children: is cross-sectional imaging necessary? Radiology 1997;202(3):829–31.

45. Lee EY. Pediatric radiology: practical imaging evaluation of infants and children. Philadelphia: Wolters Kluwer; 2017.

46. Kupeli E, Ulubay G. Bony bridge of a bifid rib. Cleve Clin J Med 2010;77(4):232–3.

47. Kurihara Y, Yakushiji YK, Matsumoto J, et al. The ribs: anatomic and radiologic considerations. Radiographics 1999;19(1):105–19 [quiz: 151–2].

48. Kaneko H, Kitoh H, Mabuchi A, et al. Isolated bifid rib: clinical and radiological findings in children. Pediatr Int 2012;54(6):820–3.

49. Kimonis VE, Mehta SG, Digiovanna JJ, et al. Radiological features in 82 patients with nevoid basal cell carcinoma (NBCC or Gorlin) syndrome. Genet Med 2004;6(6):495–502.

50. Keceli O, Coskun-Benlidayi I, Benlidayi ME, et al. An uncommon disorder with multiple skeletal anomalies: Gorlin-Goltz syndrome. Turk J Pediatr 2014;56(4):434–6.

51. Ghandhari H, Tari HV, Ameri E, et al. Vertebral, rib, and intraspinal anomalies in congenital scoliosis: a study on 202 caucasians. Eur Spine J 2015;24(7):1510–21.

52. Sharma RC, Mahajan V, Sharma NL, et al. Kindler syndrome. Int J Dermatol 2003;42(9):727–32.

53. Glass RB, Norton KI, Mitre SA, et al. Pediatric ribs: a spectrum of abnormalities. Radiographics 2002;22(1):87–104.

Cyanotic Congenital Heart Disease
Essential Primer for the Practicing Radiologist

Evan J. Zucker, MD[a],*, Jeffrey L. Koning, MD[b],
Edward Y. Lee, MD, MPH[b]

KEYWORDS

- Congenital heart disease • Cyanosis • Computed tomography angiography
- Magnetic resonance imaging • Tetralogy of Fallot • Transposition of the great arteries
- Truncus arteriosus • Tricuspid atresia

KEY POINTS

- The cyanotic congenital heart diseases are rare and complex, often with multiple anomalies, requiring timely diagnosis and urgent management in the neonatal period.
- The 3 most prevalent causes of cyanotic heart disease are tetralogy of Fallot, transposition of the great arteries, and tricuspid atresia.
- Echocardiography provides an excellent and often definitive assessment. However, CT and MR imaging are increasingly used both preoperatively and postoperatively, supplementing echocardiography and helping to reduce the need for invasive cardiac catheterization.
- With continued improvements in therapies for cyanotic congenital heart disease and longer expected life spans, it is essential for the radiologist to be familiar with the preoperative and postoperative imaging appearances and complications of these entities.

INTRODUCTION

Congenital heart disease (CHD) broadly refers to anatomic malformations of the heart or great vessels.[1] Although specific defects are rare, CHD overall is among the most common inborn anomalies, arising in 0.6% to 0.8% of neonates.[2,3] CHD may be subclassified into acyanotic and cyanotic disease, depending on whether the clinical presentation includes cyanosis, characterized by bluish discoloration of the skin or mucous membranes that is usually apparent with oxygen saturations less than 80% or deoxygenated hemoglobin concentration greater than 5 g/dL.[1,4]

Acyanotic CHD includes left-to-right shunts, in which oxygenated blood is redirected toward the right heart containing deoxygenated blood, and obstructive lesions, characterized by vessel or valvular stenosis.[5,6] In contrast, cyanotic CHD is caused by right-to-left shunts in which deoxygenated systemic venous blood is directed toward the left heart, circumventing the lungs and leading to arterial desaturation. Defects are usually multiple and include admixture of pulmonary and systemic venous return, obstruction of pulmonary blood flow, and parallel rather than in-series pulmonary and systemic circulations.[1] Although acyanotic CHD may be mild and even remit spontaneously,

Disclosures: None.
[a] Department of Radiology, Lucile Packard Children's Hospital, Stanford University School of Medicine, 725 Welch Road, Stanford, CA 94305, USA; [b] Department of Radiology, Boston Children's Hospital and Harvard Medical School, 300 Longwood Avenue, Boston, MA 02115, USA
* Corresponding author.
E-mail address: zucker@post.harvard.edu

cyanotic CHD usually presents more acutely and requires surgery.[7]

Echocardiography remains the mainstay in the imaging assessment of CHD.[8] However, in recent years, advanced noninvasive modalities such as computed tomography angiography (CTA) and magnetic resonance (MR) imaging have garnered increasing importance, helping to refine presurgical and postsurgical planning and sometimes obviate invasive procedures such as cardiac catheterization.[9]

In this article, the authors review the broad spectrum of cyanotic CHD, focusing on the most common disorders, or "5 Ts" (tetralogy of Fallot [TOF], transposition of the great arteries [TGA], tricuspid atresia [TA], total anomalous pulmonary venous connection [TAPVC], truncus arteriosus), and additional frequently encountered lesions that may present with cyanosis (hypoplastic left heart syndrome [HLHS], pulmonary atresia with intact ventricular septum [PA-IVS], double-outlet right ventricle [DORV], double-inlet left ventricle [DILV], interrupted aortic arch [IAA], Ebstein anomaly).[1,3,6,10] The burgeoning role of advanced imaging is emphasized, while clinical features and treatment considerations are highlighted.

IMAGING EVALUATION
Chest Radiography

Although rarely able to elucidate a precise diagnosis, chest radiographs (CXRs) nonetheless remain an invaluable tool in the initial imaging assessment of CHD and may be the first examination to suggest an underlying cardiovascular malformation.[11–13] A systematic approach helps to avoid overlooking potential interpretive clues.[11] Postsurgical material, support devices, and abnormal calcifications are usually well evaluated.[12–14] Situs abnormalities can be readily detected by scrutinizing the stomach, spleen, and liver position and tracheobronchial branching pattern.[11,12,15] Although complete mirror-image situs (situs inversus) is associated with no greater prevalence of CHD compared with normal situs (situs solitus), rates of CHD are significantly greater with intermediate situs variations (situs ambiguous, heterotaxy).[15] Similarly, an anomalous position of the great vessels may be visible and should raise suspicion for underlying CHD. For example, a (single) right aortic arch, which manifests on radiographs as a right aortic knob deviating the trachea leftward of its expected position (normally slightly rightward of midline), is associated with CHD in 90% of cases.[11] Finally, an abnormal position of the cardiac apex in a location other than the left hemithorax (levocardia), that is, in the right hemithorax (dextrocardia) or in

the midline (mesocardia), should prompt attention.[11] Of note, the apex position is not dependent on the anatomic arrangement of intracardiac and visceral structures.[15]

The heart size and shape should also be assessed on every radiograph, although they are nonspecific.[11] A cardiothoracic ratio (CTR), calculated as the maximal transverse heart diameter divided by the maximal transverse thoracic diameter from the inner edge of the ribs and pleura, of ≥ 0.5 is a useful indicator of cardiomegaly in older children undergoing posteroanterior (PA) radiography. However, the same measurement is not reliable in neonates, in whom prior interpretative experience often ultimately proves most useful; one indicator of left atrial enlargement is rightward deviation of an enteric tube.[11,16] Moreover, an enlarged heart may be due to extracardiac an abnormality such as anemia or an arteriovenous malformation rather than an intracardiac process or even confused with a normal thymus in neonates and infants. Although certain cardiac shapes are classically associated with specific CHDs (as described later in this review), they are neither commonly encountered nor reliable for making a definitive diagnosis.[11]

Although it can prove challenging in practice, attempt should also be made to assess the pulmonary vasculature and pulmonary blood flow. Decreased pulmonary arterial blood flow, in which the hilum and vessels appear small and the lungs appear overly radiolucent, may be seen in cyanotic CHD. Increased pulmonary arterial blood flow, in which the vessels dilate and extend to the lateral third of the lungs, may be observed in left-to-right shunts and admixture lesions.[11,14] Pulmonary arterial abnormalities must be distinguished from pulmonary venous congestion and edema, in which the vessels appear hazy and ill-defined due to pulmonary venous dilation and migration of fluid into the perivascular tissues; such findings may be seen, for example, with impaired myocardial contractility. Concomitant lung disease may obscure the pulmonary vasculature, whereas enlargement of pulmonary vessels or cardiac chambers may secondarily cause focal atelectasis or air trapping.[11]

A variety of extracardiovascular findings appreciable on CXRs should raise suspicion for CHD or an associated syndrome. Osseous features associated with CHD include sternal hypoplasia, absence, or premature fusion; pectus excavatum; scoliosis; vertebral segmentation anomalies; abnormal number and morphology of ribs; and rib notching.[11,14] In addition, a small thymus is typical of cyanotic infants subject to extreme stress and in DiGeorge syndrome, which is associated with aortic arch abnormalities.[11] Nonetheless, full characterization of any CHD requires additional imaging.

Echocardiography

Noninvasive, portable, widely available, and effectively risk free, transthoracic echocardiography (TTE), or cardiac ultrasound, is generally regarded as the first-line and most important diagnostic test in the evaluation of CHD.[11–13] In many cases, it can provide a precise anatomic roadmap, helping to reduce cardiac catheterization examination times and even sufficing for presurgical planning.[11] In the same examination, cardiac function can be assessed.[12,13] In addition, the use of Doppler techniques allows assessment of blood flow velocity and direction, in turn facilitating estimation of shunt sizes and valvular gradients. Moreover, echocardiography provides excellent imaging guidance for certain interventions, such as balloon atrial septostomy (Rashkind procedure).[11] The advent of 3-dimensional (3D) TTE, which can produce a dynamic 3D volume-rendered display of sonographic data, may also improve visualization of such structures as the interatrial septum, mitral valve, and aortoseptal continuity.[12]

Nevertheless, TTE has several limitations. It is highly operator dependent, and thus findings and measurements may not be reliably replicated between examinations.[12,13] For example, one study found a 53% rate of major or moderate diagnostic error in pediatric echocardiograms performed at adult community hospitals.[12,17] In addition, acoustic windows may be suboptimal, limiting visualization; this problem is more likely in patients who have undergone surgery or possess a large body habitus, have severe emphysema, or have narrow intercostal spaces.[12,13] Even in the best hands, TTE in general underperforms in the assessment of such structures as the thoracic aorta, pulmonary arteries, pulmonary veins, and coronary arteries, particularly with complex malformations.[9,11]

Transesophageal echocardiography (TEE) is a useful supplement to TTE and may offer new data, alter the underlying diagnosis, or provide intraoperative imaging guidance. Nevertheless, TEE is invasive, with potential risks related to anesthesia, periprocedural infection, and correct technical performance.[12,13] Moreover, TEE is still operator dependent and suffers from suboptimal visualization of such structures as the right ventricular outflow tract (RVOT), apicoposterior septum, pulmonary valve, proximal left pulmonary artery, and distal right pulmonary artery. Other limitations include restricted view planes and blind spots that may arise, for example, when implanted graft material is present.[12,13] When

echocardiography is insufficient, computed tomography (CT), MR imaging, or invasive angiography may be warranted.[11]

Radionuclide Imaging

Radionuclide (nuclear medicine) imaging allows quantification of cardiac function and shunts. However, its use has declined with the growing adoption of competing modalities such as MR imaging that can provide as accurate data with better anatomic definition and no ionizing radiation. Nevertheless, selected applications for radionuclide imaging in CHD remain. These selected applications include ventilation-perfusion lung scintigraphy to identify and quantify abnormal patterns of pulmonary blood flow in patients with anomalous pulmonary arteries and stress-rest myocardial perfusion scans to evaluate for myocardial ischemia and infarction in individuals with coronary artery abnormalities. In addition, if MR imaging is contraindicated or not tolerated, nuclear medicine techniques provide a viable alternative.[12,13] Hybrid radionuclide/anatomic imaging with combined cardiac PET/MR imaging may present novel opportunities for the assessment of CHD, although the field is currently in early stages.[18]

Computed Tomography Angiography

Multidetector computed tomography (MDCT) with angiographic technique allows rapid and exquisite anatomic assessment of the heart and great vessels in a single acquisition.[12,13] Extracardiac structures such as the lungs and airways are also optimally evaluated.[9] Postprocessing software allows multiplanar reformatting, maximum and minimum intensity projection reconstructions, and 3D volume rendering, facilitating visualization of complex CHD for diagnostic and presurgical planning purposes.[11] Electrocardiographic (ECG) gating may be used not only to minimize image degradation from cardiac motion (eg, as may be needed for coronary imaging) but also to quantify ventricular and regurgitant volumes, ventricular function, myocardial mass, cardiac output, shunt flow, and pulmonary to systemic flow ratios (Qp:Qs).[9,12,13]

Exposure to ionizing radiation is a chief drawback of CT, with increased doses when cardiac gating is used.[12,13] However, continued advances in CT technology have allowed substantial dose reduction without compromising image quality. For example, a recent study comparing prospectively ECG-gated 320-MDCT to ungated helical 64-MDCT in neonates and infants showed submillisievert (mSv) effective doses and subjectively better image quality in the 320-MDCT group, while effective doses were on average nearly 5 mSv in the 64-MDCT cohort.[19] In general, low (70–80) kilovoltage peak (kVp) settings, with concomitant increase in tube current as needed, permit substantial dose reduction (eg, 40% decrease when lowering kVp from 120 to 80). Iterative reconstruction algorithms also allow for reduced image noise at the same exposure, thus permitting possible dose decreases while maintaining image quality.[9] In addition, it should be remembered that a high-quality CT may decrease the number of runs needed in the cardiac catheterization laboratory or obviate invasive angiography altogether, thus indirectly potentially lowering overall radiation dose.[20] The theoretic risks of radiation exposure such as future cancer should also be weighed against competing risks such as surgical mortality.[9]

Additional downsides to CT include the need for intravenous line (IV) placement, administration of iodinated contrast, and possibly anesthesia to help reduce patient motion.[9,12,13] Although the risks of an idiosyncratic allergic reaction and nephrotoxicity from iodinated contrast cannot be entirely mitigated, overall, nonionic low-osmolality agents such as iohexol and iopamidol have lower rates of adverse reactions. Iso-osmolar agents such as iodixanol may be safer in premature infants and patients with known renal insufficiency.[9] Achieving optimal contrast opacification in neonates can be technically challenging in view of 2 mL/kg contrast dose limits and 10 mL/kg total fluid limits. Injection protocols should be tailored to allow an injection duration for the entire scan length, including monitoring for peak enhancement of the area of interest, moving the CT table to the starting position, prompting breath-hold (if needed), and actually performing the diagnostic scan. A foot IV may be preferred to arm injection if dense contrast in the superior vena cava (SVC) may obscure the anatomy of concern.[9] The potential risks of anesthesia, albeit uncommon, must be weighed against the potential diagnostic benefits of the scan. On the upside, anesthesia requirements for CT are typically less than those for MR imaging, which mandates MR-compatible devices that are less accessible to the anesthesiologist and usually a longer depth and duration of sedation.[9] Moreover, the rapid scan times of modern CT increasingly allow successful "awake" acquisition in patients who would have previously required anesthesia.[19] Ultimately, if functional and flow information is required, MR imaging is generally preferred to CT, unless patients are too ill to tolerate its longer scan times or MR imaging is contraindicated due to incompatible devices.[9]

MR Imaging

In use for more than 20 years, MR imaging is among the most powerful imaging tools in CHD. In a single examination, intracardiac and vascular anatomy as well as ventricular function and blood flow can be accurately assessed.[8] Images can be obtained in any plane, including capabilities for 3D visualization, without the "acoustic window" or operator-dependency limitations of echocardiography.[8,13] In addition, MR imaging has no ionizing radiation exposure, and diagnostic imaging may be obtained even without IV contrast.[12] Traditional scans for CHD include some combination of spin-echo "black-blood" sequences, gradient-echo "bright-blood" cine sequences, MR angiography (MRA), and velocity-encoded phase-contrast (PC) sequences.[8,9] Additional sequences for myocardial tissue characterization, such as perfusion, late gadolinium enhancement, and T1 mapping, are available, although less commonly needed for CHD evaluation.[9]

Traditionally, a major limitation of pediatric cardiovascular MR has been the technical expertise needed to perform a successful scan. Unique challenges in children with CHD include planning appropriate imaging planes efficiently in real-time despite complex anatomy and achieving adequate visualization of small structures in the face of high heart rates.[21] However, the landscape has changed with the advent and growing availability of 3D time-resolved (4-dimensional [4D]) flow MR imaging. This novel technique captures morphologic, function, and flow data from both intracardiac and extracardiac structures as a single 3D volumetric acquisition, performed free breathing within 10 to 15 minutes and requiring no special knowledge of the often complex CHD anatomy before the scan is performed.[22–25] Blood flow can be retrospectively quantified at any desired region of interest after the scan is performed.[22] Moreover, anesthesia requirements can be lessened compared with traditionally longer examinations requiring breath holding.[9] Although validation studies are ongoing, studies to date have shown good correlation between 4D flow and traditional sequences for quantifying ventricular volume, mass, and function as well as blood flow.[22,23,26] Workflow issues are a current drawback to 4D flow imaging, which amasses large datasets requiring long reconstruction times and specialized software; however, these shortcomings have ready opportunities for progress.[9]

The use of IV contrast agents is preferred in 4D flow acquisition, helping to improve signal-to-noise in magnitude data and reduce noise in velocity data.[23] At Stanford, the pediatric cardiovascular radiologists have for more than 3 years successfully used ferumoxytol, an ultra-small superparamagnetic iron oxide nanoparticle with a circulating half-life of 14 to 15 hours, developed for the treatment of iron-deficiency anemia, as an off-label cardiovascular imaging contrast agent in this setting.[23,27–29] The risk of acute adverse allergic reactions with ferumoxytol is likely higher than that of gadolinium-based agents; in fact, the US Food and Drug Administration strengthened warnings about the agent in March 2015.[27] Nevertheless, ferumoxytol overall has a robust safety profile when administered as a slow infusion of diluted agent and allows for reliably high image quality with lighter anesthesia requirements.[23,27] Moreover, unlike gadolinium-based agents, ferumoxytol does not a pose a known risk of nephrogenic systemic fibrosis and may be administered in patients with renal failure.[27]

Alternatives to ferumoxytol include the gadolinium-based blood pool imaging agent gadofosveset. However, in the Stanford experience, vascular enhancement is qualitatively greater with ferumoxytol than with gadofosveset.[28] Moreover, ferumoxytol permits longer acquisition times, helping to improve signal-to-noise and allowing for greater motion averaging, compared with gadofosveset, which provides adequate vascular imaging up to only 45 to 60 minutes after administration.[28–30] Finally, gadofosveset is no longer available for purchase in US markets and thus inaccessible for routine clinical use. Traditional extracellular gadolinium agents initially are taken up in the intravascular space but soon equilibrate with the extracellular space, with an elimination half-time of only 70 to 90 minutes.[31] In contrast, gadofosveset has an elimination half-time of approximately 18 hours, while ferumoxytol affects MR signal for days to months after administration.[27,31] Thus, extracellular agents are not optimal when extended preservation of vascular signal may be needed.

Several additional limitations and contraindications to MR imaging remain. Metallic devices such as pacemakers may not be MR compatible, although even scanning with some pacemakers is now possible.[12,13] Claustrophobia may be a concern in some patients but can be overcome usually with only mild sedation.[13] Prosthetic graft material and calcification are in general not optimally imaged.[12,13] Motion and respiratory artifacts have traditionally been setbacks, although novel techniques such as motion compensation and compressed sensing have made free-breathing cardiac MR imaging a possibility.[12,25] Currently,

discounting radiation exposure and patient factors, CT is in general preferred when anatomic imaging of the lungs, coronary arteries, or small pulmonary vessels is a primary goal of the examination, while MR imaging is optimal for function and flow imaging.[9]

Cardiac Catheterization

Cardiac catheterization has been considered the "gold standard" in CHD imaging for more than half a century.[12,13] Typical indications include coronary and hypoplastic pulmonary artery assessment and presurgical planning.[11] At the same time, invasive angiography allows measurement of pressure gradients as well as oxygen saturations, helping to define the direction and severity of shunts. Cardiac morphology and function are also delineated.[12,13] Because of the dynamic nature of the examination, pulmonary vascular reactivity to vasoactive agents can also be stablished.[13] In addition, some interventions can be readily performed at the time of catheterization, such as balloon atrial septostomy, valvuloplasty, and angioplasty, patent ductus arteriosus (PDA) and aortopulmonary collateral closure, and stent placement.[11,12]

Nevertheless, with continued advances in noninvasive modalities such as cardiac CT and MR imaging, the route use of cardiac catheterization has accordingly declined, particularly for less complex CHD.[12,13] Even if catheterization cannot be avoided, supplementary noninvasive imaging may at the very least shorten procedure times. In addition to its invasive nature, catheter angiography also carries risks associated with IV contrast administration (allergic reaction, renal failure), ionizing radiation exposure, arterial and venous injury, bleeding, stroke, and even mortality, albeit rare.[12,21] The radiation exposure from catheterization can be orders of magnitude higher than that of CTA; for example, in one retrospective cohort, the median effective dose for nongated chest CTA was 0.76 mSv for children less than 1 year of age, compared with 13.4 mSv for catheterization.[32] Thus, it is not surprising that catheterization at many institutions is now reserved for situations in which very accurate hemodynamic data are crucial or interventional procedures are anticipated.[21]

SPECTRUM OF CYANOTIC CONGENITAL HEART DISEASE
Tetralogy of Fallot

TOF is characterized by 4 main anatomically abnormal features: a malaligned, subaortic, membranous ventricular septal defect (VSD), an

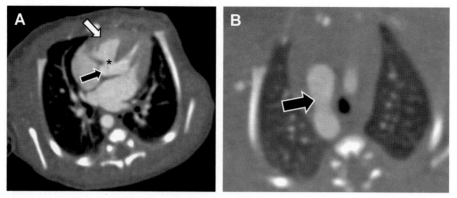

Fig. 1. TOF in a 3-day-old boy. (A) Axial CT angiogram image shows a malalignment VSD (*asterisk*) with overriding aorta (*black arrow*). The RV is hypertrophied (*white arrow*). (B) Axial CT angiogram image more superiorly shows a right aortic arch (*arrow*), a common associated finding.

overriding aorta, right ventricular hypertrophy, and pulmonary stenosis (PS), which may be valvular, subvalvular, and/or supravalvular (**Fig. 1**).[1,7–9,33] It is the most common cause of cyanotic CHD.[1,7–9] In fact, although TOF arises in only approximately 4 per 10,000 live births, TOF in fact accounts for 7% to 10% of all CHD.[1,7,8,33] The underlying pathogenesis is attributed to malposition of the conal septum in relationship to the ventricular endocardial cushion, resulting in lack of normal signaling for membranous septum formation.[33]

The anatomy in TOF is variable, and several discrete subtypes in addition to the conventional form are recognized. These subtypes include TOF with pulmonary atresia, in which the central PAs are completely discontinuous from the RVOT; TOF with major aortopulmonary collaterals (MAPCAs), in which the main pulmonary artery (MPA) is also absent or diminutive, but in addition, there are collateral vessels (MAPCAs) that typically arise from the aorta and supply the lungs (**Figs. 2 and 3**); and TOF with absent pulmonary valve, in which the pulmonic valve is rudimentary or nonexistent, leading to severe pulmonary regurgitation and pulmonary artery dilation (**Fig. 4**).[1,7–10,33]

TOF associations include a right aortic arch (25%); atrial septal defects (ASDs; 15%; referred to as "pentalogy" of Fallot); and coronary artery anomalies, most commonly the left anterior descending arising from the right coronary artery (RCA).[1] Presenting clinical features may range from an asymptomatic murmur or decreased exercise tolerance to hypercyanotic episodes, typically evident between 2 and 6 months of age.[1] In general, the degree of PS determines the onset and severity of cyanosis; with only mild RVOT obstruction, neonates may be "pink."[1,11] In patients with such mild RVOT obstruction, the resistance to

blood flowing through the pulmonary artery may be less than the resistance of blood flowing to the systemic circulation. As a result, excess blood flows from the LV to the RV, resulting in a net left-to-right shunt. Therefore, TOF patients with mild RVOT obstruction are often acyanotic (thus, called "pink tetralogy of Fallot") and may clinically present with congestive heart failure (CHF). The absent pulmonary valve form of TOF is unique in that the markedly enlarged pulmonary arteries cause tracheobronchial compression and resultant respiratory distress.[7,9,10]

The classic (although not universal) radiographic findings in TOF include a "boot-shaped heart" with elevation of the cardiac apex due to right ventricular hypertrophy, a concave MPA silhouette, and a large, right-sided aortic arch.[11,34] Pulmonary vascular markings are characteristically diminished but may be normal or engorged in "pink" patients without significant PS.[1,11] Echocardiography is the first-line imaging modality and provides an excellent assessment of the typical intracardiac anatomy in TOF, the magnitude and direction of shunting across the VSD, and the maximum velocity across the RVOT.[1,7,8] The maximum velocity can be used to estimate the pressure gradient across the RVOT via the modified Bernoulli equation, $\Delta P = 4V^2$, where ΔP is the pressure gradient in millimeters of mercury and V is the average maximum velocity is meters per second.[35] Although the main and proximal branch pulmonary arteries can be visualized, the distal pulmonary arteries are usually not well evaluated.[1]

CT offers an excellent anatomic assessment of RVOT morphology, branch pulmonary artery stenoses, and any MAPCAs, which usually arise from the thoracic aorta but may originate from the abdominal aorta or the subclavian, internal mammary, intercostal, or even coronary

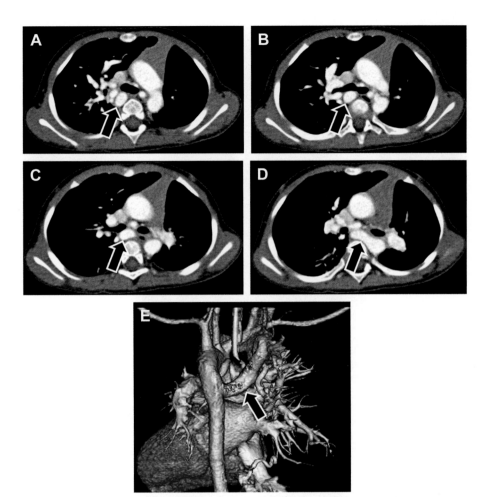

Fig. 2. TOF with pulmonary atresia and MAPCAs in a 9-month-old girl. (*A–D*) Contiguous axial CT angiogram images of the chest centered at the level of the carina demonstrate a large MAPCA coursing from the descending aorta, crossing midline to supply the right upper lobe (*arrow*). (*E*) Posterior 3D reformatted CT image demonstrates the large MAPCA (*arrow*) supplying the right upper lobe.

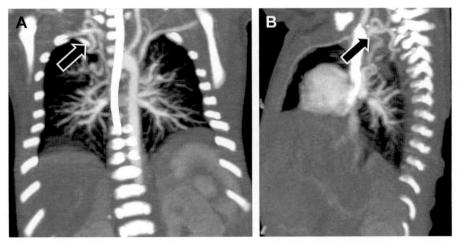

Fig. 3. TOF with pulmonary atresia and MAPCAs in a 15-day-old girl. (*A*) Coronal CT angiogram image at the level of the descending aorta demonstrates tortuous MAPCAs (*arrow*) arising from the right subclavian artery to supply the right upper lobe. (*B*) Sagittal CT angiogram image at the level of the SVC demonstrates tortuous MAPCAs from the right subclavian artery (*arrow*).

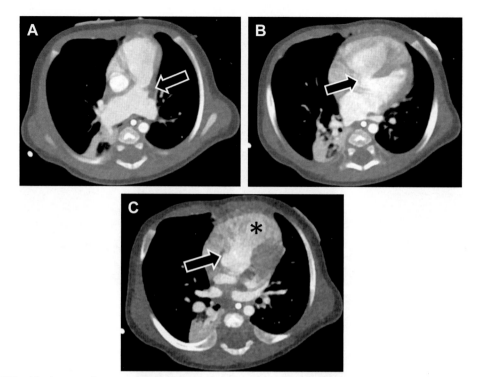

Fig. 4. TOF with absent pulmonary valve in a 53-day-old girl. (*A*) Axial CT angiogram image at the level of the MPA demonstrates focal pulmonary artery stenosis (*arrow*) and otherwise dilation of the MPA and proximal right and left pulmonary arteries. There is partial compression of the bronchi secondary to the enlarged pulmonary arteries. (*B*) Axial CT angiogram image at the level of the interventricular septum demonstrates a VSD (*arrow*). (*C*) Axial CT angiogram image at the level of the aortic root demonstrates an overriding aorta (*arrow*) and the adjacent RV (*asterisk*).

arteries.[8,9] When MAPCAs are present, it is important for presurgical planning purposes to delineate which segments of the lung are supplied by the native PAs, MAPCAs, or both.[9,36] For TOF with absent pulmonary valve, CT provides a superior assessment of tracheobronchial compression in relation to the aneurysmal pulmonary arteries.[9] In addition, CT is preferred to MR imaging for anatomic assessment when metallic stents are present.[8] Lung windows may reveal a mosaic attenuation pattern related to variations in regional lung perfusion and pulmonary hypertension.[33]

The major role of MR imaging in TOF is for postoperative assessment, when surgical material such as a conduit limits visualization.[8] A typical MR imaging exam for postoperative TOF includes evaluation of the following: right ventricular volume and function; RVOT anatomy, RVOT caliber, and peak velocity at the level of RVOT obstruction, if present; severity of pulmonary regurgitation and differential branch pulmonary artery regurgitation (quantified using PC techniques); and branch pulmonary artery stenosis (typically imaged with contrast-enhanced MRA).[8] When performed, late gadolinium enhancement imaging not

uncommonly demonstrates myocardial scarring in postoperative TOF patients, typically older with later repair, although the clinical significance is uncertain.[37] MR imaging has a well-established role in assessing the appropriate timing for pulmonary valve replacement (PVR) in patients with repaired TOF based on quantitative parameters. In the presence of a pulmonary regurgitation fraction of ≥25%, indications for valve replacement include an RV end-diastolic volume index greater than 150 mL/m^2 or Z score greater than 4, an RV/LV end-diastolic volume ratio greater than 2, a large RVOT aneurysm, right ventricular ejection fraction (EF) less than 45% to 47%, or left ventricular EF less than 55%.[38,39]

Cardiac catheterization has limited additional diagnostic utility in TOF before initial surgery. Nevertheless, it is useful for quantifying hemodynamics, delineating the central and branch pulmonary arteries and MAPCAs, and demonstrating coronary anomalies. A major and increasing role for catheterization is percutaneous PVR and exchange, obviating more invasive surgery.[8]

Initial therapy for TOF depends on the underlying anatomy. Most affected patients are at most minimally cyanotic at presentation and undergo elective surgical repair between the ages of 6 months and 1 year of age. Definitive surgical correction consists of VSD closure and relief of RVOT obstruction, which may be performed with infundibulectomy, a transannular patch, or a pulmonary artery valved conduit (usually a homograft). In patients with significant symptoms or cyanosis, a modified Blalock-Taussig (BT) shunt, typically consisting of a Gore-Tex graft from the right or left subclavian artery to the ipsilateral pulmonary artery, may be used to augment pulmonary blood flow. Other palliative procedures as bridge to surgery may include balloon pulmonary valvuloplasty or placement of an RVOT stent. In TOF with pulmonary atresia, initial maintenance of ductal flow is critical and may be accomplished via infusion of prostaglandin E_1 (PGE_1) and sometimes ductal stenting.[1,7,33,40] Treatment in the presence of MAPCAs is complex but in generally consists of multistage surgeries and catheterization to augment the pulmonary arteries and allow forward pulmonary blood flow; the use of MAPCAs to supplement the native pulmonary arteries is known as "unifocalization."[1,7,9,33,36] In TOF with absent pulmonary valve, management includes partial resection and repair of the aneurysmal pulmonary arteries.[7] After definitive repair, patients with TOF are at risk for complications ranging from RV dysfunction to arrhythmia to sudden death and require long-term monitoring (for example, to determine the timing of PVR), as previously described.[1,7,33,38]

Transposition of the Great Arteries

Although variable definitions exist in the literature, TGA in general refers to anatomy in which the aorta arises from the RV, whereas the main pulmonary artery arises from the LV (ventriculoarterial discordance). The most common form is known as complete transposition, which in addition is characterized by the following: atrial situs solitus (normal atrial position), atrioventricular discordance (right atrium [RA] connected to RV and left atrium connected to LV), D-looping of the ventricles (typically RV to the right of the LV), and the aortic valve positioned to the right of the pulmonary valve (dextro-TGA [d-TGA]) (**Fig. 5**).[1,7] TGA is rare, with an incidence 1 in 2000 to 5000 live births.[9] Nonetheless, TGA comprises 5% to 7% of all CHD and 10% of all neonatal cyanotic CHD.[1,9,10] It is the second most common cause of cyanotic CHD diagnosed by 1 year of age and the most common cyanotic CHD that presents in the first day of life.[8,11] TGA has a male predominance of 1.5 to 3:1 and arises most commonly in infants of diabetic mothers.[9,34] Other risk factors include fetal exposure to antiepileptic drugs and herbicides.[9]

TGA is usually isolated but in 10% may be associated with an extracardiac malformation or syndrome.[9,34] Symptoms depend on the anatomic subtype. When the ventricular septum is intact, patients develop cyanosis by the first week of life due to lack of mixing between the in-parallel rather than normally in-series pulmonary and systemic circulations.[1,7,11] If a VSD is present, cyanosis is typically minimal, but congestive heart failure (CHF) ensues between 4 and 8 weeks of life.[1] When a VSD is present, but there is superimposed PS, the balance of cyanosis versus CHF is directly related to the severity PS; marked PS essentially mimics an intact septum.[1]

The classic radiographic description of d-TGA is an "egg on a string." The "egg" refers to the heart, which characteristically has an enlarged and globular shape after the first few days of life (normal at birth), with an abnormally convex right atrial border and an enlarged left atrium.[11,34] The "string" refers

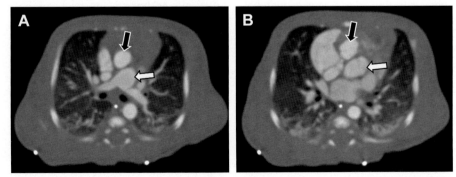

Fig. 5. d-TGA in a 7-day-old boy. (*A*) Axial CT angiogram image demonstrates the ascending aorta (*black arrow*) positioned anterior and to the right of the MPA (*white arrow*). (*B*) Axial CT angiogram image more inferiorly shows the aortic valve (*black arrow*) positioned anterior and to the right of the pulmonic valve (*white arrow*). These findings are consistent with d-TGA.

to the narrow mediastinum produced by the anteroposterior (AP) position of the great vessels and diminutive thymus due to stress.[11] Of course, the radiographic appearance is variable depending on whether the great arteries are truly superimposed as well as the size of pulmonary-systemic communication and severity of pulmonary obstruction.[34] Echocardiography is essential for preoperative diagnosis and allows detailed intracardiac assessment, including evaluation for atrioventricular and ventriculoarterial discordance, interatrial and interventricular communication, outlet valve morphology and function, and left ventricular outflow tract (LVOT) obstruction. The patency of the ductus arteriosus, coronary artery origins, and possible presence of aortic coarctation can also be evaluated.[1,8]

As in other CHD, CT provides an excellent anatomic assessment of such structures as the RVOT, branch pulmonary arteries, coronary arteries, postoperative baffles, and common sites of complications after surgery and is highly useful in the presence of metallic stent material.[8] MR imaging is also most valuable for postoperative assessment, allowing accurate quantification of biventricular function and assessment of maximum velocity at any sites of obstruction for pressure gradient estimation, in addition to anatomic evaluation.[8] The role of cardiac catheterization for TGA diagnosis has declined, except for coronary artery assessment depending on local cardiac CT expertise. However, palliative procedures, such as balloon atrial septostomy, can be performed at the time of catheterization.[1]

Initial survival in TGA depends on the presence of a shunt, allowing mixing between the systemic and pulmonary circulations, such as a patent foramen ovale (PFO), VSD, or PDA. Infusion of PGE_1 helps maintain ductus patency. With persistent cyanosis, balloon atrial septostomy is indicated. Definitive management is operative. The current surgery of choice is the arterial switch (Jatene) procedure, in which the positions of the aorta and pulmonary artery are reversed and the coronaries are reimplanted on the neoaortic root.[7,41] The Jatene procedure is often combined with pulmonary root translocation, known as the LeCompte maneuver.[42,43] In patients who present early, complete repair is preferably performed between 1 and 2 weeks of age but can be delayed until 2 to 3 months of age if there is a VSD. However, in patients who present late, pulmonary artery banding is typically needed to "train" the deconditioned LV before arterial switch.[7]

Venous/atrial switch operations such as the Senning and Mustard are no longer favored, although many living individuals have had these surgeries.[1,7,8] In these procedures, caval blood flow is redirected toward the mitral valve, whereas pulmonary venous flow is redirected toward the tricuspid valve via intraatrial baffles after atrial septal tissue removal. However, as a result, the unequipped systemic RV must pump against higher than expected pressures, leading to eventual failure; arrhythmia and baffle stenosis are also not uncommon.[7] When PS is present, a modified BT shunt may be necessary for palliation. In addition, a Rastelli-type surgical repair is typically pursued between the ages of 1 and 2; the VSD is repaired such that LV blood flow is rerouted to the aorta via an intraventricular patch and a conduit is inserted to connect the RV with the PA.[1,7]

Tricuspid Atresia

TA is characterized by agenesis or congenital absence of the tricuspid valve.[1,7,11,44] Most commonly, there is a localized fibrous thickening at the expected location of the tricuspid valve in the lower portion of the RA with a small and hypoplastic RV (**Fig. 6**).[1,7] TA is subclassified according the position of the great arteries, which may be normal, d-transposed, otherwise malposed, or have a truncus arteriosus configuration (detailed in later discussion).[1,7,11] Overall, it accounts for 1.4% of patients with CHD and is the third most common cause of cyanotic CHD and most common cause of cyanosis with left ventricular hypertrophy (LVH). Associations include a stretched PFO, VSD (usually muscular), valvar or subvalvar PS, and aortic coarctation when there is concomitant TGA. Symptoms develop in 50% of neonates

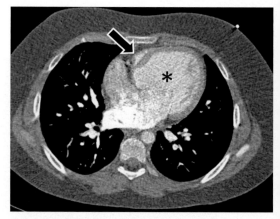

Fig. 6. TA and restrictive VSD in a 10-year-old girl after Glenn procedure. Axial ECG-gated cardiac CT angiographic image at the level of the atrioventricular groove demonstrates a severely hypoplastic RV (*arrow*) and a dilated LV (*asterisk*).

with TA by the first day of life, increasing to 80% by the first month of life.[1,7] Cyanosis is the primary presenting feature in 50% of patients by the first days of life, whereas 30% manifest with CHF within several weeks of life.[1,44] Infants with cyanosis tend to have PS or a small VSD, usually with normally related great vessels, whereas those with CHF typically have large VSDs and transposed great vessels.[1]

CXRs in TA are nonspecific and may be normal. Findings may include mild cardiomegaly due to right atrial and left ventricular enlargement and LVH. Pulmonary blood flow is variable depending on associated abnormalities but is more commonly decreased, correlating with the more common cyanotic presentation with a restrictive VSD or PS.[11,44,45] Echocardiography allows direct visualization of the atretic tricuspid valve, which appears as an echogenic band with the anterior leaflet of the would-be valve attached to the left aspect of the interatrial septum. Additional findings include biatrial and left ventricular enlargement and a small RV. Echocardiography can also help assess the presence of associated abnormalities such as transposed great arterials and aortic coarctation. Finally, as in other CHD, Doppler can be used to quantify shunts (eg, VSD) and maximum velocities at potential sites of obstruction (eg, RVOT), also allowing pulmonary artery pressure estimation.[1] Contrast echocardiography, when performed, characteristically shows serial enhancement of the RA, left atrium, LV, then RV, reflecting the complex intracardiac shunting.[1,11]

CT and MR imaging are predominantly used for postoperative monitoring but can also demonstrate the underlying morphologic abnormalities in TA. Typical findings include absence of the tricuspid valve, which is replaced by fat extending deep into the anterior atrioventricular groove. The RV is generally hypoplastic, while the LV is usually dilated and hypertrophied. Additional features may include an ASD or PFO, VSD, PDA, aortic coarctation, transposed great arteries potentially accompanied by interruption and juxtaposition of the atrial appendages, left or bilateral SVCs, and anomalous pulmonary venous return. Both techniques may be used to quantify ventricular size and function.[44,46] Cardiac catheterization is rarely necessary but in selected circumstances may be used as a problem-solving tool.[1]

Initial management in TA is usually palliative. In patients with decreased pulmonary blood flow, ductus patency is preserved via PGE$_1$ infusion, and a modified BT shunt is typically performed. In patients with increased pulmonary blood flow, CHF medical management should be optimized; in refractory cases, pulmonary artery banding

may be necessary. Although interatrial obstruction is not common, in later infancy, atrial septostomy may be needed to maintain an interatrial communication. The Fontan or Fontan-Kreutzer operation is currently the preferred definitive repair for TA, consisting of staged total cavopulmonary anastomosis and completed after 2 years of age. The first stage is palliation, as previously described. The second stage, usually performed at 6 months of age, involves an end-to-side anastomosis between the SVC and PA, known as the bidirectional Glenn procedure. The final stage involves rerouting blood flow from the inferior vena cava (IVC) to the pulmonary artery, via an extracardiac conduit or lateral tunnel. Postsurgical complications include unremitting shunts, obstruction of Fontan circuits, and systemic venous congestion, all of which are monitored by serial imaging studies.[1,7]

Truncus Arteriosus

Truncus arteriosus is characterized by a common arterial trunk (truncus) that arises from the base of the heart via a single semilunar valve and gives rise to the pulmonary, systemic, and coronary arteries, which contain mixed oxygenated/deoxygenated blood (**Fig. 7**).[7,9,10,46] The pulmonary arteries arise distal to the coronary artery origins but proximal to the first aortic branch.[9] The truncus overrides a large conal septal VSD and usually straddles the ventricles but may favor one ventricle.[7,9,10] Aside from the VSD, the atria and ventricles are typically normally formed.[10] Truncus may be further subtyped according to the Collet and Edwards classification scheme. In type I (50%–70%), a single pulmonary trunk arises from the common trunk and divides into right and left pulmonary arteries. In type II (30%–50%), there are close but separate origins of the right and left pulmonary arteries from the common trunk at its posterolateral aspect. In type III (6%–10%), the branch pulmonary arteries arise at separate locations from the common trunk or aortic arch. In type IV, neither pulmonary artery branch arises from the common trunk; this is now more appropriately characterized as a form of TOF with pulmonary atresia and VSD.[9,10]

Truncus is rare, with an estimated incidence of 5 to 15 per 100,000 live births and accounts for 1% to 2% of CHD.[9] Other findings may include a right aortic arch (30%–40%); IAA, usually between the left common carotid and left subclavian arteries (type B); supernumerary and dysplastic truncal valve leaflets; truncal valve regurgitation; and coronary anomalies.[9,10] In addition, there is an association with DiGeorge (22q11 deletion) syndrome.[9,11] Affected patients are initially

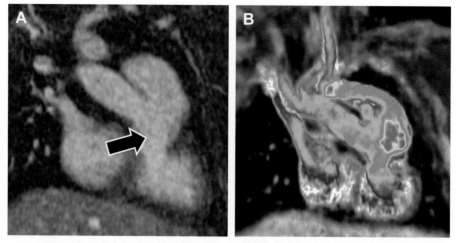

Fig. 7. Truncus arteriosus in a 2-day-old boy. (*A*) Coronal MPR image from a ferumoxytol-enhanced MRA of the chest demonstrates a common arterial trunk (*arrow*) that originates from the LV and gives rise to both great arteries. (*B*) Corresponding coronal still image from a 3D time-resolved (4D) flow dataset illustrates the flow egress pattern from the LV.

asymptomatic due to high pulmonary vascular resistance but develop stigmata of CHF within several weeks of life.[10] Cyanosis is usually minimal but more pronounced with more severe pulmonary artery stenosis.[7,10]

CXRs in truncus show prominent cardiomegaly with increased pulmonary vascularity. When a right aortic arch is also present, truncus should be strongly considered.[11,14,47] The "hilar comma" or "hilar waterfall" sign is more typical of older children with truncus and related to malposition of the pulmonary arteries; the MPA segment appears abnormally concave, whereas the right and left pulmonary arteries are more superior in position and enlarged.[11] Echocardiography allows visualization of the common arterial trunk overriding a VSD, the truncal valve and any associated regurgitation or stenosis, and sometimes the takeoff and branching pattern of the pulmonary arteries.[10] Although usually not needed preoperatively, CT or MR imaging may have added value in helping to discern the presence or absence of pulmonary arteries and MAPCAs and their branching pattern, pulmonary venous drainage, and any aortic arch anomalies in the neonate or potentially more complex anatomy in the unrepaired adult.[43,46,48–52] These modalities are routinely used for postoperative assessment of biventricular and neoaortic valvular function, pulmonary homograft patency, pulmonary regurgitation, and anatomy of the branch pulmonary arteries and aortic arch.[43,51] Cardiac catheterization is not routinely needed for diagnosis but, as in other CHD, may be used as a problem-solving tool.[10]

Patients with truncus usually undergo complete repair within the first weeks to months of life after CHF medical management is optimized. Operative management consists of VSD closure such that LV output is directed toward a neoaorta. The pulmonary arteries are separated from the common trunk and connected to the RV using a homograft. Morality rates after surgery are overall low, but the RV-PA conduit may require future replacement because of calcific degeneration or growth of the child.[7,10,40]

Total Anomalous Pulmonary Venous Connection

TAPVC (or total anomalous pulmonary venous return [TAPVR]) is characterized by anomalous drainage of all pulmonary veins to the systemic circulation. Usually, the pulmonary veins form a common confluence, which then drains into the left brachiocephalic vein (overall most common), SVC, IVC, coronary sinus, portal vein, or rarely, other locations. Less commonly, each pulmonary vein drains to the RA.[7,9,10,40] As a result, there is a left-to-right shunt of oxygenated blood back to the lungs rather than to the body.[9] TAPVC is anatomically subclassified as supradiaphragmatic (including supracardiac or cardiac levels) or infradiaphragmatic, depending on the location where the anomalous venous connection occurs. Physiologically, TAPVC may be characterized as obstructive or nonobstructive, depending on whether free flow through the pulmonary veins is impeded.[7,10]

TAPVC may also be classified according venous drainage relative to the heart. Type I (55%) is

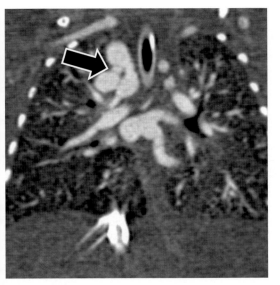

Fig. 8. TAPVC in a 3-day-old girl. Coronal CT angiogram image shows from a CT angiogram of the chest shows convergence of the pulmonary veins (*arrow*) at a right-sided SVC, consistent with supracardiac TAPVR.

supracardiac (**Fig. 8**), type II (30%) at the cardiac level, type III (13%) infracardiac or infradiaphragmatic, and type IV (mixed) with 2 or more anomalous connections.[9,34,53]

TAPVR is rare, accounting for 2% to 3% of CHD presenting in the neonatal period.[10] Although non-obstructive, supradiaphragmatic drainage is most frequent overall, in the infant, infradiaphragmatic TAPVC is most typical, commonly with obstruction.[7,10] A PFO or ASD is invariably present to allow survival. Additional associations include an underlying heterotaxy syndrome.[9,40] Neonates with obstructive TAPVC tend to present with cyanosis in the first hours to days of life. On the other hand, infants with nonobstructive TAPVC tend to develop only minimal to no cyanosis and present with CHF between the ages of 4 and 6 weeks.[10]

Radiographic findings in TAPVC depend on the level of venous drainage and the presence or absence of obstruction. The classic radiographic appearance known as the "snowman" or "figure-of-eight" sign is seen in type I TAPVC. The mediastinum is widened, related to a dilated right SVC and a left vertical vein, representing the confluence of the pulmonary veins posterior to the left atrium. These features form the "snowman" head, whereas the heart comprises the "snowman" body.[11,34] In general, cardiomegaly, increased pulmonary vascularity, and pulmonary arterial dilation are typical of supradiaphragmatic TAPVC without obstruction, whereas a small heart with pulmonary venous congestion (interstitial edema, pleural effusion) is seen in infradiaphragmatic TAPVC with obstruction.[11]

Echocardiography with Doppler is usually considered adequate for identifying the site of anomalous venous drainage as well as the presence of a PFO/ASD and RV enlargement.[10] However, CT and MR imaging may provide supplemental information when echocardiography is equivocal or acoustic windows are suboptimal, with the scan range from the thoracic inlet to the inferior edge of the liver to detect both supradiaphragmatic and infradiaphragmatic variants.[9,54] For example, with mixed TAPVR or a concurrent heterotaxy syndrome, completing arterial and venous mapping can prove difficult with echocardiography alone.[9,53] In one study of 23 neonates, ages 1 to 5, with surgically confirmed TAPVC, MDCT had perfect accuracy for detecting the drainage site of the pulmonary vein confluence, vertical vein stenosis, and vertical vein course into the systemic venous system. In contrast, echocardiography had 100% specificity but only 87%, 71%, and 0% sensitivity, respectively, for visualizing these 3 features.[54,55] Cardiac catheterization is usually not required for TAPVC diagnosis.[10]

Definitive repair for TAPVC consists of anastomosis of the common pulmonary vein to the left atrium. In neonates with obstructive TAPVC, surgery should be undertaken urgently after initial stabilization with intubation, high-pressure airway ventilation, and PGE$_1$ infusion to maintain ductal patency. In nonobstructive TAPVC, surgery can be performed on an elective or semielective basis, possibly with PFO closure, after optimal management for CHF symptoms. Serial imaging follow-up helps monitor for anastomotic obstruction.[7,10]

Hypoplastic Left Heart Syndrome

Hypoplastic left heart syndrome (HLHS) comprises a broad spectrum of anomalies involving marked underdevelopment of the left-sided structures of the heart, including the mitral and aortic valves, LV, and ascending aorta.[7,10,11,56,57] The left atrium is usually small but may be normal or increased in size (**Fig. 9**). In contrast, the right heart structures (atrium, ventricle, pulmonary arteries) are significantly dilated.[10] The pathogenesis of HLHS is still not entirely understood, although it may relate to abnormal cardiac partitioning during embryogenesis.[56]

HLHS is rare, with a reported prevalence of 1 per 5000 live births, although it represents 1.2% to 1.5% of all CHD and 7% to 9% of CHD diagnosed before the age of 1 year.[7,56,57] In fact, it is the fourth most frequent cardiac malformation to present in the first year of life. It is also the most

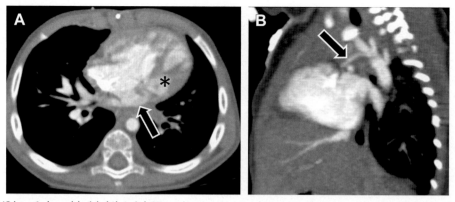

Fig. 9. HLHS in a 4-day-old girl. (*A*) Axial CT angiogram image demonstrates a hypoplastic left atrium (*arrow*) and hypoplastic LV (*asterisk*). (*B*) Sagittal CT angiogram image demonstrates a severely hypoplastic aortic root and ascending aorta (*arrow*). The cervical branch vessels were fed by a large patent ductus arteriosus and transverse ductal arch (not shown).

common type of univentricular cardiac malformation.[56] There is a male-to-female predominance of at least 2:1.[56,57] Siblings are also at an increased risk, with an HLHS prevalence of 0.5%.[57] In approximately 25% of HLHS cases, there is marked LV hypoplasia in association with other complex CHD such as DORV (described in later discussion) with mitral atresia. A PFO and PDA are commonly present, facilitating initial survival.[7,10] Other associations may include aortic coarctation, VSD, and endocardial fibroelastosis (EFE), a fibrotic thickening of the endocardium that decreases cardiac function.[56] A major extracardiac anomaly or genetic syndrome such as Turner, Noonan, Holt-Oram, or Smith-Lemli-Oplitz is seen in about 25% of HLHS patients.[57] Neonates may be asymptomatic at birth.[10,57] However, as the ductus closes, they develop initially mild cyanosis, progressing to CHF and shock within hours to days and death by 1 week if untreated.[10,11,56,57]

In the first hours of life, CXRs in neonates with HLHS are often normal, with preserved heart size and pulmonary vascularity. Within 2 days, marked cardiomegaly and both increased pulmonary arterial flow and pulmonary venous congestion are evident.[10,11] Often, chest radiographic findings belie the severity of clinical symptoms.[11] Echocardiography establishes the diagnosis and is usually sufficient for presurgical planning purposes or defining anatomic characteristics that suggest aggressive measures would be futile.[56] Important components of the assessment include the patency and size of the PFO/ASD and PDA, valvular competency, and the presence of a VSD, aortic coarctation, and associated anomalies.[10,56] Wall motion abnormalities may reflect EFE or ischemia.[56] Attempt has been made

to determine a cutoff size of the LV below which only single-ventricle palliation should be performed (mean long-axis cross-sectional area of 2.0 cm^2 in one study). However, these efforts have posed challenges, with inconsistent data.[56,58]

Preoperatively, CT and MR imaging are usually not needed. However, they may be useful to delineate associated complex malformations such as anomalous pulmonary venous return.[59] In addition, both cardiac MR imaging and CT have been used to provide estimations of LV volume, which should be more accurate than those based on echocardiography.[59,60] Another preoperative role of MR imaging is in the setting of the "hypoplastic left heart complex" in which the mitral and aortic valves are small but morphologically normal. In these patients, the presence of EFE, which is best demonstrated on MR imaging myocardial delayed (late gadolinium) enhancement sequences, is commonly used as an exclusion criterion for biventricular repair.[59] Postoperatively, advanced modalities, particularly MR imaging, have a well-established role in monitoring ventricular and valvular function and vascular anatomy.[61] Cardiac catheterization is reserved for situations in which other modalities are not diagnostic.[56]

Once considered inoperable, HLHS now has 2 treatment strategies: multistage Norwood repair and cardiac transplantation. The latter is usually unfeasible due to lack of donors. After stabilization in the intensive care unit with PGE$_1$ infusion to maintain ductal patency, the first stage of the Norwood operation is performed during week 1 of life.[7] The stage I Norwood repair consists of atrial septectomy, PDA ligation, MPA division and anastomosis to the hypoplastic aortic arch that is patch augmented, and placement of a modified BT or

Sano (RV to PA) shunt.[7,40] The second and third stages consist of a bidirectional Glenn and completion Fontan (as previously discussed), performed 6 months after stage I and 12 months after stage II, respectively.[7] Postsurgical and interstage mortalities are high; long-term morbidity and mortality data after successful stage III surgery are under study.[7,57] When cardiac transplantation is the only option due to unfavorable anatomy, nearly one-fifth of neonates die awaiting a donor heart. Even when transplantation is successful, lifelong immunosuppression is required and mandates intensive monitoring.[7,56]

Pulmonary Atresia with Intact Ventricular Septum

PA-IVS is defined by total obstruction of the pulmonary valve with 2 separate ventricles and a patent although usually hypoplastic tricuspid valve but no VSD.[7,10] The RV is usually but not universally hypoplastic and to varying degrees.[7,10,62] PA-IVS is rare, with a prevalence of 5 to 9 cases per 100,000 live births, accounting for 1% to 3% of CHD.[63,64] Associations include a coexistent PFO (common) allowing right-to-left shunting; coronary arteriovenous fistulae (10%–50%); and tricuspid regurgitation (TR; 20%), associated with marked RV dilation.[7,10,63] Neonates develop severe cyanosis, hypoxemia, and tachypnea after an initially uneventful course as the ductus closes.[10]

The characteristic radiographic appearance is known as the "wall-to-wall" heart, typified by marked cardiomegaly. However, this is generally only seen in PA-IVS patients with severe TR.[65] The heart size, pulmonary vascularity, and lungs may appear normal. Echocardiography shows a lack of forward flow from the RV to the PA. The RV is generally small in size. TR and right-to-left shunting across a PFO can also be visualized.[10] Although RV to coronary artery fistulae can be identified, they are often incompletely characterized. Typically, cardiac catheterization has been used for this purpose.[63,66] However, recent reports document the successful use of cardiac CT in identifying and characterizing these fistulae.[67] MR imaging is generally reserved for postoperative patients and can be used to monitor the timing of PVR, RV function, the presence of fibrosis, and the adequacy of repair (Fig. 10).[62,64,68] Cardiac catheterization, in addition to assessing for coronary fistulae, can be used as guidance for transcatheter pulmonary valve perforation.[10]

Management in PA-IVS is dependent on the severity of RV hypoplasia.[69] Biventricular repair is the ideal goal but generally only possible with an adequate-sized RV and absence of infundibular atresia and RV-dependent coronary circulation.[7,10] In such cases, percutaneous radiofrequency pulmonary valvotomy alone may be sufficient.[7,10,69] If a 2-ventricle repair is not possible, a single-ventricle staged Fontan procedure may be performed, as previously described. One alternative is the one-and-a-half ventricle repair consisting of only a bidirectional Glenn: SVC blood communicates via the Glenn directly with the pulmonary artery while the RV actively pumps IVC blood to the pulmonary artery.[7,10,64,69] Management algorithms for PA-IVS will likely undergo continued modifications as less invasive catheter-based therapies for this heterogeneous disorder continue to improve.[69]

Double-Outlet Right Ventricle

DORV is a type of ventriculoarterial discordance in which both the pulmonary artery and the aorta arise from the morphologic RV by at least 50% circumference (Fig. 11).[7,10,43,70–73] This rare malformation, comprising less than 1% of CHD with an estimated incidence of less than 127 per million live births, results from a failure of normal embryologic development.[10,43,70] Usually, a large VSD is present, and its location as well as the presence and severity of superimposed PS governs the clinical course in the disorder.[7,10] The VSD is usually perimembranous and subaortic but may be subpulmonic, doubly committed (related to pulmonary artery and aorta), or noncommitted (distant from the pulmonary artery and aorta).[7,10,73]

DORV itself is classified into 4 types: VSD type (24%); TOF type (36%); TGA/Taussig-Bing type (18%); and DORV noncommitted VSD type (22%).[73] These subtypes are characterized, respectively, by a VSD without PS; significant PS; a subpulmonary VSD with the LVOT oriented toward the pulmonary artery; and a noncommitted VSD.[7,10] DORV with a doubly committed VSD is effectively most similar to the TGA type. Accordingly, the clinical presentation is dependent on the type of DORV. As implied by the subcategories, the TOF and TGA types behave most similarly to TOF and TGA, respectively, as previously described. In contrast, with a subaortic VSD and no PS, DORV may present with CHF and failure to thrive, similar to a VSD.[3,6,10]

CXRs in DORV are variable and dependent on the subtype. Cardiomegaly and increased pulmonary blood flow are typical of subaortic and subpulmonary VSD, whereas normal to mildly enlarged heart size with decreased vascular markings are seen with significant PS.[10] As in other CHD, echocardiography is most useful. Pertinent features of the evaluation include biventricular size and function, VSD

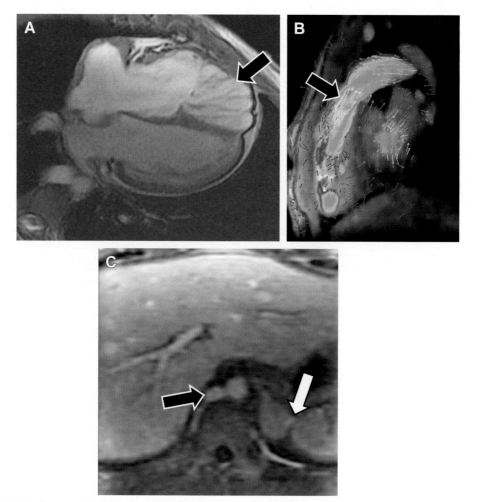

Fig. 10. PA-IVS after repair in a 12-year-old boy. (*A*) Four-chamber bright-blood cine FIESTA image shows a dilated RV with disorganized trabeculations (*arrow*), suggesting maldevelopment, compatible with the history of PA-IVS. (*B*) RVOT still image from the 4D flow sequence performed after IV gadolinium demonstrates pulmonic regurgitation (*arrow*), which was severe by quantitation. Note the backwards direction of vector flow. (*C*) Postcontrast axial-reformatted MRA in the same patient also shows azygous continuation of the IVC (*black arrow*) and polysplenia (*white arrow*).

location and size, degree of PS, position of the aorta and MPA, and in subpulmonary VSD, the presence of subaortic obstruction and coarctation.[10]

Although echocardiography is often sufficient for presurgical planning, CT or MR imaging can be very useful in depicting the precise VSD anatomy, extracardiac vasculature, and presence of collaterals, findings that may have previously required cardiac catheterization at higher radiation doses.[43,72,74] For example, in one study of 64-row MDCT versus echocardiography and cardiac catheterization, MDCT detected significantly more main and branch pulmonary artery anatomy and stenoses than did echocardiography, although fewer MAPCAs than did catheterization.[74] Another using dual-source CT with retrospective ECG-gating demonstrated better sensitivity of CT for

detecting coronary, great vessels, and other thoracoabdominal anomalies compared with echocardiography, although slightly inferior detection of intracardiac malformations.[70] MR imaging can also be used for these purposes, while also providing dynamic and functional assessment.[43,75,76] The advent of 3D printing using MR or CT datasets may also be helpful for presurgical planning.[77] Postoperatively, as sonographic windows become limited, both modalities are very useful, allowing assessment for biventricular size and function; residual VSD, valvular/subvalvular stenosis, and coarctation; and RVOT or conduit stenosis/regurgitation.[43,73] Cardiac catheterization may be needed in complex cases.[10]

Treatment also depends on the type of DORV. For DORV with a subaortic VSD and PS, VSD

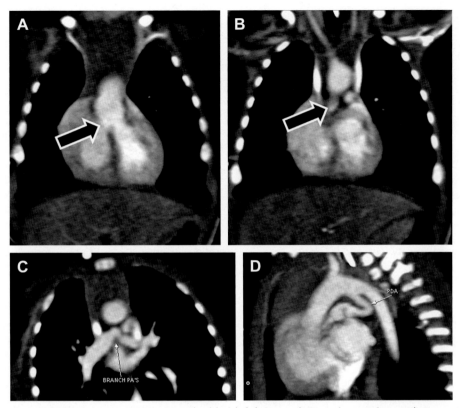

Fig. 11. DORV and pulmonary atresia in a 4-week-old girl. (*A*) Coronal CT angiogram image demonstrates a sub-aortic conus aligned with the RV with a large subaortic VSD (*arrow*). (*B*) Coronal CT angiogram image at the level of the MPA demonstrates a severely hypoplastic MPA (*arrow*). (*C*) Curved axial oblique MPR CT image at the pulmonary bifurcation demonstrates the branch pulmonary arteries with narrowing of the origin of the left pulmonary artery (labeled). (*D*) Curved sagittal oblique MPR CT image of the aortic arch demonstrates a large tortuous PDA (labeled).

closure is undertaken such that the LVOT is redirected to the aorta, after stabilization with an anti-CHF regimen. With PS, surgery mimics TOF repair. In the TGA type, an arterial switch procedure along with VSD closure and if needed coarctation repair is performed.[7,10,43] Cases with an uncommitted VSD prove challenging and require individualized management, ranging from complete repair to single-ventricle palliation with a Fontan pathway.[7,43]

Double-Inlet Left Ventricle

In DILV, greater than 50% of each AV connection is contiguous with a dominant LV.[7,10,78–80] Comprising 70% to 80% of cases, DILV is the most common of the functional single-ventricle disorders, which overall have an incidence of 5 to 10 per 100,000 live births.[79,80] Associations include TGA (70%, usually I [evo]-type), valvular/subvalvular pulmonic stenosis or atresia (66%),

subaortic obstruction, and aortic coarctation.[7,10] Concomitant DORV with both the pulmonary artery and the aorta arising from a hypoplastic RV can also occur.[7,10,81] DILV patients with PS present with hypoxemia and cyanosis as early as the neonatal period, while those without it develop CHF by several months of life with only minimal cyanosis.[10]

The chest radiographic appearance in DILV is variable depending on the underlying anatomy. Prominent cardiomegaly and increased pulmonary vascular markings are associated with increased pulmonary flow, whereas only mild cardiomegaly and decreased vascular markings are associated with decreased pulmonary flow. In addition, the left heart border may appear enlarged if there is concomitant I-TGA.[10] Echocardiography establishes the diagnosis, including absence of the ventricular septum, and can also be used to evaluate the severity of PS. As in other CHD, CT and MR imaging may supplement echocardiography in

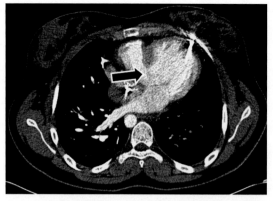

Fig. 12. DILV and TA in a 19-year-old girl after Glenn and Fontan procedures. Axial CT angiogram image at the level of the interventricular septum demonstrates a hypoplastic RV with a VSD (*arrow*).

assessing complex anatomic relationships (**Fig. 12**), particularly of the extracardiac vasculature, and overcome acoustic window limitations after surgery.[81,82] Cardiac catheterization may be needed in select cases.[10]

Management is operative but depends on the patient's age and weight, anatomy, and physiology. Initial efforts on neonatal palliation use a modified BT shunt if there is decreased pulmonary blood flow or a pulmonary artery band if there is increased flow, while correcting any aortic coarctation. Next steps include the Glenn and Fontan procedures, as previously described.[7,10] The Damus-Kaye-Stansel operation, in which the proximal PA is split near its bifurcation and connected to the side of the ascending aorta, may be needed to bypass obstruction related to PA banding.[7,10,83]

Interrupted Aortic Arch

IAA is characterized by loss of luminal continuity between the ascending and descending thoracic aorta, either complete or joined by an atretic band of fibrous tissue.[7,9,10,43,46,52] There are 3 types, according to the Celoria-Patton classification. In types A (42%), B (53%), and C (4%), respectively, the interruption occurs distal to the left subclavian artery (**Fig. 13**), between the left common carotid and subclavian arteries, and between the brachiocephalic and left common carotid arteries.[9,46,52] Each type is further subcategorized based on any additional anomalies of the subclavian arteries.[10]

IAA is rare overall, with an estimated incidence of 3 per million live births, accounting for 1% of CHD.[9,52] In most cases, associated abnormalities are present, the most common of which are PDA and VSD.[7,9,10] Other anomalies may include truncus arteriosus, an aortopulmonary window (aortic arch-pulmonary artery connection), aberrant right subclavian artery, valvar/subvalvar aortic stenosis, DORV, and a functional single ventricle.[7,9,10,43,52,71] IAA, particularly type B, also has a strong association with DiGeorge syndrome; 50% of patients with IAA have DiGeorge, and 5% to 20% of patients with DiGeorge have IAA.[9,10] In addition, IAA arises more frequently with CHARGE syndrome, which includes

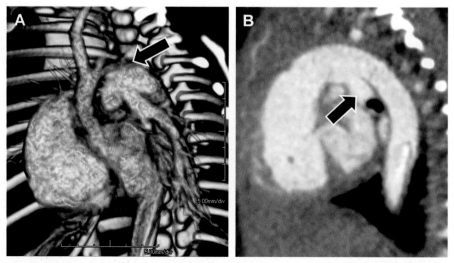

Fig. 13. IAA in a 5-day-old boy. (*A*) 3D volume-rendered image from a CT angiogram of the chest demonstrates lack of continuation of the aortic arch beyond the left subclavian artery (*arrow*), consistent with a type A IAA. The ascending aorta is small in caliber. (*B*) Sagittal CT angiogram image demonstrates reconstitution of the thoracic aorta via a PDA (*arrow*).

coloboma, heart disease, choanal atresia, retarded growth, genital hypoplasia, and ear anomalies.[9] Affected patients are initially asymptomatic in the immediate neonatal period but become cyanotic as the PDA closes, and pulmonary vascular resistance decreases.[10]

CXRs in IAA may show an enlarged heart with increased pulmonary blood flow or edema but is not specific for the diagnosis. Echocardiography provides excellent initial imaging.[10] The precise anatomy of the defect and any associated anomalies is well depicted by both CT and MR imaging.[52,84,85] Cardiac catheterization is rarely needed for diagnosis.[10]

Prompt infusion of PGE[1] is required in patients with IAA, who would otherwise die within 1 to 2 weeks of life. Definitive correction is surgical, preferably direct aortic anastomosis with patch augmentation.[7,9,10] Postsurgical complications may include operative bed aneurysm development, residual or recurrent arch or LVOT obstruction, patch leak at the site of a concomitant repaired VSD, and LV hypertrophy (**Fig. 14**).[43] Reoperation is ultimately needed in 28% of cases.[10]

Ebstein Anomaly

Ebstein anomaly is a malformation of the septal and posterior tricuspid valve leaflets, which are

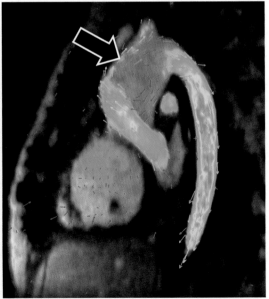

Fig. 14. IAA after repair in a 4-year-old girl. Candy cane still image from a ferumoxytol-enhanced 4D flow MR imaging exam shows relative dilation of the repaired aortic arch (*arrow*). Vectors denote the direction of blood flow.

dysplastic and displaced downward into the right ventricular cavity, usually with associated TR.[7,11,86–94] The severity of the disease is governed by the magnitude of tricuspid valve displacement, which results in a large portion of the RV being continuous with a dilated RA, so-called atrialization of the RV.[7,11,86,92] Ebstein anomaly is rare, with a prevalence of 5.2 per 100,000 births, comprising 0.3% to 1% of CHD, although it accounts for approximately 40% of congenital tricuspid valve malformations.[7,87,92,94] Most cases are sporadic, although there are links to maternal benzodiazepine and lithium exposure.[95] A PFO or ostium secundum ASD is invariably present.[7,86] PS or atresia may also occur.[7] Because of decreased RV outflow, RA pressure increases, with resultant right-to-left shunting via the atrial level communication. As a result, neonates present with cyanosis. CHF may also be present.[11] However, the clinical course of Ebstein anomaly is variable; milder forms may be only incidentally detected during adulthood due to nonspecific symptoms such as fatigue.[94]

Severe cases of Ebstein anomaly are characterized by an enlarged, "box-shaped" or "balloon-shaped" heart due to a markedly dilated RA (**Fig. 15**).[11,86,95] Echocardiography can be used to visualize the apically displaced tricuspid leaflet. The disorder is established when the distance from the septal leaflet of the tricuspid valve to the anterior leaflet of the mitral valve is greater than 15 mm in children less than 14 years old or greater than 20 mm in adults. Alternatively, a distance indexed to body surface area greater than 0.8 mm/cm^2 is also considered diagnostic. Echocardiography can also assess for right ventricular function and any associated TR.[86,88,95] The addition of 3D echocardiography may assist in differentiating Ebstein anomaly from tricuspid valvar dysplasia in which RV volumes are greater with a different clinical course.[89]

ECG-gated cardiac CT can be used to depict the anatomy and provide an assessment of cardiac chamber size and function when echocardiography is inadequate, and MR imaging is not possible.[91,93] It may also be useful for assessment of postoperative complications such as thromboembolism related to the Fontan procedure.[96] In addition to anatomic and functional assessment, MR imaging allows for quantitative estimation of TR severity using through-plane MR imaging velocity mapping (PC).[86,90,92,94] A plane is prescribed to transect the regurgitant jet on its immediate atrial side, with typical velocity encoding in the range of 250 cm/s. Cross-sectional dimensions of the jet more than 6 × 6 mm suggest severe TR.[92]

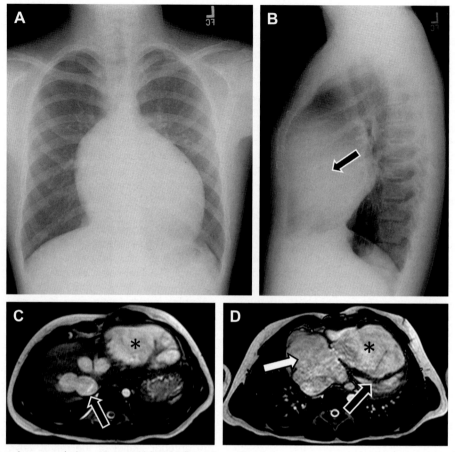

Fig. 15. Ebstein anomaly in a 12-year-old girl after tricuspid valve repair and annuloplasty at age 8. (*A*) Frontal CXR demonstrates a boxed-shaped heart consistent with Ebstein anomaly. (*B*) Lateral radiograph of the chest shows dehiscence of the annuloplasty ring (*black arrow*). (*C*) Axial balanced FFE (white blood) image at the level of the diaphragm from a cardiac MR imaging exam in the same patient demonstrates dilated hepatic veins and a dilated intrahepatic IVC (*arrow*) as well as an atrialized RV (*asterisk*). (*D*) Axial balanced FFE image at the level of the mid tricuspid valve demonstrates a dilated RA (*white arrow*), atrialized RV (*asterisk*), and bowed interventricular septum (*black arrow*).

Cardiac catheterization is usually not needed, although it may be used for preoperative coronary assessment and occasionally pressure measurements.[95]

Management in Ebstein anomaly is variable depending on the severity of the malformation.[94] Nonsurgical approaches are more common in asymptomatic patients.[86] Even neonates with cyanosis often do not need treatment unless hypoxemic, for which temporary PGE$_1$ infusion may be helpful. If they develop severe TR, closure of the tricuspid valve (Starnes procedure) and a modified BT shunt may be needed.[7] Surgical options in teenagers and adults include tricuspid valve replacement (possibly prosthetic) or repair and plication/isolation of the deformed RV.[7,94] The cone reconstruction, a type of circumferential tricuspid valve repair, has had promising results in recent reports.[97] Patients with Ebstein anomaly are also prone to arrhythmias, particularly Wolff-Parkinson-White syndrome, which may respond to catheter ablation therapy.[7,97]

SUMMARY

The cyanotic congenital heart diseases represented are a rare and heterogeneous yet often pressing spectrum of disorders with complex anomalies requiring prompt neonatal intervention. Radiographic findings are generally nonspecific but may assist in the determination of heart size and relative pulmonary blood flow. Echocardiography is mandatory with little downside and provides an excellent overall assessment of intracardiac morphology, function, and flow. However, recent years have seen a burgeoning role for CT and

MR imaging in the evaluation of cyanotic CHD, particularly for visualization of the extracardiac vasculature and postoperative monitoring, helping to obviate invasive cardiac catheterization or decrease procedure times. At the same time, continued technological innovations have allowed ever-lower ionizing radiation and contrast doses and anesthesia requirements for these advanced noninvasive modalities with better image quality. With ongoing progress in therapies for cyanotic CHD and more patients living to later adult years, the role of CT and MR imaging will likely only continue to expand.

REFERENCES

1. Rao PS. Diagnosis and management of cyanotic congenital heart disease: part I. Indian J Pediatr 2009;76(1):57–70.
2. Hughes D, Siegel MJ. MRI of complex cyanotic congenital heart disease: pre- and post surgical considerations. Int J Cardiovasc Imaging 2010; 26(Suppl 2):333–43.
3. Rao PS. Consensus on timing of intervention for common congenital heart diseases: part I - acyanotic heart defects. Indian J Pediatr 2013;80(1):32–8.
4. Strobel AM, Lu le N. The critically ill infant with congenital heart disease. Emerg Med Clin North Am 2015;33(3):501–18.
5. Syamasundar Rao P. Diagnosis and management of acyanotic heart disease: part I – obstructive lesions. Indian J Pediatr 2005;72(6):496–502.
6. Syamasundar Rao P. Diagnosis and management of acyanotic heart disease: part II – left-to-right shunt lesions. Indian J Pediatr 2005;72(6):503–12.
7. Rao PS. Consensus on timing of intervention for common congenital heart diseases: part II - cyanotic heart defects. Indian J Pediatr 2013;80(8):663–74.
8. Puranik R, Muthurangu V, Celermajer DS, et al. Congenital heart disease and multi-modality imaging. Heart Lung Circ 2010;19(3):133–44.
9. Chan FP, Hanneman K. Computed tomography and magnetic resonance imaging in neonates with congenital cardiovascular disease. Semin Ultrasound CT MR 2015;36(2):146–60.
10. Syamasundar Rao P. Diagnosis and management of cyanotic congenital heart disease: part II. Indian J Pediatr 2009;76(3):297–308.
11. Schweigmann G, Gassner I, Maurer K. Imaging the neonatal heart–essentials for the radiologist. Eur J Radiol 2006;60(2):159–70.
12. Ho VB. ACR appropriateness criteria on suspected congenital heart disease in adults. J Am Coll Radiol 2008;5(2):97–104.
13. Ho VB. Radiologic evaluation of suspected congenital heart disease in adults. Am Fam Physician 2009; 80(6):597–602.
14. Steiner RM, Gross GW, Flicker S, et al. Congenital heart disease in the adult patient: the value of plain film chest radiology. J Thorac Imaging 1995;10(1):1–25.
15. Applegate KE, Goske MJ, Pierce G, et al. Situs revisited: imaging of the heterotaxy syndrome. Radiographics 1999;19(4):837–52.
16. Zaman MJ, Sanders J, Crook AM, et al. Cardiothoracic ratio within the "normal" range independently predicts mortality in patients undergoing coronary angiography. Heart 2007;93(4):491–4.
17. Stanger P, Silverman NH, Foster E. Diagnostic accuracy of pediatric echocardiograms performed in adult laboratories. Am J Cardiol 1999;83(6):908–14.
18. Saeed M, Van TA, Krug R, et al. Cardiac MR imaging: current status and future direction. Cardiovasc Diagn Ther 2015;5(4):290–310.
19. Jadhav SP, Golriz F, Atweh LA, et al. CT angiography of neonates and infants: comparison of radiation dose and image quality of target mode prospectively ECG-gated 320-MDCT and ungated helical 64-MDCT. AJR Am J Roentgenol 2015;204(2):W184–91.
20. Chan FP. CTA for surgical planning of neonatal repair of pulmonary atresia with major aortopulmonary collateral arteries. 2016. Available at: https://health.siemens.com/ct_applications/somatomsessions/index.php/cta-for-surgical-planning-of-neonatal-repair-of-pulmonary-atresia-with-major-aortopulmonary-collateral-arteries/. Accessed August 29, 2016.
21. Bailliard F, Hughes ML, Taylor AM. Introduction to cardiac imaging in infants and children: techniques, potential, and role in the imaging work-up of various cardiac malformations and other pediatric heart conditions. Eur J Radiol 2008; 68(2):191–8.
22. Gabbour M, Rigsby C, Markl M, et al. Comparison of 4D flow and 2D PC MRI blood flow quantification in children and young adults with congenital heart disease. J Cardiovasc Magn Reson 2013;15(Suppl 1):E90.
23. Hanneman K, Kino A, Cheng JY, et al. Assessment of the precision and reproducibility of ventricular volume, function, and mass measurements with ferumoxytol-enhanced 4D flow MRI. J Magn Reson Imaging 2016;44(2):383–92.
24. Vasanawala SS, Hanneman K, Alley MT, et al. Congenital heart disease assessment with 4D flow MRI. J Magn Reson Imaging 2015;42(4):870–86.
25. Cheng JY, Hanneman K, Zhang T, et al. Comprehensive motion-compensated highly accelerated 4D flow MRI with ferumoxytol enhancement for pediatric congenital heart disease. J Magn Reson Imaging 2016;43(6):1355–68.
26. Hsiao A, Yousaf U, Alley MT, et al. Improved quantification and mapping of anomalous pulmonary venous flow with four-dimensional phase-contrast MRI and interactive streamline rendering. J Magn Reson Imaging 2015;42(6):1765–76.

27. Vasanawala SS, Nguyen KL, Hope MD, et al. Safety and technique of ferumoxytol administration for MRI. Magn Reson Med 2016;75(5):2107–11.

28. Ruangwattanapaisarn N, Hsiao A, Vasanawala SS. Ferumoxytol as an off-label contrast agent in body 3T MR angiography: a pilot study in children. Pediatr Radiol 2015;45(6):831–9.

29. Ning P, Zucker EJ, Wong P, et al. Hemodynamic safety and efficacy of ferumoxytol as an intravenous contrast agents in pediatric patients and young adults. Magn Reson Imaging 2016;34(2):152–8.

30. Goyen M. Gadofosveset-enhanced magnetic resonance angiography. Vasc Health Risk Manag 2008; 4(1):1–9.

31. Rigsby CK, Popescu AR, Nelson P, et al. Safety of blood pool contrast agent administration in children and young adults. AJR Am J Roentgenol 2015; 205(5):1114–20.

32. Watson TG, Mah E, Joseph Schoepf U, et al. Effective radiation dose in computed tomographic angiography of the chest and diagnostic cardiac catheterization in pediatric patients. Pediatr Cardiol 2013;34(3):518–24.

33. Gartner RD, Sutton NJ, Weinstein S, et al. MRI and computed tomography of cardiac and pulmonary complications of tetralogy of Fallot in adults. J Thorac Imaging 2010;25(2):183–90.

34. Ferguson EC, Krishnamurthy R, Oldham SA. Classic imaging signs of congenital cardiovascular abnormalities. Radiographics 2007;27(5):1323–34.

35. Yock PG, Popp RL. Noninvasive estimation of right ventricular systolic pressure by Doppler ultrasound in patients with tricuspid regurgitation. Circulation 1984;70(4):657–62.

36. Malhotra SP, Hanley FL. Surgical management of pulmonary atresia with ventricular septal defect and major aortopulmonary collaterals: a protocol-based approach. Semin Thorac Cardiovasc Surg Pediatr Card Surg Annu 2009;145–51.

37. Preim U, Sommer P, Hoffmann J, et al. Delayed enhancement imaging in a contemporary patient cohort following correction of tetralogy of Fallot. Cardiol Young 2015;25(7):1268–75.

38. Geva T. Repaired tetralogy of Fallot: the roles of cardiovascular magnetic resonance in evaluating pathophysiology and for pulmonary valve replacement decision support. J Cardiovasc Magn Reson 2011; 13:9.

39. Saremi F, Gera A, Ho SY, et al. CT and MR imaging of the pulmonary valve. Radiographics 2014;34(1): 51–71.

40. Gaca AM, Jaggers JJ, Dudley LT, et al. Repair of congenital heart disease: a primer–Part 2. Radiology 2008;248(1):44–60.

41. Gaca AM, Jaggers JJ, Dudley LT, et al. Repair of congenital heart disease: a primer-part 1. Radiology 2008;247(3):617–31.

42. Yoon DW, Kim TH, Shim MS, et al. Pulmonary root translocation with the Lecompte maneuver: for transposition of the great arteries with ventricular septal defect and pulmonary stenosis. Korean J Thorac Cardiovasc Surg 2015;48(5):351–4.

43. Frank L, Dillman JR, Parish V, et al. Cardiovascular MR imaging of conotruncal anomalies. Radiographics 2010;30(4):1069–94.

44. Burns SK, Spindola-Franco H. Tricuspid atresia. Chapter 35. In: White CS, Haramati LB, Chen JJ-S, et al, editors. Rotations in radiology: cardiac imaging. New York: Oxford University Press; 2014. p. 179–82.

45. Elliott LP, Van Mierop LHS, Gleason DC, et al. The roentgenology of tricuspid atresia. Semin Roentgenol 1968;3(4):399–409.

46. Goo HW. Cardiac MDCT in children: CT technology overview and interpretation. Radiol Clin North Am 2011;49:997–1010.

47. Hallermann FJ, Kincaid OW, Tsakiris AG, et al. Persistent truncus arteriosus. A radiographic and angiocardiographic study. Am J Roentgenol Radium Ther Nucl Med 1969;107(4):827–34.

48. Hong SH, Kim YM, Lee CK, et al. 3D MDCT angiography for the preoperative assessment of truncus arteriosus. Clin Imaging 2015;39(6):938–44.

49. Koplay M, Cimen D, Sivri M, et al. Truncus arteriosus: diagnosis with dual-source computed tomography angiography and low radiation dose. World J Radiol 2014;6(11):886–9.

50. Borges CP. Diagnosis of truncus arteriosus using flash CT scanning. 2012. Available at: https://health.siemens.com/ct_applications/somatomsessions/index.php/diagnosis-of-truncus-arteriosus-using-flash-ct-scanning/. Accessed August 29, 2016.

51. Agrawal R, Ghoshhajra B, Kovacina B, et al. Truncus arteriosus. MGH Cardiovascular Images eNewsletter 2012;(45). Available at: http://www.massgeneral.org/imaging/news/cv-newsletter/march_2012/. Accessed August 29, 2016.

52. Kimura-Hayama ET, Meléndez G, Mendizábal AL, et al. Uncommon congenital and acquired aortic diseases: role of multidetector CT angiography. Radiographics 2010;30(1):79–98.

53. Vyas HV, Greenberg SB, Krishnamurthy R. MR imaging and CT evaluation of congenital pulmonary vein abnormalities in neonates and infants. Radiographics 2012;32(1):87–98.

54. Katre R, Burns SK, Murillo H, et al. Anomalous pulmonary venous connections. Semin Ultrasound CT MR 2012;33(6):485–99.

55. Oh KH, Choo KS, Lim SJ, et al. Multidetector CT evaluation of total anomalous pulmonary venous connections: comparison with echocardiography. Pediatr Radiol 2009;39(9):950–4.

56. Bardo DM, Frankel DG, Applegate KE, et al. Hypoplastic left heart syndrome. Radiographics 2001; 21(3):705–17.

57. Connor JA, Thiagarajan R. Hypoplastic left heart syndrome. Orphanet J Rare Dis 2007;2:23.

58. Parsons MK, Moreau GA, Graham TP Jr, et al. Echocardiographic estimation of critical left ventricular size in infants with isolated aortic valve stenosis. J Am Coll Cardiol 1991;18(4):1049–55.

59. Fonseca BM. Perioperative imaging in hypoplastic left heart syndrome. Semin Cardiothorac Vasc Anesth 2013;17(2):117–27.

60. Kim HJ, Goo HW, Park SH, et al. Left ventricle volume measured by cardiac CT in an infant with a small left ventricle: a new and accurate method in determining uni- or biventricular repair. Pediatr Radiol 2013;43(2):243–6.

61. Muthurangu V, Taylor AM, Hegde SR, et al. Cardiac magnetic resonance imaging after stage I Norwood operation for hypoplastic left heart syndrome. Circulation 2005;112(21):3256–63.

62. Bautista-Hernandez V, Hasan BS, Harrild DM, et al. Late pulmonary valve replacement in patients with pulmonary atresia and intact ventricular septum: a case-matched study. Ann Thorac Surg 2011;91(2):555–60.

63. Kleinman CS. The echocardiographic assessment of pulmonary atresia with intact ventricular septum. Catheter Cardiovasc Interv 2006;68(1):131–5.

64. Uribe S, Bächler P, Valverde I, et al. Hemodynamic assessment in patients with one-and-a-half ventricle repair revealed by four-dimensional flow magnetic resonance imaging. Pediatr Cardiol 2013;34(2):447–51.

65. Freedom RM, Jaeggi E, Perrin D, et al. The "wall-to-wall" heart in the patient with pulmonary atresia and intact ventricular septum. Cardiol Young 2006;16(1):18–29.

66. Ono M, Otake S, Fukushima N, et al. Huge right ventricle-right coronary artery fistula compromising right ventricular function in a patient with pulmonary atresia and intact ventricular septum: a case report. J Thorac Cardiovasc Surg 2001;122(5):1030–2.

67. Hascoet S, Combelles S, Acar P. Cardiac computed tomography of multiple coronary arteries to right ventricle fistulas in a newborn with pulmonary atresia and intact ventricular septum. Can J Cardiol 2014;30(2):247.e7-9.

68. Liang XC, Lam WW, Cheung EW, et al. Restrictive right ventricular physiology and right ventricular fibrosis as assessed by cardiac magnetic resonance and exercise capacity after biventricular repair of pulmonary atresia and intact ventricular septum. Clin Cardiol 2010;33(2):104–10.

69. Alwi M. Management algorithm in pulmonary atresia with intact ventricular septum. Catheter Cardiovasc Interv 2006;67(5):679–86.

70. Shi K, Yang ZG, Chen J, et al. Assessment of double outlet right ventricle associated with multiple malformations in pediatric patients using retrospective ECG-gated dual-source computed tomography. PLoS One 2015;10(6):e0130987.

71. Goo HW, Park IS, Ko JK. CT of congenital heart disease: normal anatomy and typical pathologic conditions. Radiographics 2003;23 Spec No:S147–65.

72. Chen SJ, Lin MT, Liu KL, et al. Usefulness of 3D reconstructed computed tomography imaging for double outlet right ventricle. J Formos Med Assoc 2008;107(5):371–80.

73. Saremi F, Ho SY, Cabrera JA, et al. Right ventricular outflow tract imaging with CT and MRI: part 1, morphology. AJR Am J Roentgenol 2013;200(1):W39–50.

74. Chandrashekhar G, Sodhi KS, Saxena AK, et al. Correlation of 64 row MDCT, echocardiography and cardiac catheterization angiography in assessment of pulmonary arterial anatomy in children with cyanotic congenital heart disease. Eur J Radiol 2012;81(12):4211–7.

75. Yoo SJ, Lim TH, Park IS, et al. MR anatomy of ventricular septal defect in double-outlet right ventricle with situs solitus and atrioventricular concordance. Radiology 1991;181(2):501–5.

76. Mayo JR, Roberson D, Sommerhoff B, et al. MR imaging of double outlet right ventricle. J Comput Assist Tomogr 1990;14(3):336–9.

77. Bharati A, Garekar S, Agarwal V, et al. MRA-based 3D-printed heart model—an effective tool in the pre-surgical planning of DORV. BJR Case Rep 2016;2:20150436.

78. Cook AC, Anderson RH. The anatomy of hearts with double inlet ventricle. Cardiol Young 2006;16(Suppl 1):22–6.

79. Agir AA, Celikyurt U, Karauzum K, et al. Clinical ventricular tachycardia and surgical epicardial ICD implantation in a patient with a Fontan operation for double-inlet left ventricle. Cardiovasc J Afr 2014;25(6):e6–10.

80. Güvenç O, Sayqi M, Şenqül FS, et al. Double inlet left ventricle-ventriculoarterial discordance without surgical treatment. Pediatr Int 2016;58(6):509–11.

81. Beekmana RP, Roest AA, Helbing WA, et al. Spin echo MRI in the evaluation of hearts with a double outlet right ventricle: usefulness and limitations. Magn Reson Imaging 2000;18(3):245–53.

82. Ito D, Shiraishi J, Noritake K, et al. Multidetector computed tomography demonstrates double-inlet, double-outlet right ventricle. Intern Med 2011;50(18):2053–4.

83. Mazur W, Siegel MJ, Miszalski-Jamka T, et al. CT atlas of adult congenital heart disease. London: Springer-Verlag; 2013.

84. Shirani S, Soleymanzadeh M. Diagnosis of aortic interruption by CT angiography. Pol J Radiol 2013;78(1):72–4.

85. Garcipérez de Vargas FJ, Marcos G, Mogollón MV, et al. Isolated interrupted aortic arch in an adult male. J Vasc Surg 2013;58(5):1399.

86. Malik SB, Kwan D, Shah AB, et al. The right atrium: gateway to the heart—anatomic and pathologic imaging findings. Radiographics 2015;35(1):14–31.

87. Negoi RI, Ispas AT, Ghiorghiu I, et al. Complex Ebstein's malformation: defining preoperative cardiac anatomy and function. J Card Surg 2013;28(1):70–81.

88. Kerst G, Kaulitz R, Sieverding L, et al. Images in cardiovascular medicine. Ebstein's malformation with imperforate tricuspid valve. Circulation 2007;115(6):e177–8.

89. Bharucha T, Anderson RH, Lim ZS, et al. Multiplanar review of three-dimensional echocardiography gives new insights into the morphology of Ebstein's malformation. Cardiol Young 2010;20(1):49–53.

90. Choi YH, Park JH, Choe YH, et al. MR imaging of Ebstein's anomaly of the tricuspid valve. AJR Am J Roentgenol 1994;163(3):539–43.

91. Zikria JF, Dillon EH, Epstein NF. Common CTA features of Ebstein anomaly in a middle-aged woman with a heart murmur and dyspnea on exertion. J Cardiovasc Comput Tomogr 2012;6(6):431–2.

92. Kilner PJ. Imaging congenital heart disease in adults. Br J Radiol 2011;84 Spec No 3:S258–68.

93. Garrett JS, Schiller NB, Botvinick EH, et al. Cine-computed tomography of Ebstein anomaly. J Comput Assist Tomogr 1986;10(4):664–6.

94. Beerepoot JP, Woodard PK. Case 71: Ebstein anomaly. Radiology 2004;231(3):747–51.

95. Attenhofer Jost CH, Connolly HM, Dearani JA, et al. Ebstein's anomaly. Circulation 2007;115(2):277–85.

96. Kardos M. Detection of right ventricle thrombosis in patient with Ebstein anomaly of tricuspid valve after Fontan procedure by CT. J Cardiovasc Comput Tomogr 2014;8(3):248–9.

97. Reddin G, Poterucha JT, Dearani JA, et al. Cone reconstruction of atypical Ebstein anomaly associated with right ventricular apical hypoplasia. Tex Heart Inst J 2016;43(1):78–80.

Neonatal Gastrointestinal Emergencies
Step-by-Step Approach

A. Luana Stanescu, MD[a], Mark C. Liszewski, MD[b],
Edward Y. Lee, MD, MPH[c,d], Grace S. Phillips, MD[a],*

KEYWORDS

- Neonatal • Gastrointestinal • Intestinal atresia • Malrotation • Tracheoesophageal fistula
- Pyloric stenosis • Hirschsprung disease • Meconium ileus

KEY POINTS

- Neonatal gastrointestinal emergencies comprise 2 main categories, those affecting the upper gastrointestinal tract and those affecting the lower gastrointestinal tract.
- Imaging approach is guided by a combination of prenatal history, presenting signs and symptoms, and abdominal radiographs, which help to differentiate upper from lower gastrointestinal emergencies.
- Although a handful of neonatal gastrointestinal emergencies have a diagnostic appearance on radiographs, more commonly either an upper gastrointestinal series or a contrast enema is necessary for definitive diagnosis.
- With a few exceptions, ultrasound, computed tomography, and MR imaging are typically reserved for problem solving in this population.

INTRODUCTION

Neonatal gastrointestinal emergencies arise from a constellation of varied abnormalities that can occur anywhere along the alimentary tract, from the esophagus to the colon. In some conditions, the underlying cause may be suggested by prenatal imaging. More frequently, the patient presents emergently and requires a combination of a careful history and physical examination, and correlative imaging for an accurate diagnosis. A correct, timely diagnosis is essential for minimizing potential mortality and morbidity in this population. The authors review the most common causes of gastrointestinal emergencies in neonates (**Box 1**), with an emphasis on imaging techniques and algorithms, and radiological features.

IMAGING MODALITIES AND TECHNIQUES
Radiography

Radiography is generally the first step in the imaging assessment of neonates with a suspected gastrointestinal emergency. A single supine anteroposterior (AP) view of the abdomen is often the first examination performed. The addition of a second view, either a left lateral decubitus or a cross-table lateral view, can often assist in the evaluation

Disclosure Statement: The authors have nothing to disclose.
[a] Department of Radiology, Seattle Children's Hospital, University of Washington School of Medicine, 4800 Sand Point Way Northeast, Seattle, WA 98105, USA; [b] Division of Pediatric Radiology, Montefiore Medical Center, Albert Einstein College of Medicine, 111 East 210th Street, Bronx, NY 10467, USA; [c] Division of Thoracic Imaging, Department of Radiology, Boston Children's Hospital, Harvard Medical School, 300 Longwood Avenue, Boston, MA 02115, USA; [d] Pulmonary Division, Department of Medicine, Boston Children's Hospital, Harvard Medical School, 300 Longwood Avenue, Boston, MA 02115, USA
* Corresponding author.
E-mail address: grace.phillips@seattlechildrens.org

Radiol Clin N Am 55 (2017) 717–739
http://dx.doi.org/10.1016/j.rcl.2017.02.010
0033-8389/17/© 2017 Elsevier Inc. All rights reserved.

radiologic.theclinics.com

> **Box 1**
> **Causes of gastrointestinal emergencies in neonates**
>
> Causes of upper gastrointestinal emergencies
> - Esophageal atresia and tracheoesophageal fistula
> - Pyloric atresia
> - Hypertrophic pyloric stenosis
> - Duodenal atresia
> - Duodenal web and stenosis
> - Malrotation and midgut volvulus
>
> Causes of lower gastrointestinal emergencies
> - Jejunoileal atresia
> - Meconium ileus
> - Meconium peritonitis
> - Colonic atresia
> - Functional immaturity of the colon
> - Hirschsprung disease
> - Anorectal malformations
> - Bowel duplication cysts
> - Necrotizing enterocolitis

for ectopic air, air-fluid levels, and rectal gas. Care should be taken to minimize artifact from overlying monitoring equipment and comfort pads to allow for the most optimal radiographic evaluation of the child and minimize radiation dose.[1,2]

Fluoroscopy

Upper gastrointestinal series (UGI) are performed when there is concern for abnormalities of the esophagus, stomach, or proximal small bowel. The patient ingests barium or water-soluble contrast under fluoroscopic monitoring. The patient is typically first positioned in the left lateral decubitus position, and a solid column view of the esophagus is obtained. The positioning on the patient's left side facilitates control of the administered contrast bolus, which typically pools in the gastric fundus in the left lateral decubitus position. An AP view of the esophagus is then obtained in the supine position. Subsequently, the patient is placed in the right decubitus position to study the gastric outlet. When the second portion of the duodenum is filled with contrast, the patient is then placed supine to evaluate the duodenal-jejunal junction, or ligament of Treitz. The patient may then be placed again in the right lateral position to fully distend all parts of the duodenum. A final frontal radiograph may be obtained to assess

the distribution of contrast throughout the opacified portions of bowel. Patient radiation exposure should be minimized by using intermittent pulsed fluoroscopy, appropriate collimation, limiting digital magnification, minimizing the distance between the patient and the image intensifier, and removing the antiscatter grid.

Contrast enema examinations are performed when there is a concern for abnormalities of the rectum, colon, or distal small bowel. Contrast is instilled retrograde via a catheter placed within the rectum. Water-soluble contrast may be used if there is concern for perforation or a surgical abdomen. The examination typically begins with the patient in the decubitus position, and a lateral view of the distended rectum is obtained. The patient is then placed supine, and contrast is followed through the remainder of the colon. Oblique views are often helpful for visualizing all portions of the colon, particularly the sigmoid colon, and splenic and hepatic flexures. The examination is typically terminated once the cecum or distal small bowel is visualized; in patients with a competent ileocecal valve, the distal small bowel may not fill. As in the upper GI examination, an effort to minimize patient radiation exposure should be made, using the shortest fluoroscopy time with the lowest radiation dose possible to achieve a diagnostic quality examination.

Ultrasound, Computed Tomography, and MR Imaging

Ultrasound utilization in neonatal gastrointestinal emergencies has increased over the last decades, particularly in centers with specific expertise. However, the routine use of ultrasound in the diagnosis of most neonatal gastrointestinal emergencies is not universally accepted. The exception is pyloric stenosis, where the sensitivity and specificity of ultrasound approach 100%.[3–5] Sonography can serve as a complementary imaging tool in the evaluation of patients with necrotizing enterocolitis (NEC), providing a real-time cross-sectional examination of bowel loop anatomy and function as well as depiction of free fluid.[5–7] Ultrasound has been used in the evaluation of suspected intestinal malrotation to assess the anatomic relationship of the superior mesenteric artery (SMA) and vein as well as the presence of volvulus; however, upper GI examination remains the current standard of care to exclude malrotation.[5] In neonates with cystic abdominal masses, sonography can help delineate wall structure and cyst content to aid in the diagnosis of bowel duplication cysts, meconium pseudocysts, and mesenteric cysts.

Computed tomography (CT) and magnetic resonance (MR) imaging have a limited role in the evaluation of neonates with gastrointestinal emergencies. These modalities are typically reserved as problem-solving tools in complicated cases. The potential need for anesthesia, the radiation dose in CT, and the relatively long duration of studies for MR examinations are substantial limiting factors. MR imaging without sedation may play a larger role in the future, as fast MR imaging techniques advance. For example, high-resolution MR imaging without sedation was recently shown to be feasible in neonates up to 4 months of age with anorectal malformations (ARMs).[8]

IMAGING EVALUATION APPROACH
Upper Gastrointestinal Emergencies

The approach to imaging a neonate with an upper gastrointestinal (GI) emergency is typically dictated by the presenting signs and symptoms and the prenatal imaging findings, when pertinent.[9] With the exception of suspected pyloric stenosis, abdominal radiographs are the initial imaging test used to evaluate a suspected upper GI emergency. Radiographs should include an abdominal series, consisting of a single supine AP abdominal radiograph and a cross-table lateral or left lateral decubitus AP view.[10] Radiographs alone are sufficient for the diagnosis of several upper GI abnormalities. For example, a gasless abdomen is diagnostic of isolated esophageal atresia (EA) or esophageal atresia with proximal tracheoesophageal fistula (Gross types A and B). The radiographic finding of a "double bubble" is often sufficient to diagnose duodenal atresia without the need for an upper GI.[10] Similarly, the radiographic finding of a "triple bubble" in proximal jejunal atresia may be sufficient for diagnosis.[10] The finding of a "single bubble" is frequently sufficient to diagnose antral or pyloric atresia, although caution should be applied because these entities are very rare, and a delayed film or a film after the instillation of a small (10 mL) amount of air via nasogastric tube may reveal the presence of distal air.[10]

Several other upper GI emergencies cannot be diagnosed based on radiographs alone, and further imaging with an upper GI series is needed. Perhaps most importantly, abdominal radiographs in a child presenting with bilious emesis due to intestinal malrotation with midgut volvulus may demonstrate signs of obstruction, but can be normal. Therefore, an urgent upper GI is indicated in a child with bilious emesis and suspected malrotation, even when radiographs are normal. In addition, when the bowel gas pattern suggests an upper intestinal obstruction of unclear cause, such as in the case of a

"single" or "double" bubble with distal gas, an upper GI is the next step in the imaging evaluation.[10]

UPPER GASTROINTESTINAL EMERGENCIES
Esophageal Atresia/Tracheoesophageal Fistula

EA, with or without tracheoesophageal fistula (TEF), is the most common congenital anomaly of the esophagus, with an incidence of 1 in 2500 to 1 in 3000 live births.[11] The Gross classification system describes 5 types: type A) EA without TEF, type B) EA with a proximal TEF, type C) EA with a distal TEF, type D) EA with both proximal and distal TEF (**Fig. 1**), and type E) TEF without EA. Gross type C is by far the most common, comprising 85%.[12] There is a high rate of other anomalies associated with EA and TEF, which may involve the cardiovascular, musculoskeletal, gastrointestinal, or genitourinary systems, among others. Associated anomalies are most often seen in isolated EA without TEF, with an incidence of approximately 65%.[12] The term VACTERL refers to a constellation of 3 or more anomalies involving the vertebral, anorectal, cardiac, tracheal, esophageal, renal, and limb systems in the absence of a chromosomal aberration.

EA may be suspected on prenatal sonography with the combination of polyhydramnios and an

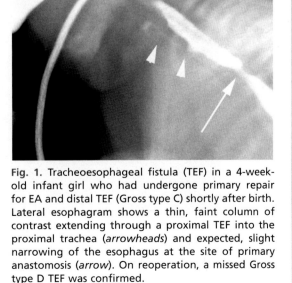

Fig. 1. Tracheoesophageal fistula (TEF) in a 4-week-old infant girl who had undergone primary repair for EA and distal TEF (Gross type C) shortly after birth. Lateral esophagram shows a thin, faint column of contrast extending through a proximal TEF into the proximal trachea (*arrowheads*) and expected, slight narrowing of the esophagus at the site of primary anastomosis (*arrow*). On reoperation, a missed Gross type D TEF was confirmed.

absent stomach bubble. In the absence of a pre-natal diagnosis, affected pediatric patients typically become symptomatic shortly after birth with an inability to feed, drooling, and cyanotic or apneic episodes while feeding.[12] The diagnosis is strongly suggested by the inability to pass a nasogastric tube. Radiograph may show an absence of bowel gas in neonates with pure EA or EA with proximal TEF (Gross types A and B). Bowel gas can be seen with a distal TEF by 4 hours of life.[13] Bronchoscopy is considered the gold standard for detecting TEF in the setting of EA.[14,15] Because of the potential for aspiration in EA, preoperative upper GI is typically avoided.[16] CT has been studied in the preoperative management of patients with EA, although a recent review has concluded that its utility is controversial, and that careful surgical technique can compensate for the absence of a preoperative CT.[17] Following primary repair, the most common early and late complications, respectively, include leak, occurring in 15% to 20% of patients, and stricture formation, occurring in 30% to 40% (Fig. 2).[12]

Pyloric Atresia

Pyloric atresia is a rare entity, with an estimated incidence of 1 in 100,000 births and constituting approximately 1% of all intestinal atresias.[18] Pyloric atresia may be seen in isolation, which portends a good prognosis. Up to 55% of patients with pyloric atresia may have associated anomalies, most commonly epidermolysis bullosa (Fig. 3) and multiple intestinal atresias, both of which are associated with substantial mortality and morbidity.[19] Three types of pyloric atresia are described: type A consisting of a web, which may be multiple; type B, consisting of a cord of solid tissue in place of the pylorus; and type C, in which there is a gap between the stomach and duodenum. Treatment is surgical and depends on the type of pyloric atresia.

On prenatal sonography or MR, the diagnosis of pyloric atresia may be suggested by the presence of polyhydramnios, a persistently dilated stomach, and absence of duodenal or other intestinal dilation.[20] In addition, the associated condition of epidermolysis bullosa may be suggested with

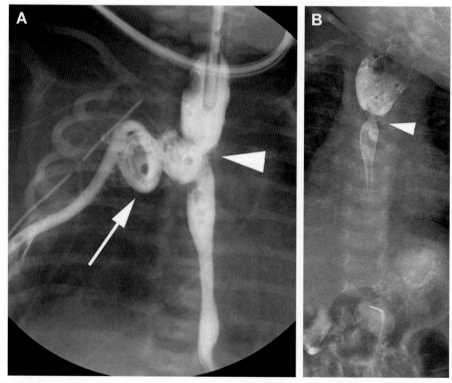

Fig. 2. Leak and stricture after esophageal atresia (EA) repair in an 8-day-old infant boy who had undergone primary repair of EA on the first day of life. (A) Frontal esophagram shows an irregular stream of contrast (arrow) draining into a pigtail pleural catheter, near the anastomotic site (arrowhead), consistent with leak. (B) Follow-up frontal esophagram obtained at 5 weeks of age shows stenosis (arrowhead) at the site of anastomosis and dilation of the more proximal esophagus, consistent with stricture.

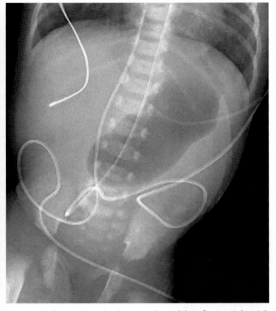

Fig. 3. Pyloric atresia in a 1-day-old infant girl with prenatal history of polyhydramnios and postnatal diagnosis of epidermolysis bullosa. Frontal radiograph shows gaseous distention of the stomach and no distal air, most consistent with pyloric atresia.

the imaging findings of layering debris in the amniotic fluid and deficiency of the bilateral external ears.[20] Postnatally, the radiographic diagnosis of pyloric atresia may be made by the identification of a "single bubble" or gaseous distention of the stomach with a complete absence of distal air.

Hypertrophic Pyloric Stenosis

Hypertrophic pyloric stenosis (HPS) refers to the abnormal thickening and elongation of the pyloric sphincter musculature, with resultant gastric outlet obstruction. The exact cause of HPS is unknown, but appears related to a combination of environmental and genetic factors. Infants typically present between 2 and 12 weeks of age with projectile, nonbilious emesis.[21] Historically, on physical examination, patients presented with a palpable "olive" representing the thickened pyloric channel, although with earlier diagnosis this finding has become less prevalent.[22] The incidence of HPS is between 2 and 5 per 1000 live births.[23] Risk factors for HPS include primiparity, male gender, birth at 28 to 36 weeks' gestational age, and early postnatal erythromycin exposure.[21] In addition, 5 genetic loci have been identified that are associated with HPS.[21]

Historically, upper GI was used to diagnose HPS. Fluoroscopic findings of HPS (**Fig. 4**)

include the "string sign," representing the narrowed pyloric channel, an abnormal impression from the enlarged pylorus upon the contrast column of the antrum or duodenum, referred to as the "shoulder" and "mushroom" signs, respectively, and hyperperistalsis of the stomach with essentially no egress of contrast. However, sonography is now the gold standard in the diagnosis of HPS (see **Fig. 4**), with a sensitivity that approaches 100%,[21] and the added benefit of avoiding ionizing radiation. Sonographic diagnostic criteria for HPS include a single muscular wall thickness greater than or equal to 3 mm, and a pyloric length of greater than or equal to 15 mm.[24] Visualization of the pylorus may be hampered by an overdistended stomach, which can sometimes be ameliorated by right lateral decubitus positioning.[21] Corroborative evidence of HPS includes the failure of gastric contents to pass through the pyloric channel during real-time imaging. False positives can occur in the setting of pylorospasm. Equivocal cases may benefit from repeat imaging.[21]

DUODENAL OBSTRUCTION
Duodenal Atresia

Duodenal atresia is a complete obstruction of the duodenum related to the embryologic failure of recanalization and has an incidence of 1 in 10,000 births. Although duodenal atresia may occur in isolation, there is a known association with trisomy 21. The diagnosis is often made prenatally by the sonographic findings of polyhydramnios and a "double bubble" representing the fluid-filled, dilated stomach and duodenum. In the absence of a known prenatal diagnosis, neonates may present with bilious or nonbilious emesis. Radiographs are diagnostic when a "double bubble" is seen, with gaseous distention of the dilated stomach and duodenum, with an absence of more distal air (**Fig. 5**). On rare occasion, as described by Latzman and colleagues,[25] more distal air may be seen in patients with duodenal atresia and anomalous biliary ducts that span the atretic duodenal segment. In this setting, upper GI may be indicated for definitive diagnosis.

Duodenal Stenosis and Duodenal Web

Duodenal stenosis and duodenal web are both partial duodenal obstructions. Duodenal stenosis implies incomplete recanalization of the duodenum, with persistent narrowing of the second segment. Duodenal web consists of a persistent, partially obstructing membrane, also typically in the second segment at the level of the ampulla

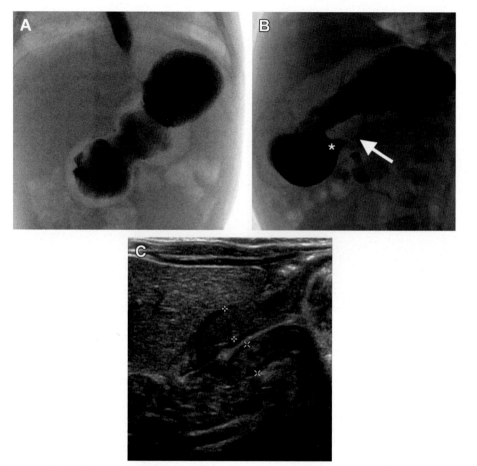

Fig. 4. Hypertrophic pyloric stenosis (HPS) in a 7-week-old girl with nonbilious emesis. (*A*) Frontal image from an upper GI series shows hyperperistalsis of the stomach. (*B*) Lateral view from the upper GI series shows beaking of the contrast column at the antrum (*asterisk*) and a "string sign" (*arrow*) from contrast within the severely narrowed pyloric channel, consistent with HPS. (*C*) Correlative transverse sonogram from the same patient shows pronounced pyloric muscular wall thickening (*cursors*) up to 7.7 mm and elongation of the pyloric channel up to 26 mm.

of Vater.[26] Duodenal stenosis can be suggested by upper GI with the finding of persistent luminal narrowing of the second segment of the duodenum. The characteristic fluoroscopic findings of a duodenal web are a "windsock" deformity, with dilation of the segment proximal to the level of the stenosis, and bulging of the web into the nondilated segment (**Fig. 6**). A similar finding has also been reported sonographically, although the more distal segment must be fluid or gas filled to reliably distinguish a web from duodenal atresia.[26] Importantly, it can be difficult to distinguish these 2 entities from other causes of partial or complete duodenal obstruction, such as malrotation with volvulus. Furthermore, duodenal stenosis and web can be seen in association with malrotation, annular pancreas, and preduodenal portal vein.

Malrotation

Malrotation refers to the incomplete rotation of the bowel during embryologic development, that causes an abnormal fixation of the duodenojejunal junction and/or cecum within the peritoneum. The estimated incidence of malrotation is 1 in 500.[27,28] Pediatric patients with malrotation are at risk for the potentially devastating complication of midgut volvulus and resultant intestinal ischemia, particularly when the mesenteric pedicle that extends from the duodenojejunal junction to the cecum is shortened. Associated Ladd's bands, or peritoneal bands that attempt to fix the cecum, may also serve as a source for duodenal obstruction. Although most patients (75%) present as newborns, up to 10% may present after the first year of life.[28–30] Classic symptoms are bilious emesis and abdominal distention,[31] although atypical

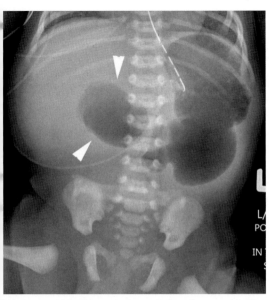

Fig. 5. Duodenal atresia in an infant boy on his first day of life. Frontal abdominal radiograph shows a characteristic "double bubble," with gaseous distention of both the stomach and the duodenum (*arrowheads*), consistent with duodenal atresia. Also noted is a nasogastric tube tip located in the proximal stomach.

symptoms such as pain, nonbilious emesis, hypovolemia, and gastrointestinal bleeding may also occur.[32] Malrotation is virtually always present in patients with congenital diaphragmatic hernia,

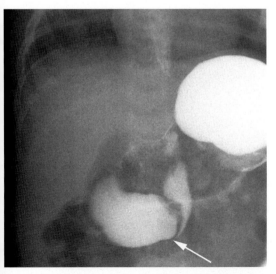

Fig. 6. Duodenal web in an 18-day-old infant boy with a prenatal history of polyhydramnios and several days of increasing emesis. Frontal image from an upper GI series shows abnormal dilation of the proximal duodenum, which protrudes into a nondilated distal portion of the duodenum, outlining a thin membrane (*arrow*), consistent with a duodenal web.

oomphalocele, and gastroschisis. There is also a high association of approximately 90% with heterotaxy syndromes.[33] There is a known association of malrotation with various syndromes as well as with other congenital disorders of the gastrointestinal system, including duodenal or jejunal atresia/stenosis, annular pancreas, Hirschsprung disease, and intussusception.[34]

Upper GI is considered the gold standard in the diagnosis of malrotation and midgut volvulus. Upper GI is 93% to 100% sensitive for the diagnosis of malrotation[27,28,35,36] and 56% to 79% sensitive for the diagnosis of volvulus.[27,36] False positives may occur in young children due to inherent laxity of ligaments, which persists up to 4 years of age, with the possibility of displacement of the duodenojejunal junction by an overdistended stomach, dilated bowel loops, or splenomegaly.[34] Accurate diagnosis rests upon meticulous technique, with full opacification of all portions of the duodenum on both the frontal and the lateral projections. Multiple investigators in particular have emphasized the importance of a true lateral projection.[27,32,34,37] Findings that are associated with an abnormal position of the duodenojejunal junction include a dilated duodenum (**Fig. 7**), a "corkscrew" appearance of the duodenum (**Fig. 8**), an abnormally anteriorly displaced third portion of the duodenum on the lateral projection, and jejunum located within the right upper quadrant or midline.[37] Of note, 2% of normal patients have jejunum located in the right upper quadrant, and some patients with malrotation may have jejunum located within the left upper quadrant.[27] In equivocal cases of suspected malrotation, a small bowel follow through (SBFT) or barium enema may be performed to document the cecal position, and thus, assess the length of mesenteric fixation. In 80% of patients with malrotation, the cecal position is abnormal.[29]

Several studies have focused on the sonographic features of malrotation. Ultrasound in malrotation may demonstrate an inverted relationship between the SMA and the superior mesenteric vein (SMV) with the SMA abnormally located to the right of the SMV, or the SMV may reside directly anterior to the SMA.[38] Ultrasound can show an intraperitoneal third portion of the duodenum that does not traverse posterior to the SMA. In midgut volvulus, a "whirlpool" sign may be seen, representing the twisted mesenteric vessels.[39] However, many investigators have concluded that because of the more frequent false positives and false negatives compared with upper GI series, sonography is not the test of choice for excluding malrotation or midgut volvulus.[40,41]

Pearls, pitfalls and variants: upper gastrointestinal emergencies

- Contrast studies in the setting of EA are potentially dangerous. Bronchoscopy is the gold standard for detection of tracheoesophageal fistulas.
- Pyloric atresia is a rare entity that may be seen in isolation or with other congenital anomalies, most commonly epidermolysis bullosa.
- Borderline cases of hypertrophic pyloric stenosis on sonography may benefit from repeat imaging if there are persistent symptoms.
- Duodenal web and stenosis can be associated with malrotation, annular pancreas, and preduodenal portal vein.
- Meticulous upper GI series technique is the cornerstone for accurate diagnosis of malrotation, with full visualization of the duodenal course on both frontal and lateral projections. False positives may still occur because of ligamentous laxity that persists up to 4 years of age.
- Upper GI series is still preferred over ultrasound in the diagnosis of malrotation.

Low Gastrointestinal Emergencies

Low gastrointestinal emergencies typically involve the small bowel and the colon in neonates presenting with bilious vomiting or failure to pass meconium in the first 24 to 48 hours of life as well as variable degrees of abdominal distension depending on the lesion location. Differential diagnosis commonly includes jejunoileal atresia/stenosis, meconium ileus, functional immaturity of the colon, and Hirschsprung disease.[9] Colonic atresia/stenosis and ARMs may also cause low intestinal obstruction, but are less common. Many of the low gastrointestinal emergencies have similar findings on abdominal radiographs, typically demonstrating numerous dilated bowel loops. Water-soluble contrast enema can help differentiate these clinical entities by localizing the level of obstruction and may also have a therapeutic effect in specific clinical entities (**Table 1**). Meconium peritonitis and meconium pseudocysts are the result of bowel perforation in utero and have imaging findings that differ from the other low gastrointestinal emergencies.

SMALL BOWEL INVOLVEMENT
Jejunoileal Atresia

Jejunoileal atresia is encountered in approximately 1 in 5000 neonates,[42] representing 46%

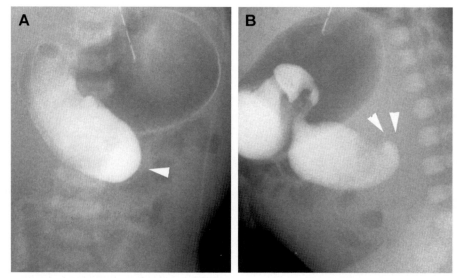

Fig. 7. Malrotation with volvulus in a 2-day-old infant boy with bilious emesis. (*A*) Frontal image from an upper GI series demonstrates abnormal dilation of the first and second portions of the duodenum with an abrupt cutoff (*arrowhead*) of the contrast column. (*B*) Lateral image from the upper GI series again displays abnormal dilation of the first and second portions of the duodenum with abrupt beaking (*arrowheads*) of the contrast column. Malrotation with volvulus was confirmed at surgery.

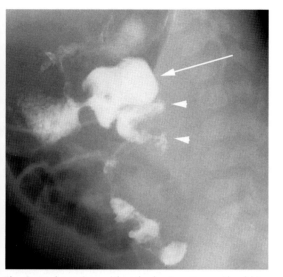

Fig. 8. Malrotation with volvulus in a 2-month-old infant boy with bilious emesis. Lateral image from an upper GI series shows dilation of the first and second portions of the duodenum (*arrow*), and a "corkscrew" appearance of the more distal duodenum (*arrowheads*), characteristic of malrotation with volvulus.

to 73% of intestinal atresias.[43,44] The cause is thought to be related to a late in utero mesenteric ischemic insult affecting one or multiple already-formed bowel loops, in contradistinction to duodenal atresia, which is caused by a failure in bowel recanalization during early fetal development. Congenital cardiac or chromosomal anomalies are infrequently associated with jejunoileal atresia as compared with duodenal atresias being present in less than 10% of the cases. Cystic fibrosis (CF) is encountered in up to 20% of the neonates with jejunoileal atresia, and abdominal wall defects like gastroschisis and omphaloceles are seen in up to 17% of the cases, likely representing predisposing factors.[43,45,46] Pathologic findings in jejunoileal atresia are complex, with 4 patterns demonstrating different prognostic and therapeutic implications identified in the Grosfeld classification: type I (mucosal web), type II (fibrous cord), type III a (mesenteric gap defect), type III b (apple peel), and type IV (multiple atresias).[47,48] Small bowel stenosis with focal narrowing of the bowel lumen without associated mesenteric

Table 1
Differentiating imaging features in common causes of distal bowel obstruction

	Radiographs	Contrast Enema: Colon	Contrast Enema: Small Bowel
Distal jejunal and ileal atresia	• Multiple dilated bowel loops, too many to count • Air-fluid levels present • Meconium peritonitis/meconium pseudocyst with calcifications in cases of in utero perforation	Microcolon only if: • Distal • Occurred early in gestation Normal sized colon if: • Proximal • Occurred late	• Small-caliber terminal ileum • No meconium pellets
Meconium ileus	• Multiple dilated bowel loops, too many to count • No air-fluid levels • Bubbly pattern	• Always microcolon	• Large-caliber terminal ileum • Filled with meconium pellets
Functional immaturity of the colon	Multiple dilated bowel loops, too many to count	• Normal caliber or small left colon with smooth transition • Multiple filling defects consistent with meconium plugs • Normal rectosigmoid ratio	• Normal-caliber terminal ileum
Hirschsprung disease (short and long segment)	Multiple dilated bowel loops, too many to count	• Cone-shaped zone of transition • Irregular contractions • Altered rectosigmoid ratio	• Easy reflux of contrast in dilated terminal ileum
Hirschsprung disease (total aganglionosis)	Multiple dilated bowel loops, too many to count	• Normal caliber • Short, comma-shaped colon • Microcolon	• Intraluminal calcifications may be present in terminal ileum

defect is rare, with a ratio of approximately 1/20 relative to atresia.[49]

Imaging findings depend on the timing of the in utero insult and the level of obstruction. Few dilated small bowel loops on abdominal radiographs are suggestive of a proximal level of obstruction in the jejunum (**Fig. 9**). Multiple dilated bowel loops with air fluid levels are typically seen with more distal obstruction, in either the distal jejunum or the ileum. Given difficulties in differentiating small and large bowel loops in neonates on radiography, the finding of multiple dilated bowel loops entails a broad differential diagnosis, including distal jejunal or ileal atresia, meconium ileus, colonic atresia, Hirschsprung disease, and meconium plug syndrome. Water-soluble contrast enema is used to exclude coexisting colonic atresia as well as to potentially identify the level of small bowel obstruction. As colonic caliber depends on the amount of enteric secretions passing through, a microcolon is present in distal ileal atresia and in the setting of early vascular insult, whereas in jejunal or proximal ileal atresia as well as with late ischemic event, the colonic caliber may be normal. Contrast enema can also identify the position of the cecum when evaluating for malrotation. Upper GI series has limited utility in cases with clinical and radiologic findings suggestive of distal bowel obstruction.

Approximately 10% of neonates with small bowel atresia develop in utero perforation of the dilated bowel proximal to the atretic segment with subsequent meconium peritonitis and meconium pseudocysts.[47]

Meconium Ileus

Meconium ileus is caused by thick inspissated meconium obstructing the terminal ileum. Meconium ileus is frequently due to CF, which is eventually diagnosed in up to 90% of patients with meconium ileus, and up to 15% of CF patients present as infants with meconium ileus.[50–52] Abdominal radiographs demonstrate a distal obstructive bowel gas pattern characterized by multiple dilated bowel loops with a "soap bubble" appearance (Neuhauser sign) due to meconium admixed with air (**Fig. 10**). The pasty consistency of thick meconium precludes the formation of air-fluid levels typical for obstruction, which is a useful diagnostic clue when present.[53] Water-soluble contrast enema with hyperosmolar agents may be diagnostic as well as therapeutic. Contrast enema typically demonstrates an unused, small-caliber microcolon. Contrast refluxed into terminal ileum outlines multiple filling defects consistent with meconium pellets (see **Fig. 10**). Interestingly, the success rate of disimpaction with contrast enema was noted to decrease over the last 20 years from a historic high rate of up to 83% to approximately 39%. These changes are attributed to reluctance to repeat enemas multiple times, possible decrease in radiologist experience, and use of lower osmolarity contrast agents to decrease risk of perforation.[54,55]

Half of the patients with meconium ileus typically show evidence of in utero complications, with either bowel necrosis or volvulus leading to perforation, with meconium peritonitis or meconium pseudocyst formation. Contrast enemas are not

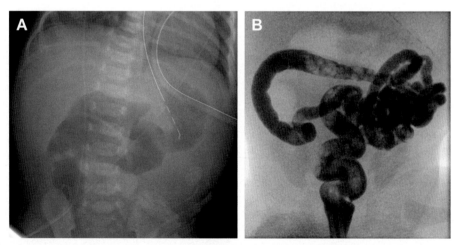

Fig. 9. Jejunal atresia in newborn girl with abdominal distention. (*A*) Abdominal radiograph shows a few dilated bowel loops in the upper abdomen. (*B*) Water-soluble contrast enema demonstrates normal rectosigmoid ratio with diffusely small caliber of the colon. There is opacification of multiple nondilated small bowel loops located primarily in the left hemiabdomen and no contrast reflux into the dilated air-filled small bowel loops, suggestive of proximal small bowel obstruction. Three areas of jejunal atresias were found at surgery.

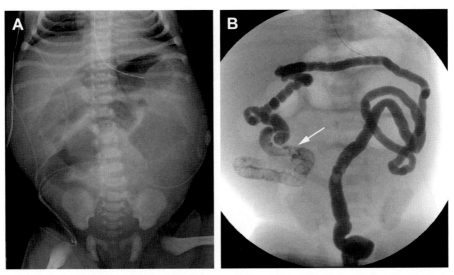

Fig. 10. Meconium ileus in newborn girl with abdominal distention. (A) Abdominal radiograph demonstrates multiple dilated proximal as well as distal bowel loops, containing dense bubbly material representing meconium admixed with air producing a "soap bubble" appearance. (B) Water-soluble contrast enema demonstrates a redundant microcolon. Contrast opacifies the terminal ileum, which is distended with multiple filling defects (arrow) consistent with meconium pellets. Findings are suggestive of meconium ileus, confirmed at surgery.

indicated in these patients. Treatment is surgical, consisting of bowel resection and reanastomosis.

With increased survival of extremely premature low-birth-weight neonates, meconium-related ileus has been described as a rare new clinical entity in these patients, the underlying cause hypothesized as a combination of viscid meconium and functional bowel immaturity.[56,57] Bowel obstruction develops in the first or second week of life; an important radiologic finding that allows the differentiation from NEC is the absence of pneumatosis.[56] Imaging findings are similar to uncomplicated meconium ileus, and hyperosmolar enemas may be successful in up to 80% of these patients.[58]

Meconium Peritonitis

Meconium peritonitis is an aseptic chemical peritonitis resulting from intrauterine bowel perforation. The meconium spilled in the peritoneal cavity leads to an intense inflammatory reaction with fibrotic tissue formation and rapid (hours to days) calcification.[59] Common causes include meconium ileus, seen in up to 40% of the cases,[60] small and large bowel atresia, volvulus, and intussusception.[61] Meconium peritonitis may be generalized, with diffuse calcifications spread throughout the peritoneal cavity or cystic in cases with persistent bowel leakage leading to thick walled meconium pseudocyst formation. Peritoneal calcifications are the most common imaging finding (Fig. 11), whereas ascites, dilated bowel

loops, and the presence of meconium pseudocyst are highly predictive of the need for neonatal surgical treatment.[62] Meconium pseudocysts contain complex echogenic material on ultrasound, with linear calcifications along the walls that may be seen both on radiographs and ultrasound (Fig. 12).[63,64] Giant pseudocysts can lead to massive abdominal distension with ascites and cardiopulmonary complications.[65]

LARGE BOWEL INVOLVEMENT
Colonic Atresia

Colonic atresia is rare, representing only approximately 2% to 15% of bowel atresias.[66] Cause is thought to be a vascular insult, similar to jejunoileal bowel atresia, sharing the same pathologic findings reflected by the Grosfeld classification.[43] The right and transverse colon are more commonly affected than the left.[43,66,67]

Bowel rotation and fixation anomalies are present in most patients with colonic atresia, likely representing either a predisposing factor or a consequence of colonic atresia.[67] Hirschsprung disease is diagnosed in approximately 10% of the cases and should be excluded before surgical repair.[66,68]

Abdominal radiographs reflect a pattern of distal bowel obstruction, with multiple dilated bowel loops with air-fluid levels (Fig. 13). When present, massive dilation of the proximal colon represents a helpful diagnostic clue. Contrast enema can show a short blind-ending microcolon with no

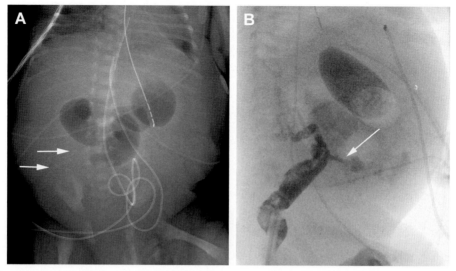

Fig. 11. Meconium peritonitis in a 2-day-old 30-week premature boy with abdominal distension. (*A*) Abdominal radiograph demonstrates moderate gaseous distention of the stomach, duodenum, and a proximal jejunal loop, with the so-called triple bubble sign. Scattered calcifications (*arrows*) are present throughout the abdomen, suggestive of meconium peritonitis. (*B*) Water-soluble contrast enema shows a normal rectosigmoid ratio with frank contrast extravasation in the region of the sigmoid (*arrow*), consistent with perforation that was confirmed at surgery. Multiple small bowel type I atretic segments were also found at surgery, the most proximal being just distal to the ligament of Treitz.

contrast reflux in the dilated proximal colon (see **Fig. 13**).

Functional Immaturity of the Colon

Functional immaturity of the colon unifies previously described small left colon syndrome and meconium plug, both characterized by benign transient colonic dysmotility thought to be related to delayed maturation of myenteric plexuses. The pathophysiology remains unclear, but it has been associated with maternal diabetes and magnesium sulfate administration in preeclamptic

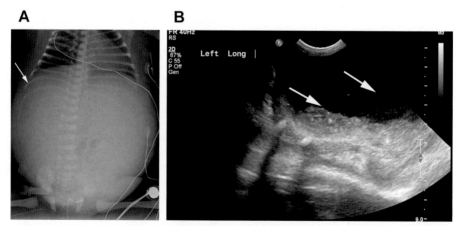

Fig. 12. Meconium pseudocyst in a 35-week-old premature newborn girl with abdominal distention. (*A*) Abdominal radiograph demonstrates paucity of bowel gas with centralization of the bowel loops. There is marked abdominal distention with peripheral linear calcifications in the right upper quadrant (*arrow*) suggestive of peritoneal calcifications. There is also diffuse abdominal and chest wall edema. (*B*) Gray-scale ultrasound image of the left hemiabdomen demonstrates a complex cystic mass, largely anechoic, with layering echogenic debris (*arrows*), found to be filling the abdomen and pelvis. A large meconium pseudocyst was found at surgery, incorporating a mesenteric volvulus of the terminal ileum, with evidence for in utero perforation.

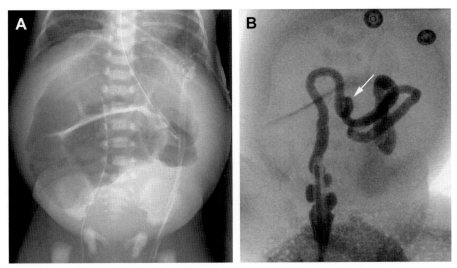

Fig. 13. Colonic atresia in a newborn girl with distended abdomen. (*A*) Abdominal radiograph shows severe gaseous distention of multiple bowel loops. (*B*) Water-soluble contrast enema demonstrates diffusely small caliber of the colon, consistent with unused microcolon, which is blind ending (*arrow*) in the upper abdomen.

mothers.[69] Radiographs demonstrate a distal bowel obstruction pattern (**Fig. 14**). Water-soluble contrast enema most often demonstrates large filling defects throughout the colon, representing meconium plugs. The colon may be normal in caliber. If the abnormality is limited to the left colon, the descending colon typically has a small caliber, with a smooth transition point at the splenic flexure (see **Fig. 14**). Contrast enema is therapeutic in most cases, with evacuation of meconium plugs and resolution of obstruction. A normal caliber of the rectum can often help differentiate this entity from Hirschsprung disease. However, recent studies have shown that up to 13% of patients diagnosed with functional immaturity of the colon were found to have underlying Hirschsprung disease,[69,70] whereas in a smaller series of patients, this association was present

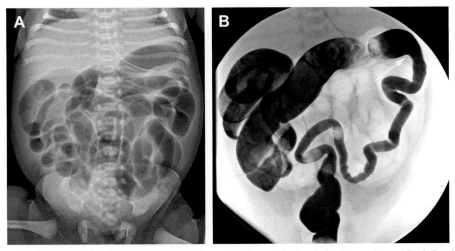

Fig. 14. Functional immaturity of the colon in a 1-day-old infant girl of a diabetic mother with abdominal distension, not passing stool since birth. (*A*) Abdominal radiograph shows multiple distended bowel loops throughout the abdomen. (*B*) Water-soluble contrast enema shows a small left colon with a smooth transition at the splenic flexure (*arrow*) to a slightly dilated proximal colon containing a large filling defect consistent with meconium plug. Smaller filling defects are seen in the dilated, opacified terminal ileum as well as in the distal colon.

in 38% of the cases.[71] Given these findings, persistent symptoms should prompt rectal biopsy in this patient group.

Hirschsprung Disease

Hirschsprung disease is present in approximately 1/5000 live births and occurs as a result of arrested distal migration of vagal neural crest cells.[72] The absence of parasympathetic plexuses in the affected bowel causes incomplete distension and spasmodic contractions, leading to functional obstruction with upstream bowel dilation. The length of aganglionic bowel is variable, but always extends proximally from the rectum in a contiguous manner. Hirschsprung disease is more common in males (male to female ratio is 4:1) and can be associated with trisomy 21 as well as other defects in neural crest migration (neurocristopathies).

Radiographs in Hirschsprung disease demonstrate multiple dilated bowel loops, with identical findings to other causes of distal bowel obstruction. Full-thickness rectal biopsy is the gold standard for diagnosing as well as confirming Hirschsprung disease, although water-soluble contrast enema can be diagnostic in a large number of cases (**Figs. 15** and **16**). On enema, a transition zone and/or an altered rectosigmoid ratio of less than 1 provide a diagnostic sensitivity of 75% to 85% and a specificity of 95% to 96%.[73] A

characteristic cone-shaped area of transition between aganglionic, relatively small-caliber bowel and proximal distended bowel filled with stool is best seen on lateral view during early filling; however, it may be less apparent in neonates because it tends to develop with time. Irregular contractions with saw-tooth appearance of the mucosa are pathognomonic, but present in only approximately 20% of the cases.[72]

Depending on the length of bowel involvement, 4 types of Hirschsprung disease may be encountered.[74] The ultrashort segment is rare, involving only up to 4 cm of the distal rectum, and could be easily missed if the rectal tube is in a deep position.[72,74] Short-segment Hirschsprung disease extends up to the midsigmoid colon and represents the most common form, present in up to 80% of the cases, whereas long segment Hirschsprung disease extends proximal to the midsigmoid without involving the whole colon. Total colonic aganglionosis may extend to the terminal ileum, with variable caliber and appearance of the colon, which may be normal, shortened with a comma shape, or diffusely small in caliber (microcolon). The presence of right lower quadrant intraluminal calcifications along the terminal ileum in the presence of a microcolon can help differentiate these cases from meconium ileus and should prompt a rectal biopsy.[75] Allergy to cow milk protein involves primarily the rectum and can

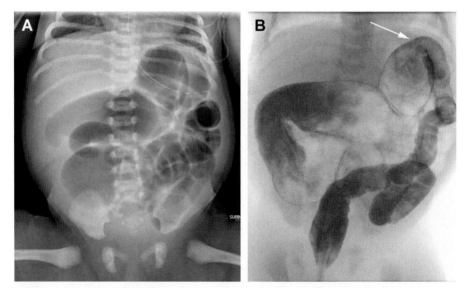

Fig. 15. Long segment Hirschsprung disease in a 2-day-old male infant with abdominal distension. (*A*) Abdominal radiograph demonstrates multiple dilated bowel loops throughout the abdomen with no gas seen in the rectum, suggestive of distal bowel obstruction. (*B*) Water-soluble contrast enema obtained the same day demonstrates normal relative diameters of the rectum and sigmoid, with small-caliber left colon with an abrupt transition (*arrow*) to the dilated upstream colon in the region of the splenic flexure. Multiple filling defects are seen throughout the colon. Findings were initially thought to represent functional immaturity of the left colon (meconium plug syndrome), while biopsy showed long segment Hirschsprung up to the splenic flexure.

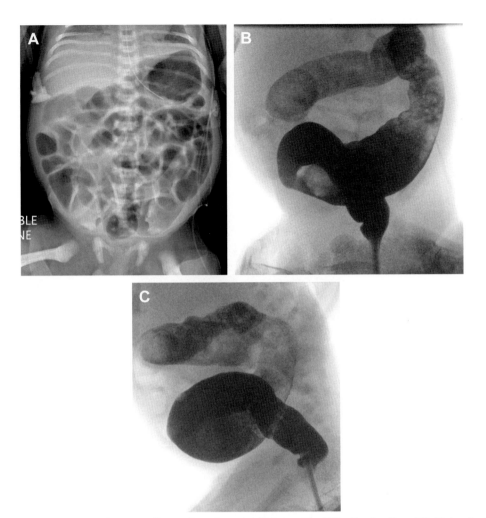

Fig. 16. Short-segment Hirschsprung disease in a 4-week-old boy with difficulty stooling. (*A*) Abdominal radiograph shows multiple dilated bowel loops. (*B, C*) Water-soluble contrast enema shows altered rectosigmoid ratio, with substantial dilation of the proximal sigmoid extending up to the level of the middescending colon. Transition point is likely at the junction of the proximal and midsigmoid colon. There are multiple filling defects throughout the colon representing stool.

mimic short segment Hirschsprung disease, with irregular rectal mucosa causing luminal narrowing. Presentation is however late as compared with Hirschsprung, and reflects the timing of transition to cow milk feeding.

Anorectal Malformations

ARMs are relatively rare, with a reported incidence of 3/10,000 live births,[76] and include a wide spectrum of abnormalities involving the anus and distal rectum as well as the urogenital tract, most commonly resulting from abnormal development of the urorectal septum. The anus is frequently imperforated, while the distal bowel ends blindly or through a fistulous connection with the urogenital tract or perineum (**Fig. 17**). Associated

congenital anomalies are present in up to 70% of the cases, with spine and urinary tract most frequently involved.[77] ARMs are currently classified based on the presence and location of fistulous connections and can be differentiated into specific types based on gender.[78] Surgical management consists of posterior sagittal anorectoplasty first described by deVries and Pena,[79] with a perineal approach repair in the first days of life for fistulous connections below or at the level of the levator muscle. High fistulous connections require a staged laparotomy or laparoscopic approach, with initial colostomy followed by later reconstruction.[77,78]

Imaging plays a crucial role in the diagnosis and management of neonates with ARMs. In the first 2 days of life, imaging evaluation aims to

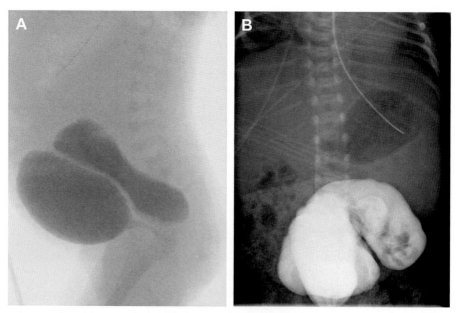

Fig. 17. ARM in a 10-day-old boy with imperforated anus after colostomy with high-output mucous fistula concerning for urine. (*A, B*) Cystourethrogram shows contrast that was instilled into the bladder passed into the rectosigmoid colon, consistent with rectovesical fistula.

characterize the ARM and detect possible associated anomalies. Radiographs of the spine and pelvis as well as ultrasound evaluation of the abdomen, pelvis, and spine are performed.[77] High-resolution perineal ultrasound may be used to delineate the location of the rectal pouch relative to the anus, and possible fistulous tracts.[80] A voiding cystourethrogram is recommended in all patients with abnormal renal or bladder findings given the high association with vesicoureteral reflux.

In patients who undergo colostomy, high-pressure distal colostography or MR imaging is performed before final repair to delineate the anatomy and fistulas. A recent study by Thomeer and colleagues[8] demonstrated that high-resolution MR imaging without sedation is feasible up to 4 months of age, is more accurate than colostography, and avoids the risk of perforation encountered with this technique.

Bowel Duplication Cysts

Intestinal duplication cysts are rare congenital anomalies with an unknown incidence. They can arise along any segment of the gastrointestinal tract from mouth to anus, most commonly seen along the ileum and at the ileocecal valve.[81] The cause remains controversial, with several hypotheses, including recanalization defects, and the split notochord syndrome being still debated.[82,83] Cystic duplications are present in up to 86% of cases, typically arising from the mesenteric

side of the bowel wall. Tubular type duplication cysts are more rare and may be located within the bowel wall. Clinical presentation is variable depending on size and structure, ranging from an asymptomatic, incidentally detected abdominal mass to life-threatening surgical complications.[84] Gastric mucosa is present in up to half of the cystic type, predisposing to hemorrhage, ulcer, and perforation.[81] Up to a third of the patients may have a complicated neonatal presentation with volvulus or intussusception.[81] Most cases present by the age of 2, with an increased proportion being now detected on prenatal ultrasound.[85]

Associated spinal defects, congenital lung lesions, and cardiac anomalies are present in approximately 30% of the patients, warranting careful investigation, potentially with fetal MR imaging.[85] Imaging modality of choice is ultrasound (**Fig. 18**). Classic sonographic features reflect the layered bowel wall structure of the duplication cysts, with a hyperechogenic mucosa, hypoechoic muscularis, and echogenic serosa, sometimes difficult to identify in large cysts with stretched wall. Peristalsis is also a useful sign when present.[86,87] Differential diagnosis includes mesenteric inclusion cysts, lymphangiomas, and ovarian cysts in females.

Necrotizing Enterocolitis

NEC is a life-threatening inflammatory intestinal disease that has emerged over the last decades as the most common neonatal gastrointestinal

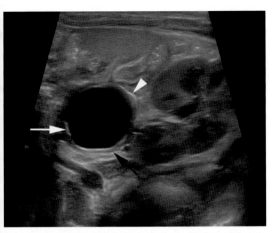

Fig. 18. Bowel duplication cyst in a 19-day-old male infant diagnosed prenatally with a left abdominal cyst. Transverse gray-scale ultrasound image shows a predominantly anechoic round structure medial to the left renal hilum and anterior to the aorta, containing minimal echogenic debris. The wall demonstrates a typical layered appearance, with hyperechoic mucosa and submucosa (*white arrow*), hypoechoic muscularis propria (*black arrow*), and a partially visualized hyperechogenic serosa (*arrowhead*), consistent with gut signature appearance, characteristic for enteric duplication cysts. Surgery was performed, confirming the diagnosis.

emergency, being one of the leading causes of death in neonatal intensive care units.[88] The cause remains unclear, with multiple factors, including immature bowel function, hypoxia/ischemia, and disruption of gut microbiota likely involved.[6,88–91] NEC is encountered primarily in premature infants, with up to 10% to 15% of those with birth weight less than 1500 g affected.[6,92,93] NEC in full-term neonates accounts for approximately 10% to 25% of cases, occurring usually in association with an underlying congenital condition such as heart disease and endocrine disorders[94] or in the presence of risk factors like sepsis or hypotension. Congenital heart disease is involved in up to 66% of these cases, with specific clinical entities like hypoplastic left heart syndrome particularly predisposing patients to alterations of the mesenteric blood supply.[94–97]

Clinical presentation of NEC in premature infants is variable and often nonspecific with bradycardia, lethargy, and mottling difficult to differentiate from other abnormalities such as neonatal sepsis.[98] The classic clinical signs include abdominal distension, feeding intolerance, and bloody stools. Time of NEC presentation depends on associated risk factors: although in premature infants it may occur in the second or third week of life,[99] term neonates tend to present

earlier, during the first week of life.[100] Therapeutic decisions are based on a staging system initially proposed in 1978 by Bell and colleagues,[101] using systemic, abdominal, and radiologic criteria. Prompt medical treatment can limit disease progression in up to 60% of patients, whereas 20% to 40% will progress to bowel necrosis with perforation requiring surgical treatment.[98]

Imaging plays an essential role in the management of patients with NEC, typically used at the time of diagnosis as well as during disease evolution, allowing early detection of confirmatory diagnostic signs as well as of potential complications. Radiography and ultrasound are the main imaging modalities used, with abdominal radiographs remaining the imaging modality of choice (**Box 2**). Contrast enema, CT, and MR imaging have been evaluated for potential use but have not proven to be reliable imaging methods in this clinical setting.[6,102–104]

The radiographic findings in NEC include abnormal bowel gas pattern, pneumatosis, portal venous gas, and pneumoperitoneum (**Box 3, Fig. 19**). In an attempt to standardize the verbiage used in radiology reports describing findings in NEC, Coursey and colleagues[105] proposed a 10-point scale meant to reflect the correlation of radiologic signs with disease severity.

The bowel gas pattern can evolve from diffuse nonspecific gaseous distension, an early sign that may precede clinical manifestations by several hours,[6,106] to a fixed dilated loop of bowel, so-called persistent loop sign, thought to be an impending sign of perforation highly predictive for the need of surgical intervention or a completely gasless abdomen.[107,108] Pneumatosis in a neonate is essentially pathognomonic for NEC and confirms the clinical suspicion when present. Pneumatosis is most frequently seen in the right lower quadrant within distal small bowel

---

Box 2
Imaging techniques in necrotizing enterocolitis

Radiography

- Abdominal radiographs 2 views, supine and dependent view (cross-table lateral or left lateral decubitus)

Ultrasound

- Gray-scale imaging to evaluate for free air, free fluid, portal venous gas, and bowel wall thickening, thinning, pneumatosis, and peristalsis
- Color flow of the bowel wall to detect potential ischemia

and proximal colonic walls.[6] Portal venous gas is a later finding in disease evolution indicating progression to severe disease.[102] Although portal venous gas is not an absolute indication for surgery, its presence is significantly associated with eventual need for surgery according to He and colleagues.[108] Pneumoperitoneum is a sign of full-thickness bowel necrosis with perforation and is an absolute indication for surgery.[6,109]

Ultrasound has emerged as a potentially valuable imaging tool in the diagnosis of NEC as well as in predicting outcomes (**Box 4**). In imaging centers with specific expertise in bowel ultrasound for NEC, ultrasound can detect pneumatosis, portal venous gas, and pneumoperitoneum with at least a similar sensitivity as radiographs.[6,110] Unlike radiographs, ultrasound can directly evaluate bowel wall thickness, peristalsis and fluid collections in real time. Specific ultrasound findings, such as increased bowel thickness greater than 2.8 mm or significant thinning less than 1.1 mm, absent peristalsis, absent perfusion, and complex free fluid, have been associated with adverse outcomes.[108,110]

The differential diagnosis for NEC includes other conditions that can present with bowel distension

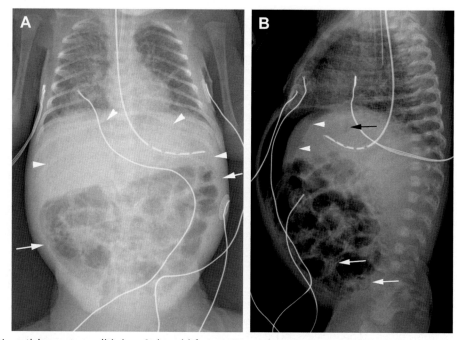

Fig. 19. Necrotizing enterocolitis in a 9-day-old former 27-week premature girl with abdominal distention and hemodynamic instability. Supine (*A*) and lateral (*B*) chest and abdominal radiographs show that there are multiple dilated bowel loops with cystic as well as linear lucencies along the bowel walls in the right lower quadrant as well as in the left upper quadrant, consistent with pneumatosis (*arrows*). There is a large pneumoperitoneum, with the so-called football sign (*arrowheads*). Trace portal venous gas also noted (*black arrow* on *B*). Coarse reticular opacities are visualized in bilateral lungs, compatible with developing chronic lung disease. Incidental note is made of an endotracheal tube, which is malpositioned, with tip in the right main stem bronchus.

Box 4
Ultrasound imaging findings in necrotizing enterocolitis

Pneumatosis

- Hyperechoic foci in the bowel wall

Portal venous gas

- Intraluminal echogenic foci in the main portal vein and branches

Pneumoperitoneum

- Echogenic shadowing air visualized outside the bowel
- Large amount may be difficult to differentiate from bowel gas

Free fluid

- Simple
- Complex: low level echoes or septations suggest perforation

Bowel wall

- Thickness: normal range 1.1 to 2.6 mm[111]
- Echogenicity: increased, may reflect edema, hemorrhage, or inflammation
- Peristalsis: absent in advanced stages
- Perfusion: initial hyperemia may evolve to absence in advanced stages

Pearls, pitfalls and variants: Lower gastrointestinal emergencies

- Small bowel atresia is not always associated with a microcolon. A normal-sized colon will be present if the vascular insult occurred late in gestation or affects the proximal small bowel.
- A microcolon will always be present in meconium ileus.
- Meconium-related ileus in low-birth-weight neonates can present in the second week of life, with a similar timing as necrotizing enterocolitis (NEC). The absence of pneumatosis and the lack of typical clinical signs help differentiate these clinical entities.
- NEC in preterm neonates presents in the second or third week of life, whereas NEC in term neonates with associated cardiac or endocrine comorbidities typically have an earlier presentation in the first week of life.
- Although a normal rectal caliber on contrast enema may help differentiate functional colonic immaturity from Hirschsprung disease, persistent symptoms should prompt rectal biopsy.
- In older children, allergy to cow milk may mimic short-segment Hirschsprung disease on contrast enema.

or increased bowel content that could mimic pneumatosis, including sepsis, meconium disease of prematurity, nonspecific feeding intolerance, and Hirschsprung disease.[98,111]

Surgical methods for treating NEC include laparotomy with resection of ischemic bowel, and primary peritoneal drainage without laparotomy. Despite many advances of modern neonatal care, mortality from surgical NEC in preterm neonates remains high, up to 34%,[93] and survivors are affected by significant complications and comorbidities, including sepsis, short bowel syndrome, and adhesions.

SUMMARY

Given the substantial overlap in signs and symptoms of many of the discussed common causes of gastrointestinal emergencies in neonates, imaging plays an important role in the diagnosis. With a step-by-step approach, one may confidently make a timely and accurate imaging diagnosis in the setting of a neonatal gastrointestinal emergency, which in turn, can lead to optimal patient care.

REFERENCES

1. Rattan AS, Cohen MD. Removal of comfort pads underneath babies: a method of reducing radiation exposure to neonates. Acad Radiol 2013;20(10): 1297–300.
2. Jiang X, Baad M, Reiser I, et al. Effect of comfort pads and incubator design on neonatal radiography. Pediatr Radiol 2016;46(1):112–8.
3. Hernanz-Schulman M, Sells LL, Ambrosino MM, et al. Hypertrophic pyloric stenosis in the infant without a palpable olive: accuracy of sonographic diagnosis. Radiology 1994;193(3):771–6.
4. Stunden RJ, LeQuesne GW, Little KE. The improved ultrasound diagnosis of hypertrophic pyloric stenosis. Pediatr Radiol 1986;16(3):200–5.
5. Hiorns MP. Gastrointestinal tract imaging in children: current techniques. Pediatr Radiol 2011;41(1):42–54.
6. Epelman M, Daneman A, Navarro OM, et al. Necrotizing enterocolitis: review of state-of-the-art imaging findings with pathologic correlation. Radiographics 2007;27(2):285–305.
7. Anupindi SA, Halverson M, Khwaja A, et al. Common and uncommon applications of bowel ultrasound with pathologic correlation in

children. AJR Am J Roentgenol 2014;202(5): 946–59.

8. Thomeer MG, Devos A, Lequin M, et al. High resolution MRI for preoperative work-up of neonates with an anorectal malformation: a direct comparison with distal pressure colostography/fistulography. Eur Radiol 2015;25(12):3472–9.

9. Vinocur DN, Lee EY, Eisenberg RL. Neonatal intestinal obstruction. AJR Am J Roentgenol 2012; 198(1):W1–10.

10. Maxfield CM, Bartz BH, Shaffer JL. A pattern-based approach to bowel obstruction in the newborn. Pediatr Radiol 2013;43(3):318–29.

11. Spitz L. Esophageal atresia and tracheoesophageal malformations. In: Ashcraft KW, Holcomb G, Murphy JP, editors. Pediatric surgery. 4th edition. Philadelphia: Elsevier Saunders; 2005. p. 352–70.

12. Pinheiro PF, Simoes E, Silva AC, et al. Current knowledge on esophageal atresia. World J Gastroenterol 2012;18(28):3662–72.

13. Gedicke MM, Gopal M, Spicer R. A gasless abdomen does not exclude distal tracheoesophageal fistula: the value of a repeat x-ray. J Pediatr Surg 2007;42(3):576–7.

14. Guo W, Li Y, Jiao A, et al. Tracheoesophageal fistula after primary repair of type C esophageal atresia in the neonatal period: recurrent or missed second congenital fistula. J Pediatr Surg 2010; 45(12):2351–5.

15. McDuffie LA, Wakeman D, Warner BW. Diagnosis of esophageal atresia with tracheoesophageal fistula: is there a need for gastrointestinal contrast? J Pediatr 2010;156(5):852.

16. Gopal M, Woodward M. Potential hazards of contrast study diagnosis of esophageal atresia. J Pediatr Surg 2007;42(6):E9–10.

17. Garge S, Rao KL, Bawa M. The role of preoperative CT scan in patients with tracheoesophageal fistula: a review. J Pediatr Surg 2013;48(9):1966–71.

18. Ilce Z, Erdogan E, Kara C, et al. Pyloric atresia: 15-year review from a single institution. J Pediatr Surg 2003;38(11):1581–4.

19. Al-Salem AH. Congenital pyloric atresia and associated anomalies. Pediatr Surg Int 2007;23(6): 559–63.

20. Merrow AC, Frischer JS, Lucky AW. Pyloric atresia with epidermolysis bullosa: fetal MRI diagnosis with postnatal correlation. Pediatr Radiol 2013; 43(12):1656–61.

21. Ranells JD, Carver JD, Kirby RS. Infantile hypertrophic pyloric stenosis: epidemiology, genetics, and clinical update. Adv Pediatr 2011;58(1):195–206.

22. Glatstein M, Carbell G, Boddu SK, et al. The changing clinical presentation of hypertrophic pyloric stenosis: the experience of a large, tertiary care pediatric hospital. Clin Pediatr (Phila) 2011;50(3):192–5.

23. MacMahon B. The continuing enigma of pyloric stenosis of infancy: a review. Epidemiology 2006; 17(2):195–201.

24. Iqbal CW, Rivard DC, Mortellaro VE, et al. Evaluation of ultrasonographic parameters in the diagnosis of pyloric stenosis relative to patient age and size. J Pediatr Surg 2012;47(8):1542–7.

25. Latzman JM, Levin TL, Nafday SM. Duodenal atresia: not always a double bubble. Pediatr Radiol 2014;44(8):1031–4.

26. Yoon CH, Goo HW, Kim EA, et al. Sonographic windsock sign of a duodenal web. Pediatr Radiol 2001;31(12):856–7.

27. Sizemore AW, Rabbani KZ, Ladd A, et al. Diagnostic performance of the upper gastrointestinal series in the evaluation of children with clinically suspected malrotation. Pediatr Radiol 2008;38(5):518–28.

28. Torres AM, Ziegler MM. Malrotation of the intestine. World J Surg 1993;17(3):326–31.

29. Strouse PJ. Disorders of intestinal rotation and fixation ("malrotation"). Pediatr Radiol 2004;34(11): 837–51.

30. Spigland N, Brandt ML, Yazbeck S. Malrotation presenting beyond the neonatal period. J Pediatr Surg 1990;25(11):1139–42.

31. Stephens LR, Donoghue V, Gillick J. Radiological versus clinical evidence of malrotation, a tortuous tale–10-year review. Eur J Pediatr Surg 2012; 22(3):238–42.

32. Marine MB, Karmazyn B. Imaging of malrotation in the neonate. Semin Ultrasound CT MR 2014;35(6): 555–70.

33. Newman B, Koppolu R, Murphy D, et al. Heterotaxy syndromes and abnormal bowel rotation. Pediatr Radiol 2014;44(5):542–51.

34. Applegate KE, Anderson JM, Klatte EC. Intestinal malrotation in children: a problem-solving approach to the upper gastrointestinal series. Radiographics 2006;26(5):1485–500.

35. Lin JN, Lou CC, Wang KL. Intestinal malrotation and midgut volvulus: a 15-year review. J Formos Med Assoc 1995;94(4):178–81.

36. Seashore JH, Touloukian RJ. Midgut volvulus. An ever-present threat. Arch Pediatr Adolesc Med 1994;148(1):43–6.

37. Tang V, Daneman A, Navarro OM, et al. Disorders of midgut rotation: making the correct diagnosis on UGI series in difficult cases. Pediatr Radiol 2013;43(9):1093–102.

38. Weinberger E, Winters WD, Liddell RM, et al. Sonographic diagnosis of intestinal malrotation in infants: importance of the relative positions of the superior mesenteric vein and artery. AJR Am J Roentgenol 1992;159(4):825–8.

39. Pracros JP, Sann L, Genin G, et al. Ultrasound diagnosis of midgut volvulus: the "whirlpool" sign. Pediatr Radiol 1992;22(1):18–20.

40. Quail MA. Question 2. Is Doppler ultrasound superior to upper gastrointestinal contrast study for the diagnosis of malrotation? Arch Dis Child 2011; 96(3):317–8.

41. Karmazyn B. Duodenum between the aorta and the SMA does not exclude malrotation. Pediatr Radiol 2013;43(1):121–2.

42. Ashcraft KW, Holcomb GW, Murphy JP, et al. Ashcraft's pediatric surgery. 6th edition. London; New York: Saunders/Elsevier; 2014.

43. Dalla Vecchia LK, Grosfeld JL, West KW, et al. Intestinal atresia and stenosis: a 25-year experience with 277 cases. Arch Surg 1998;133(5):490–6 [discussion: 6–7].

44. Verma A, Rattan KN, Yadav R. Neonatal intestinal obstruction: a 15 year experience in a tertiary care hospital. J Clin Diagn Res 2016;10(2):SC10–3.

45. Kumaran N, Shankar KR, Lloyd DA, et al. Trends in the management and outcome of jejuno-ileal atresia. Eur J Pediatr Surg 2002;12(3):163–7.

46. Best KE, Tennant PW, Addor MC, et al. Epidemiology of small intestinal atresia in Europe: a register-based study. Arch Dis Child Fetal Neonatal Ed 2012;97(5):F353–8.

47. Pediatric surgery. 4th edition. Chicago: Year Book Medical Publishers; 1986.

48. Grosfeld JL, Ballantine TV, Shoemaker R. Operative management of intestinal atresia and stenosis based on pathologic findings. J Pediatr Surg 1979;14(3):368–75.

49. Gosche JR, Vick L, Boulanger SC, et al. Midgut abnormalities. Surg Clin North Am 2006;86(2):285–99, viii.

50. Milla PJ. Cystic fibrosis: present and future. Digestion 1998;59(5):579–88.

51. Haber HP. Cystic fibrosis in children and young adults: findings on routine abdominal sonography. AJR Am J Roentgenol 2007;189(1):89–99.

52. Chang PT, Lee EY, Restrepo R, et al. Gastrointestinal tract filling defects in pediatric patients. AJR Am J Roentgenol 2014;203(1):W3–13.

53. Hernanz-Schulman M. Part 7. Duodenum and Small Intestine. Congenital and Neonatal Abnormalities. Cafey's Pediatric Diagnostic Imaging, Elsevier Saunders; 2013. p. 1057–106.

54. Copeland DR, St Peter SD, Sharp SW, et al. Diminishing role of contrast enema in simple meconium ileus. J Pediatr Surg 2009;44(11):2130–2.

55. Carlyle BE, Borowitz DS, Glick PL. A review of pathophysiology and management of fetuses and neonates with meconium ileus for the pediatric surgeon. J Pediatr Surg 2012;47(4):772–81.

56. Paradiso VF, Briganti V, Oriolo L, et al. Meconium obstruction in absence of cystic fibrosis in low birth weight infants: an emerging challenge from increasing survival. Ital J Pediatr 2011;37:55.

57. Emil S, Nguyen T, Sills J, et al. Meconium obstruction in extremely low-birth-weight neonates: guidelines for diagnosis and management. J Pediatr Surg 2004;39(5):731–7.

58. Shinohara T, Tsuda M, Koyama N. Management of meconium-related ileus in very low-birthweight infants. Pediatr Int 2007;49(5):641–4.

59. Berrocal T, Lamas M, Gutieerrez J, et al. Congenital anomalies of the small intestine, colon, and rectum. Radiographics 1999;19(5):1219–36.

60. Dirkes K, Crombleholme TM, Craigo SD, et al. The natural history of meconium peritonitis diagnosed in utero. J Pediatr Surg 1995;30(7):979–82.

61. Nam SH, Kim SC, Kim DY, et al. Experience with meconium peritonitis. J Pediatr Surg 2007;42(11): 1822–5.

62. Shyu MK, Shih JC, Lee CN, et al. Correlation of prenatal ultrasound and postnatal outcome in meconium peritonitis. Fetal Diagn Ther 2003; 18(4):255–61.

63. Chandler JC, Gauderer MW. The neonate with an abdominal mass. Pediatr Clin North Am 2004; 51(4):979–97, ix.

64. Wootton-Gorges SL, Thomas KB, Harned RK, et al. Giant cystic abdominal masses in children. Pediatr Radiol 2005;35(12):1277–88.

65. Eckoldt F, Heling KS, Woderich R, et al. Meconium peritonitis and pseudo-cyst formation: prenatal diagnosis and post-natal course. Prenat Diagn 2003;23(11):904–8.

66. Adams SD, Stanton MP. Malrotation and intestinal atresias. Early Hum Dev 2014;90(12):921–5.

67. Etensel B, Temir G, Karkiner A, et al. Atresia of the colon. J Pediatr Surg 2005;40(8):1258–68.

68. Williams MD, Burrington JD. Hirschsprung's disease complicating colon atresia. J Pediatr Surg 1993;28(4):637–9.

69. Cuenca AG, Ali AS, Kays DW, et al. "Pulling the plug"–management of meconium plug syndrome in neonates. J Surg Res 2012;175(2):e43–6.

70. Keckler SJ, St Peter SD, Spilde TL, et al. Current significance of meconium plug syndrome. J Pediatr Surg 2008;43(5):896–8.

71. Burge D, Drewett M. Meconium plug obstruction. Pediatr Surg Int 2004;20(2):108–10.

72. Blickman JG, Parker BR, Barnes PD. Pediatric radiology: the requisites. 3rd edition. Mosby; 2009.

73. Putnam LR, John SD, Greenfield SA, et al. The utility of the contrast enema in neonates with suspected Hirschsprung disease. J Pediatr Surg 2015;50(6):963–6.

74. Provenzale J, Nelson R, Vinson E. Duke radiology case review: imaging, differential diagnosis, and discussion. 2nd edition. LWW; 2011.

75. Cowles RA, Berdon WE, Holt PD, et al. Neonatal intestinal obstruction simulating meconium ileus in infants with long-segment intestinal aganglionosis: radiographic findings that prompt the need for rectal biopsy. Pediatr Radiol 2006;36(2):133–7.

76. Wijers CH, van Rooij IA, Marcelis CL, et al. Genetic and nongenetic etiology of nonsyndromic anorectal malformations: a systematic review. Birth Defects Res C Embryo Today 2014;102(4):382–400.

77. Alamo L, Meyrat BJ, Meuwly JY, et al. Anorectal malformations: finding the pathway out of the labyrinth. Radiographics 2013;33(2):491–512.

78. Levitt MA, Pena A. Anorectal malformations. Orphanet J Rare Dis 2007;2:33.

79. deVries PA, Pena A. Posterior sagittal anorectoplasty. J Pediatr Surg 1982;17(5):638–43.

80. Niedzielski JK. Invertography versus ultrasonography and distal colostography for the determination of bowel-skin distance in children with anorectal malformations. Eur J Pediatr Surg 2005;15(4): 262–7.

81. Puligandla PS, Nguyen LT, St-Vil D, et al. Gastrointestinal duplications. J Pediatr Surg 2003;38(5): 740–4.

82. Bentley JF, Smith JR. Developmental posterior enteric remnants and spinal malformations: the split notochord syndrome. Arch Dis Child 1960; 35:76–86.

83. Iyer CP, Mahour GH. Duplications of the alimentary tract in infants and children. J Pediatr Surg 1995; 30(9):1267–70.

84. Stern LE, Warner BW. Gastrointestinal duplications. Semin Pediatr Surg 2000;9(3):135–40.

85. Laje P, Flake AW, Adzick NS. Prenatal diagnosis and postnatal resection of intraabdominal enteric duplications. J Pediatr Surg 2010;45(7):1554–8.

86. Segal SR, Sherman NH, Rosenberg HK, et al. Ultrasonographic features of gastrointestinal duplications. J Ultrasound Med 1994;13(11):863–70.

87. Kangarloo H, Sample WF, Hansen G, et al. Ultrasonic evaluation of abdominal gastrointestinal tract duplication in children. Radiology 1979;131(1): 191–4.

88. Zani A, Pierro A. Necrotizing enterocolitis: controversies and challenges. F1000Res 2015;4. Available at: https://www.ncbi.nlm.nih.gov/pubmed/26918125.

89. Chen Y, Chang KT, Lian DW, et al. The role of ischemia in necrotizing enterocolitis. J Pediatr Surg 2016;51(8):1255–61.

90. Nowicki PT. Ischemia and necrotizing enterocolitis: where, when, and how. Semin Pediatr Surg 2005; 14(3):152–8.

91. Ballance WA, Dahms BB, Shenker N, et al. Pathology of neonatal necrotizing enterocolitis: a ten-year experience. J Pediatr 1990;117(1 Pt 2):S6–13.

92. Neu J, Walker WA. Necrotizing enterocolitis. N Engl J Med 2011;364(3):255–64.

93. Murthy K, Yanowitz TD, DiGeronimo R, et al. Short-term outcomes for preterm infants with surgical necrotizing enterocolitis. J Perinatol 2014;34(10): 736–40.

94. Bolisetty S, Lui K. Necrotizing enterocolitis in full-term neonates. J Paediatr Child Health 2001; 37(4):413–4.

95. Giannone PJ, Luce WA, Nankervis CA, et al. Necrotizing enterocolitis in neonates with congenital heart disease. Life Sci 2008;82(7–8):341–7.

96. Harrison AM, Davis S, Reid JR, et al. Neonates with hypoplastic left heart syndrome have ultrasound evidence of abnormal superior mesenteric artery perfusion before and after modified Norwood procedure. Pediatr Crit Care Med 2005;6(4):445–7.

97. Polin RA, Pollack PF, Barlow B, et al. Necrotizing enterocolitis in term infants. J Pediatr 1976;89(3): 460–2.

98. Dominguez KM, Moss RL. Necrotizing enterocolitis. Clin Perinatol 2012;39(2):387–401.

99. Kliegman RM, Fanaroff AA. Neonatal necrotizing enterocolitis: a nine-year experience. Am J Dis Child 1981;135(7):603–7.

100. Maayan-Metzger A, Itzchak A, Mazkereth R, et al. Necrotizing enterocolitis in full-term infants: case-control study and review of the literature. J Perinatol 2004;24(8):494–9.

101. Bell MJ, Ternberg JL, Feigin RD, et al. Neonatal necrotizing enterocolitis. Therapeutic decisions based upon clinical staging. Ann Surg 1978; 187(1):1–7.

102. Coursey CA, Hollingsworth CL, Wriston C, et al. Radiographic predictors of disease severity in neonates and infants with necrotizing enterocolitis. AJR Am J Roentgenol 2009;193(5):1408–13.

103. Kao SC, Smith WL, Franken EA Jr, et al. Contrast enema diagnosis of necrotizing enterocolitis. Pediatr Radiol 1992;22(2):115–7.

104. Maalouf EF, Fagbemi A, Duggan PJ, et al. Magnetic resonance imaging of intestinal necrosis in preterm infants. Pediatrics 2000;105(3 Pt 1): 510–4.

105. Coursey CA, Hollingsworth CL, Gaca AM, et al. Radiologists' agreement when using a 10-point scale to report abdominal radiographic findings of necrotizing enterocolitis in neonates and infants. AJR Am J Roentgenol 2008;191(1):190–7.

106. Daneman A, Woodward S, de Silva M. The radiology of neonatal necrotizing enterocolitis (NEC). A review of 47 cases and the literature. Pediatr Radiol 1978;7(2):70–7.

107. Wexler HA. The persistent loop sign in neonatal necrotizing enterocolitis: a new indication for surgical intervention? Radiology 1978;126(1):201–4.

108. He Y, Zhong Y, Yu J, et al. Ultrasonography and radiography findings predicted the need for surgery in patients with necrotising enterocolitis without pneumoperitoneum. Acta Paediatr 2016; 105(4):e151–5.

109. Buonomo C. The radiology of necrotizing enterocolitis. Radiol Clin North Am 1999;37(6):1187–98, vii.

110. Silva CT, Daneman A, Navarro OM, et al. Correlation of sonographic findings and outcome in necrotizing enterocolitis. Pediatr Radiol 2007; 37(3):274–82.

111. Faingold R, Daneman A, Tomlinson G, et al. Necrotizing enterocolitis: assessment of bowel viability with color doppler US. Radiology 2005;235(2): 587–94.

Pediatric Hepatobiliary Neoplasms
An Overview and Update

Ali Yikilmaz, MD[a],*, Michael George, MD, MFA[b],
Edward Y. Lee, MD, MPH[b]

KEYWORDS

- Children • Neoplasms • Liver • Radiology • Radiography • Ultrasonography
- Computed tomography • MR Imaging

KEY POINTS

- The most commonly encountered malignant tumors of the liver are hepatoblastoma in infants and young children and fibrolamellar carcinoma and hepatocellular carcinoma in older children.
- Infantile hepatic hemangioma is the most commonly encountered liver tumor with typical imaging findings in infants.
- Serum alpha-fetoprotein level is typically increased in children with hepatoblastoma and hepatocellular carcinoma.
- Rhabdomyosarcoma is the main malignant tumor involving the biliary tree in the pediatric population, and often presents as an intraductal mass with a grape-like or branching pattern.
- The most common site of origin of liver metastases in children with solid tumors is neuroblastoma, followed by Wilms tumor.

INTRODUCTION

Hepatobiliary neoplasms constitute a wide range of liver tumors in children (**Box 1**). Primary hepatic neoplasms account for 1% to 4% of all solid tumors of childhood with approximately two-thirds of the primary hepatic neoplasms being malignant (**Fig. 1**). The incidence rate of malignant primary hepatic neoplasms is 1.5 per 1 million annually, resulting in 100 to 150 new cases every year in the United States.[1–3] The most common cause of metastatic disease of the liver is neuroblastoma, followed by Wilms tumor.[4] Rhabdomyosarcoma arising from the biliary tree is rare, accounting for approximately 1% of all rhabdomyosarcomas in childhood. The age of the patient, underlying

hepatic disease, and laboratory tests are helpful when evaluating the imaging studies of children with hepatobiliary tumors (**Table 1**).

Recent advances in chemotherapy options, surgical approaches and transplant options for unresectable tumors, and collaboration between international pediatric oncology groups have refined the management of hepatobiliary neoplasm in pediatric patients. Accurate radiologic interpretation, correlated with supportive demographic data and laboratory findings, is critical to the diagnosis and proper treatment of hepatobiliary tumors in the pediatric population. This review article provides an overview and update on imaging strategy and characteristic imaging findings of hepatobiliary neoplasms in infants and children.

Disclosure: The authors have nothing to disclose.
[a] Department of Radiology, Goztepe Research and Training Hospital, Istanbul Medeniyet University, Dr. Erkin Street, Kadikoy, Istanbul 34722, Turkey; [b] Department of Radiology, Boston Children's Hospital, Harvard Medical School, 300 Longwood Avenue, Boston, MA 02115, USA
* Corresponding author.
E-mail addresses: dryikilmaz@yahoo.com; ali.yikilmaz@medeniyet.edu.tr

Radiol Clin N Am 55 (2017) 741–766
http://dx.doi.org/10.1016/j.rcl.2017.02.003

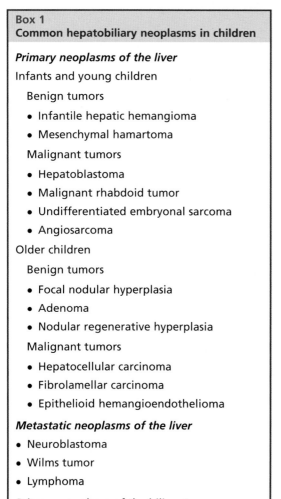

Box 1
Common hepatobiliary neoplasms in children

Primary neoplasms of the liver

Infants and young children

Benign tumors

- Infantile hepatic hemangioma
- Mesenchymal hamartoma

Malignant tumors

- Hepatoblastoma
- Malignant rhabdoid tumor
- Undifferentiated embryonal sarcoma
- Angiosarcoma

Older children

Benign tumors

- Focal nodular hyperplasia
- Adenoma
- Nodular regenerative hyperplasia

Malignant tumors

- Hepatocellular carcinoma
- Fibrolamellar carcinoma
- Epithelioid hemangioendothelioma

Metastatic neoplasms of the liver

- Neuroblastoma
- Wilms tumor
- Lymphoma

Primary neoplasm of the biliary tree

- Rhabdomyosarcoma

IMAGING EVALUATION STRATEGY

Various non-invasive imaging modalities are currently available to image tumors of the liver and biliary tract in children. Each imaging modality provides complementary information, which, when taken as a whole, allows the radiologist to diagnose and stage the tumor and determine the most effective course of management.

Ultrasonography (US) is usually the first imaging modality used to exclude a hepatobiliary mass in the pediatric population. If there is no mass in the liver on US, no further imaging is necessary. If a mass is found, then magnetic resonance (MR) imaging of the abdomen should be subsequently performed. Computed tomography (CT) of the abdomen should only be considered if MR imaging is not available or contraindicated. If the characterization of the mass yields a benign lesion, the stability of the lesion can be monitored by US or MR imaging. If the CT or MR imaging yields a malignant mass, CT of the chest should be performed to evaluate for the presence of metastatic lung disease. A biopsy of the primary liver tumor should then be completed in order to determine histopathologic diagnosis.[2]

IMAGING MODALITY AND TECHNIQUE
Radiography

Radiographs may provide useful information by providing a global view of the abdomen and excluding other potential causes for the patients' symptoms. They may demonstrate the extent of the large hepatobiliary tumors and their mass effect on adjacent intra-abdominal structures, guiding the investigation toward the organ of interest or additional modalities. Calcifications, when present

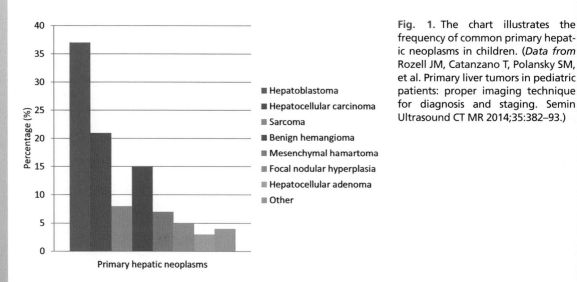

Fig. 1. The chart illustrates the frequency of common primary hepatic neoplasms in children. (*Data from* Rozell JM, Catanzano T, Polansky SM, et al. Primary liver tumors in pediatric patients: proper imaging technique for diagnosis and staging. Semin Ultrasound CT MR 2014;35:382–93.)

Primary hepatic neoplasms

- Hepatoblastoma
- Hepatocellular carcinoma
- Sarcoma
- Benign hemangioma
- Mesenchymal hamartoma
- Focal nodular hyperplasia
- Hepatocellular adenoma
- Other

Table 1
Overview of hepatobiliary neoplasms in children

Tumor Type	Presenting Age	Gender	Laboratory Findings	Typical Imaging Findings	Pearls and Pitfalls	What Referring Physicians Want to Know
IHH	• 0–8 wk • Not present at birth	F>>M	—	• Homogeneous, hypervascular mass on US, CT, and MR imaging • Peripheral enhancement during the arterial phase imaging with subsequent fill-in and homogeneous preservation of the contrast during delayed phases	Large tumors may not show a homogeneous enhancement because of lack of enhancement centrally	• Confirmation of diagnosis based on imaging features without a need of biopsy • Association of compartment syndrome or prominent arteriovenous shunting • Screening of the liver by US is necessary only when the number of cutaneous hemangiomas is 5 or more
Congenital hemangioma	Fully formed at birth	F = M	—	Similar to IHH; presence of calcification, heterogeneity, visible vessels, and ill-defined borders may help to differentiate from IHH	—	—
Mesenchymal hamartoma	• Antenatal • 0–2 y	M>F	—	• Large size • Mixed solid and cystic mass	Predominantly solid tumors may be misinterpreted as hepatoblastoma, whereas predominantly cystic tumors may be misinterpreted as congenital biliary cysts	• Mass effect on the adjacent structures especially when large • Conversion to undifferentiated embryonal sarcoma
FNH	2–5 y	F>>M	—	• Homogeneous mass with lobulated contours (no capsule) • Hypoechoic halo	Small lesions (<31 mm) may not show the characteristic US findings; therefore, an MR imaging study should	• Confirmation of diagnosis based on imaging features without a need of biopsy

(continued on next page)

Table 1
(continued)

Tumor Type	Presenting Age	Gender	Laboratory Findings	Typical Imaging Findings	Pearls and Pitfalls	What Referring Physicians Want to Know
				• Avid, homogeneous enhancement during the arterial phase without associated washout pattern • Enhancement during hepatocyte phase • Central scar • Dendritic or spoke-wheel vessel pattern on color Doppler US or CEUS • Feeding artery	be the diagnostic method • Unlike the central scar of fibrolamellar carcinoma, the scar is hypointense on T1-weighted MR images, hyperintense on T2-weighted MR images, enhances during portal venous phase images and delayed-phase images, and does not enhance during the hepatocyte phase images	• Differentiation from metastatic disease after completion of the chemotherapy, radiotherapy, or bone marrow transplant
Hepatic adenoma	Teenage	F>>M	—	—	A percutaneous biopsy should not be performed because of the potential risk of hemorrhage	• Malignant transformation to HCC • Association with many diseases, including glycogen storage disease • Genetic subgroups show distinct imaging findings
Hepatoblastoma	0–3 y	M>F	Marked increase of serum alpha-fetoprotein level	Heterogeneous mass with calcification	Imaging findings may be similar in transitional liver cell tumor, which carries features of both hepatoblastoma and HCC and reflects the continuum between these 2 tumors	Pre-treatment assessment of tumor extension (PRETEXT) system staging

Tumor	Age	Sex				
Malignant rhabdoid tumor	0–2 y	M = F	—	Aggressive behavior	—	—
Undifferentiated embryonal sarcoma	6–10 y	M = F	—	• Paradoxic cystic appearance of solid tumor on CT and MR imaging because of myxoid component • 18F-FDG uptake on PET/CT	US can confirm the solid tumor although it appears cystic on CT and MR imaging	—
Angiosarcoma	3 y	F>M	—	Multifocal areas of contrast pooling on CT, MR, and DSA	Imaging features of IHH and angiosarcoma may overlap	Conversion from IHH to angiosarcoma
HCC	>5 y	M>F	Marked increase of serum alpha-fetoprotein	—	Imaging findings may be similar in transitional liver cell tumor, which carries features of both hepatoblastoma and HCC and reflects the continuum between these 2 tumors	Pre-treatment assessment of tumor extension (PRETEXT) system staging
Fibrolamellar carcinoma	>10 y	M = F	—	No washout on dynamic CT or MR imaging	May resemble FNH; however: • Enhancement is more heterogeneous • Central scar is hypointense on both T1-weighted and T2-weighted MR images and does not enhance	Pre-treatment assessment of tumor extension (PRETEXT) system staging
Epithelioid hemangioendothelioma	>10 y	F>M	—	• Multifocal involvement • Retraction of the capsule • Lollipop sign • Target sign • Peripheral enhancement	Peripheral enhancement and target sign may cause misinterpretation of the lesions as metastasis	—
Biliary rhabdomyosarcoma	2–5 y	M>F	Increased level of conjugated bilirubin	Intraductal infiltrative mass showing grape-like or branching pattern	Should be differentiated from congenital biliary cysts by its solid nature	—

Abbreviations: CEUS, contrast-enhanced ultrasonography; CT, computed tomography; DSA, digital subtraction angiogram; F, female; FDG, fluorodeoxyglucose; FNH, focal nodular hyperplasia; HCC, hepatocellular carcinoma; IHH, infantile hepatic hemangioma; M, male; PRETEXT, Pretreatment Assessment of Tumor Extension; US, ultrasonography.

in hepatic neoplasms, may be detected on radiograph depending on their size and location.

Ultrasonography

US is usually the initial non-invasive imaging modality in the evaluation of a child with a known or suspected hepatobiliary tumor. US affords many advantages, such as lack of ionizing radiation, low cost, and availability. Contrast-enhanced US (CEUS) is currently emerging as a promising method to detect and characterize liver tumors.[5] Intraoperative US can delineate the tumor extension and may be helpful in the operative planning for hepatectomy.[6]

Computed Tomography

Previously, CT had been widely used for the characterization, staging, and surgical planning of hepatic tumors in the pediatric population. However, with recent advances in MR imaging, the diagnostic role of CT has been diminished. Radiation exposure is a significant limitation to CT, especially given the need for multiphasic studies and the increased radiosensitivity of children. Only when MRI is not available, CT becomes an acceptable substitute in the pediatric patients who requires characterization of hepatic neoplasms. For evaluation of lung metastasis from hepatic neoplasms, CT can effectively detect and monitor pulmonary nodules, and remains the gold-standard for the evaluation of metastatic lung disease.

For oral contrast used for CT imaging in pediatric patients with hepatic neoplasms, dilute iodine-based or barium-based contrast agent is the most commonly used oral contrast of choice, which can be administered by mouth or through a nasogastric tube if necessary. Iodine-based contrast agents are preferred in small children because of the risk of tracheobronchial aspiration. For the administration of intravenous contrast material, a nonionic, low-osmolar contrast agent with a concentration between 240 and 400 mg I/mL is preferred by the use of a power injector or hand injection depending on the size and stability of the intravenous catheter. The amount of contrast material is 2 mL/kg (up to a dose of 125 mL).[7]

For imaging liver tumors with CT, a dual-phase scanning during the arterial and portal venous phases (particularly for preoperative evaluation) or single phase scanning during the portal venous phase is recommended. The arterial phase can be acquired by using intravenous bolus tracking from diaphragm to iliac crest and portal venous phase from symphysis pubis to diaphragm. Because higher spatial resolution is needed in children due to their small body size, thinnest possible collimation allowing limited noise should be chosen depending on the vendor and the type of CT scanner. Automatic tube current modulation technique should be preferred in multidetector CT scanners which helps to lower the overall radiation dose.[8]

MR Imaging

MR imaging is currently the imaging modality of choice for the evaluation of hepatobiliary tumors in the pediatric population. Hardware and software advances as well as the introduction of hepatobiliary-specific contrast agents have significantly improved the efficacy of MR imaging with respect to the characterization, staging and assessment of resectability of the hepatobiliary neoplasms. Lack of ionizing radiation is the major advantage of MR imaging and allows for multiphase imaging assessment.

General anesthesia or sedation is typically required for children less than 5 years of age when MR imaging is performed for assessment of hepatic neoplasms. During the scanning, appropriate coil (cardiac, head, spinal, etc.) should be chosen according to the size of the pediatric patient. Many MR imaging protocols for the evaluation of liver tumors have been proposed.[2,9–11] A complete protocol for the imaging of liver tumors may include: 1) coronal T2-weighted echo-planar fast spin echo sequence and axial T2-weighted fast spin echo sequence with fat suppression for the detection of tumors, fluid, and edema; 2) axial T1-weighted fast spin echo sequence for the detection of fat and blood products; 3) axial T1-weighted sequence in-/opposed phase for the detection of intracellular fat; 4) axial diffusion-weighted MR imaging for detection of high cellularity in the mass; 5) axial 2D time of flight for the assessment of vasculature; 6) axial precontrast and postcontrast T1-weighted spoiled gradient echo in the arterial, portal venous, and delayed venous phases for dynamic evaluation of enhancement; 7) axial and coronal T1-weighted spoiled gradient echo sequence in the hepatocyte phase for the detection of hepatocyte function in the tumor; 8) and coronal T2-weighted 3D fast spin echo sequences for evaluation of the biliary tree as a cholangiogram.

The two most commonly used hepatobiliary-specific agents are gadoxetate disodium (Gd-EOB-DTPA) and gadobenate dimeglumine (Gd-BOPTA). The functioning hepatocytes take up these agents in varying degrees, which are then excreted in the bile. Gadolinium-based contrast agents are initially distributed in the extracellular space and are then taken up by the hepatocytes, which allows them to exhibit dual imaging capability. After the dynamic MR imaging study, hepatocyte phase imaging can be performed between 60 and 120 minutes of imaging using Gd-BOPTA and between 10 and 60 minutes using Gd-EOB-DTPA. The current recommended dose of Gd-BOPTA is 0.1 mmol/kg and 0.025 mmol/kg for Gd-EOB-DTPA.[12,13] The dynamic phase of Gd-BOPTA is identical to that of the extracellular contrast agents.[10] During the dynamic MR imaging of Gd-EOB-DTPA, however, the liver parenchyma starts enhancing 90 seconds after the injection and the vessels lose their signal during the delayed phases.[12,13]

SPECTRUM OF IMAGING FINDINGS
Benign Hepatic Tumors in Infants and Young Children

Infantile hepatic hemangiomas
The most commonly encountered hemangioma of the liver is infantile hepatic hemangioma (IHH), which is the counterpart of the soft tissue infantile hemangioma. These are benign tumors of vascular endothelium, and classified under the category of benign vascular tumors according to the updated classification of The International Society for the Study of Vascular Anomalies (ISSVA) in 2014.[14] There is increased risk of liver involvement if an infant has 5 or more cutaneous infantile hemangiomas.[15]

Infantile hemangiomas are typically not present at birth and present during the first 8 weeks of life. The lesions grow rapidly during early childhood (proliferative phase), gradually involute, and regress by the age of 5-9 years (involution phase). Half of all infantile hemangiomas completely involute by the age of 5 years, and 90% by the age of 9 years.[16,17]

Characteristic imaging features of IHH typically obviate tissue diagnosis (**Fig. 2**). Large lesions may show necrosis, intralesional hemorrhage, and thrombosis, and may cause heterogeneity of the mass. On US, focal lesions usually present as a hypoechoic spherical mass with well-defined contours and vascularity. The typical hyperechoic appearance of adult-type hemangiomas can be seen, but is less common in the pediatric population. The CT and MR features of IHH are similar to those of their cutaneous counterparts. The lesions appear hypodense on CT, hypointense on T1-weighted MR images, and hyperintense on T2-weighted MR images. The hyperintensity on T2-weighted MR images is less pronounced than that of venous malformations. On dynamic CT and MR images, there is peripheral enhancement during the arterial phase, followed by centripetal or uniform enhancement during the delayed phase. Flow voids may be seen due to arteriovenous shunts. Diffuse hemangiomatosis is characterized with extensive involvement of the liver

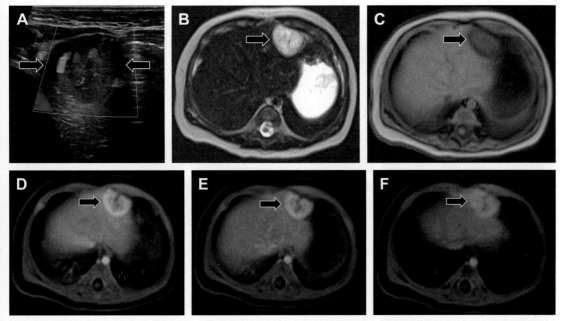

Fig. 2. Infantile hemangioma in a 6-month-old girl. (*A*) There is a hyperechoic, solid mass (*arrows*) in the left lobe of the liver with prominent internal vascularity on color Doppler ultrasonography. (*B*) The mass (*arrow*) is hyperintense on T2-weighted MR image but not as high as fluid signal. (*C*) The lesion (*arrow*) is hypointense on T1-weighted MR image, the periphery being darker as a rim. The hepatic mass (*arrow*) shows avid peripheral enhancement during the arterial phase MR image (*D*), slightly advanced centripetal enhancement (*arrow*) during the portal venous phase MR image (*E*), and persistent enhancement during delayed-phase MR image (4 minutes) with advanced central enhancement. However, there is still a small nonenhancing core of the mass (*arrow*), likely representing scar tissue (*F*). (*Courtesy of* Selim Doganay, MD, Turkey.)

associated with massive hepatomegaly and secondary mass effect. The arteriovenous shunts in diffuse hemangiomatosis or large IHHs may be hemodynamically significant, with subsequent narrowing of the aorta below the level of the celiac truncus.[18–20]

Congenital hemangiomas of the liver and IHH may have overlapping clinical and pathologic features (**Fig. 3**). Congenital hemangiomas are less infrequent than IHHs and, unlike IHHs, they lack glucose transferase-1 protein on histology. They are classified into three by the most recent ISSVA classification: noninvoluting congenital hemangioma (NICH), rapidly involuting congenital hemangioma (RICH), and partially involuting congenital hemangioma (PICH). They are usually considered as RICH when they involve the liver. All congenital forms are present at birth and fully grown and they do not show further growth after birth. As their nomenclature implies, NICH do not show any regression, whereas RICH regresses before the age of 14 months and PICH regresses rapidly with residual tumor.[21]

The radiological features of IHH and congenital hemangiomas of the liver are similar and an imaging-based differentiation may not be possible. However, presence of calcification, heterogeneity, visible vessels, and ill-defined borders favor the diagnosis of congenital hemangioma over IHH.[22]

Mesenchymal hamartoma

Mesenchymal hamartomas of the liver are the second most common benign tumors in childhood. They typically present before 2 years of age (85% before 3 years of age and 95% before 5 years of age); however, some of the affected patients may be diagnosed in the antenatal or perinatal period.[1,23,24] Children with mesenchymal hamartoma usually present with abdominal distension or a palpable mass.

Imaging typically demonstrates a large mass (up to 30 cm) with variable solid (stromal) and cystic components (**Fig. 4**). The cysts appear anechoic on US, whereas the solid portions appear hyperechoic. Intraoperative aspiration of the cystic components by US guidance improves the surgical technique by decreasing the size of the tumor. On CT, demonstration of a multilocular low-attenuation cystic mass with enhancing septae and solid component is typical. Calcification is rare, and peripheral if present. On MR imaging, the cystic components appear hypointense on T1-weighted MR images

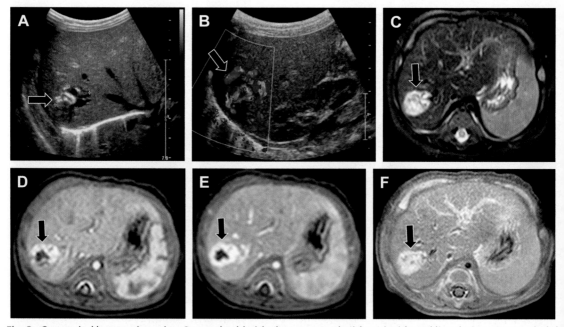

Fig. 3. Congenital hemangioma in a 2-month-old girl who presented with an incidental liver lesion. Gray-scale (*A*) and color Doppler (*B*) ultrasonography images demonstrate a hypervascular mass (*arrow*) in the right lobe of the liver consisting of gross calcification. (*C*) The mass (*arrow*) is heterogeneously hyperintense on T2-weighted MR images due to flow voids and calcification. On dynamic series, the lesion (*arrow*) shows strong peripheral enhancement during the arterial phase (*D*), centripetal fill-in during the portal venous phase (*E*), and homogeneous enhancement during the delayed-phase (*F*).

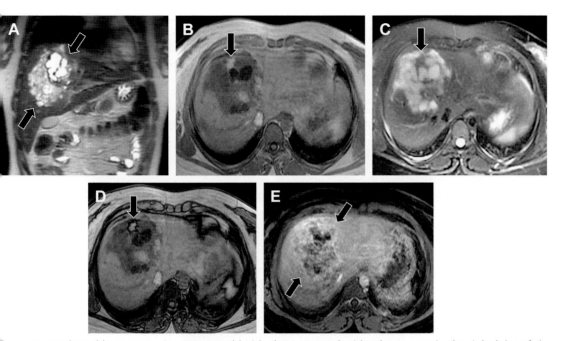

Fig. 4. Mesenchymal hamartoma in a 15-year-old girl who presented with a large mass in the right lobe of the liver. (*A*) The lesion (*arrows*) appears as a complex mass with mixed solid and cystic components on coronal T2-weighted MR image. (*B*) The lesion is generally hypointense on T1-weighted gradient in-phase MR image associated with internal hyperintense foci representing gross fat (*arrow*). (*C*) The hyperintense focus seen in (*B*) demonstrates signal loss on fat-saturated T2-weighted MR image consistent with gross fat (*arrow*). (*D*) Typical rimlike signal loss around the focus of fat (*arrow*) is seen on out-phase image. (*E*) There is heterogeneous enhancement of the mass (*arrows*) after gadolinium administration.

and hyperintense on T2-weighted MR images which has been called a Swiss cheese appearance (**Fig. 5**). As on CT, the solid component and septae show mild contrast enhancement on MR imaging.[20,24,25]

Malignant Hepatic Tumors in Infants and Young Children

Hepatoblastoma

Hepatoblastoma is the most common malignant primary hepatic tumor in childhood. The majority of hepatoblastomas occur in the first 2 years of life. They present with a rapidly growing abdominal mass, hepatomegaly, pain, anorexia, and weight loss. Precocious puberty is a rare presentation of pediatric patients with hepatoblastoma which is secondary to secretion of chorionic gonadotropins. They are most commonly sporadic, but are also associated with Li-Fraumeni syndrome, Beckwith-Wiedemann syndrome, type 1a glycogen storage disease, trisomy 18, and familial adenomatous polyposis.[2,17,20]

Although not specific, increased serum alpha-fetoprotein level is the cardinal tumor marker in pediatric patients with hepatoblastoma. Approximately, 90% of pediatric patients with hepatoblastoma present with an elevation of the serum alpha-fetoprotein. Although serum alpha-fetoprotein may be elevated to some degree in other liver tumors, they do not exceed the level of 10^4 ng/dL (except hepatocellular carcinoma [HCC]). Therefore, marked increase (>10^4 ng/dL) of the serum alpha-fetoprotein level narrows the differential diagnosis to hepatoblastoma and HCC only.[17]

On imaging, there is usually a large (>12 cm in 80% of cases), heterogeneous mass with well-defined contours (**Fig. 6**).[20] However, multifocal or infiltrative involvement may also be seen (**Fig. 7**). Heterogeneity is more common in mixed-type tumors. US usually demonstrates a heterogeneous mass on a background of normal-appearing liver parenchyma. On CT, the mass appears hypodense and shows heterogeneous contrast enhancement which may be accompanied with hyperdense areas of hemorrhage and calcification (50%). When present, calcifications usually appear coarse and chunky.[26] On MR imaging, a typical hepatoblastoma appears hypointense on T1-weighted MR images, and heterogeneously hyperintense on T2-weighted MR images. Hemorrhage may appear as focal areas of T1 hyperintensity. After

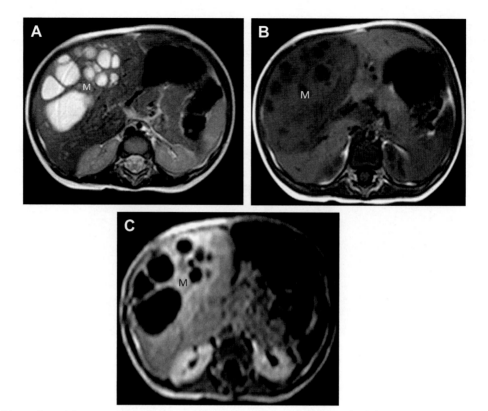

Fig. 5. Mesenchymal hamartoma in an 11-month-old boy who presented with abdominal distention. There is a large, mixed solid and multicystic mass (M) occupying the right lobe of the liver. The solid portion appears slightly hyperintense on T2-weighted MR image (A), hypointense on T1-weighted MR image (B) compared to the liver parenchyma, and slightly enhances during the portal venous phase (C). Note the typical Swiss cheese appearance of the hepatic mesenchymal hamartoma.

gadolinium injection, hepatoblastoma usually shows avid contrast enhancement and may have focal nonenhancing areas representing tumor necrosis. Hepatoblastoma typically does not show contrast enhancement during the hepatobiliary phase; however, a few cases of hepatoblastoma were reported to show enhancement during the hepatobiliary phase, suggesting the presence of functioning hepatocytes in the tumor.[26–28]

The International Childhood Liver Tumor Strategy Group (SIOPEL) designed the Pretreatment Assessment of Tumor Extension (PRETEXT) system for staging and risk stratification in liver tumors, particularly hepatoblastoma and HCC. The PRETEXT classification is based on the well-known Couinaud system of segmentation of the liver. The liver segments are grouped into 4 sections: segments 2 and 3 (left lateral section), segments 4a and 4b (left medial section), segments 5 and 8 (right anterior section), and segments 6 and 7 (right posterior section).

The PRETEXT classification is defined as: 1) PRETEXT I: one section is involved and three adjoining sections are free; 2) PRETEXT II: one or two sections are involved, but two adjoining sections are free; PRETEXT III: two or three sections are involved, and no two adjoining sections are free; and 4) PRETEXT IV: all four sections are involved. The stage of the pediatric patients with hepatoblastoma correlates closely with prognosis and survival.[28,29]

Malignant rhabdoid tumor
Similar to its counterparts in central nervous system and kidney, malignant rhabdoid tumor (MRT) of the liver is a highly aggressive tumor of childhood with a high mortality. Pediatric patients with MRT of the liver usually present with a rapidly growing abdominal mass. The mean age for MRT at diagnosis is 2 years, with a range of 0 to 324 months.[30–32]

There are no specific imaging findings of MRT of the liver because of the rarity of the disease. On imaging, there is usually a heterogeneous solid mass, sometimes accompanied by cystic components. Periportal hypodensity (periportal collar sign), periportal lymphadenopathy, and calcification may be seen on CT. There may be multiple

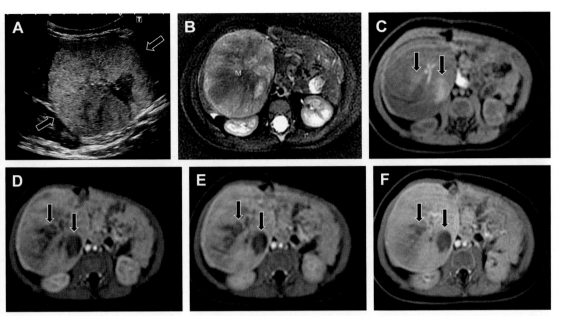

Fig. 6. A 7-month-old girl who presented with a palpable mass in the right lower quadrant and increased alpha-fetoprotein levels (>20,000 ng/mL). (*A*) There is a large, heterogeneous, solid, exophytic mass (*arrows*) originating from segments 5 and 6 of the liver on sagittal ultrasonography image. (*B*) The mass (M) is heterogeneous with mixed signal on axial T2-weighted fat-saturated MR image. On precontrast (*C*), arterial phase (*D*), portal venous phase (*E*), and delayed phase (5 minutes) (*F*) T1-weighted 3D gradient-echo images, the lesion (*arrows*) appears heterogeneous with central and peripheral focal areas of nonenhancing T1-hyperintense areas in the tumor in keeping with areas of necrosis with high protein content. The tumor shows strong contrast enhancement which starts during the arterial phase and increases gradually during the dynamic series until the delayed phase.

masses in the liver at the time of diagnosis. The most common site of metastasis is the lung.[30–32]

Undifferentiated embryonal sarcoma

Undifferentiated embryonal sarcoma (UES) is the third most common hepatic malignancy of mesenchymal origin, accounting for 6% of all pediatric liver tumors and 10–15% of all malignant pediatric liver tumors. UES of the liver is thought to be the malignant counterpart of mesenchymal hamartoma based on documentation of malignant degeneration.[1,25]

UES typically occurs in children 6–10 years of age. No gender predilection is described. Abdominal pain, discomfort, and weight loss are the most common symptoms in affected pediatric patients. The prognosis is poor due to the aggressive behavior of the tumor.[33]

UES of the liver is usually a single and well-circumscribed lesion, mainly due to a fibrous pseudocapsule formed by compression of the liver parenchyma. It consists of both solid and cystic components. The solid component appears sarcomatoid with a myxoid background.[33] On US, there is usually a large (>10 cm at diagnosis) heterogeneous solid mass. However, paradoxically, UES typically appears as a cystic

mass on CT and MR imaging because of its myxoid stroma which is a similar imaging feature of myxoid sarcoma and synovial sarcoma. On MR imaging, the signal intensity is similar to that of fluid as being hypointense on T1-weighted MR images and hyperintense on T2-weighted MR images. There is mild enhancement of the solid portions and in the periphery of the lesion, which becomes more pronounced during the delayed phases.[34] Peripheral contrast enhancement reflects the presence of the pseudocapsule formation. 18F-fluorodeoxyglucose (FDG) PET/CT can demonstrate pathologic tumor necrosis and is very helpful in monitoring treatment response.[35]

Angiosarcoma

Angiosarcoma is a high-grade malignant tumor of the liver derived from endothelial cells. They are more common in adults; however, the same type of tumor occurs rarely in children. The mean presenting age is 3 years (range, 2 months to 15 years). The prognosis is poor with a survival of 6 months to 2 years after initial diagnosis.[36] Although IHH is known to be a safe tumor, malignant transformation of IHH to angiosarcoma has been documented in the literature.[37,38]

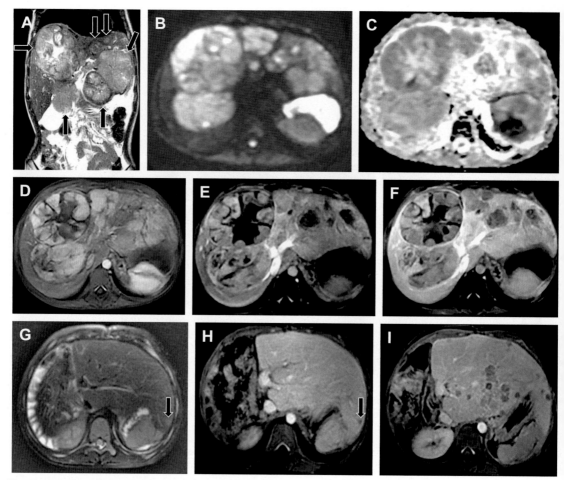

Fig. 7. Multifocal hepatoblastoma in a 7-year-old boy who presented with increased serum alpha-fetoprotein levels and multiple liver masses. There are multiple, heterogeneous, hyperintense, masses (*arrows*) in varying degrees diffusely involving the liver on coronal T2-weighted MR images (*A*) and showing restricted diffusion on diffusion-weighted imaging (*B*) and apparent diffusion coefficient map (*C*) MR images. The lesions show avid heterogeneous enhancement during the arterial phase (*D*), and partial washout during the portal venous (*E*) and delayed venous phases (*F*). Large nonenhancing area, likely representing necrosis, becomes more evident during the venous phases. An allogenic liver transplant from the mother was performed a few weeks after the MR imaging study. The patient showed recovery for the following 5 months, but then presented with increased serum alpha-protein levels and repeated dedicated ultrasonography studies did not reveal any mass in the liver or in the abdomen. Therefore, an MR imaging study was performed. At MR imaging, a single 5-mm nodule (*arrow*) was detected in the periphery of the liver as hyperintense on axial fat-saturated T2-weighted MR images (*G*) and nonenhancing on postcontrast MR images (*H*). (*I*) Follow-up MR imaging after 2 months demonstrates multiple additional nodules in the allograft liver during portal venous phase images.

The imaging findings of angiosarcoma in children have been reported anecdotally. Angiosarcomas may present as a large solitary mass, multiple nodules, a mixed pattern of dominant mass with nodules, or as a diffuse infiltrating micronodular tumor. Gray-scale US findings are nonspecific; however, on CEUS, there is characteristic peripheral irregular rimlike enhancement during the arterial phase, which decreases during the portal venous phase, and washes out completely during the delayed phase.[39] On CT, the lesion appears hypodense; areas of increased density typically represent hemorrhage. On MR imaging, the tumor is usually hypointense on T1-weighted MR images and hyperintense on T2-weighted MR images. Hemorrhage within the tumor may appear hyperintense on T1-weighted MR images. Both dynamic MR imaging and CT demonstrate heterogeneous enhancement during the arterial phase which progresses during delayed phases. Catheter angiogram findings reflect the changes on dynamic studies; focal areas of contrast pooling may be seen within the lesions.[40]

Benign Hepatic Tumors in Older Children

Focal nodular hyperplasia

Focal nodular hyperplasia (FNH) is a rare tumor which is characterized by normally functioning hepatocytes with disorganized biliary ducts. It comprises 2% of all primary hepatic tumors in children. Most FNH occur between 2–5 years of age, although it can occur at any age. There is a 5 to 8-fold female predominance. Affected patients are typically asymptomatic, and diagnosed during the work-up of other clinical conditions.[1,20,25]

It is widely accepted that FNHs develop in response to increased blood flow due to an underlying congenital vascular malformation or vascular injury. The occurrence of FNH after completion of chemotherapy, radiotherapy, or bone marrow transplant for other malignancy is well documented. The incidence of FNH in these pediatric patients is 78% (225-fold), whereas it is only 0.45% in healthy children.[41] In two-thirds of these cases, the lesions are solitary, however, multiple FNH lesions and association with other liver tumors may also occur. Tumor size varies from a few millimeters to more than 20 cm.[41]

The majority of FNHs appear hypoechoic on US; however, they may be isoechoic and hyperechoic.[42] Delineation of isoechoic tumors may be difficult; in this case, recognizing indirect signs of compression adjacent to the mass are helpful clues for the diagnosis. A hypoechoic halo is present in 32% of cases.[43] The tumor is supplied by the hepatic arterial blood and drains into hepatic veins independent of portal vasculature. On color-coded Doppler US and CEUS, demonstration of the enlarged central feeding artery and the draining veins in the periphery of the lesion is typical. Multiple centrifugal arteries may demonstrate a dendritic or spoke-wheel pattern on both color-coded US and CEUS. The CEUS is highly specific for the diagnosis of FNH, with good interobserver agreement; however, its diagnostic sensitivity is much better when the tumor size is below 31 mm.[42,44,45] On spectral Doppler US imaging, there is low-resistance flow within FNHs.

On CT, there is typically avid enhancement of the mass during the arterial phase and the enhancement persists during portal venous phase and delayed phase as the mass becomes isodense with the adjacent liver parenchyma. Enlarged central feeding arteries may be demonstrated during the arterial phase (Fig. 8).

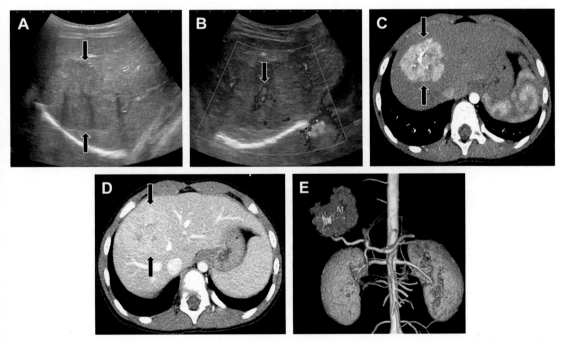

Fig. 8. Focal nodular hyperplasia in a 4-year-old girl. (A) Ultrasonography of the liver shows a slightly hypoechoic mass with lobulated contours (arrows). (B) On Doppler ultrasonography, there is vascularity in the center of the mass (arrow). On CT, the mass (arrows) shows avid heterogeneous enhancement during the arterial phase associated with central feeding arteries (C) and continues to show a more homogeneous enhancement during the portal venous phase becoming isodense with the parenchyma of the liver (D). (E) 3D volume-rendered CT angiogram shows the hypervascular tumor associated with central feeding artery originating from the hepatic artery.

MR imaging is a problem-solving method for detecting and characterizing FNH. Typical MR imaging findings of FNH include homogeneity, signal intensity similar to that of the liver, absence of capsule (lobulated contours), presence of central scar, and enhancement during the hepatocyte phase.[46,47] FNH appears isointense to slightly hypointense on T1-weighted and T2-weighted MR images, and enhances homogeneously. On dynamic MR imaging, the lesion enhances strongly during the arterial phase and early portal venous phase, becomes isointense to slightly hyperintense compared to the adjacent liver parenchyma during the late portal venous and delayed phase without showing a wash-out pattern (**Fig. 9**). Enhancement during the hepatocyte phase using Gd-EOB-DTPA or Gd-BOPTA is a characteristic feature of FNH that can reliably differentiate FNH from other benign and malignant tumors of the liver (**Fig. 10**). More than 95% of the FNHs show strong contrast enhancement during the arterial phase and more than 90% demonstrate enhancement during the hepatobiliary phase.[48]

A central scar is seen in 80% of the cases on MR imaging, and is typically hypointense on T1-weighted MR images and hyperintense on T2-weighted MR images. The scar enhances during the portal venous phase and delayed phases using extracellular contrast agents and conversely does not enhance during the hepatocyte phase using hepatocyte specific contrast agents.[47]

Hepatic adenoma

Hepatic adenoma is a rare benign tumor in childhood, accounting for 2–4% of all liver tumors. It is much more common in adults with the typical presentation in healthy young women with a history of oral contraceptives. In children, it is most commonly encountered in the teenage period with an 8 to 10-fold female dominance; however, it can occur at any age, including perinatal period.[49] The size of the lesion varies from a few centimeters to 16 cm.[50]

Hepatic adenoma may occur in healthy children or in association with precocious puberty, Fanconi anemia, glycogen storage diseases types 1 and 3, familial adenomatous polyposis coli, type 1 diabetes mellitus, tyrosinemia, and anabolic steroid use.[51] Although most of the affected pediatric patients are asymptomatic, they may present with rupture and intraperitoneal bleeding. Although rare, malignant transformation to HCC is another important potential complication.

US findings of hepatic adenoma are nonspecific and the lesion usually appears as a single or multiple heterogeneous mass depending on the presence of fat, hemorrhage, and necrosis. Hepatic adenoma is usually hypodense on CT because of the fat content; however, areas of hemorrhage appear hyperdense.[34] On MR imaging, the lesion appears isointense to slightly

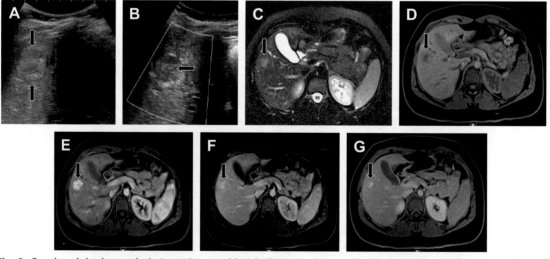

Fig. 9. Focal nodular hyperplasia in a 13-year-old girl. There is a hyperechoic heterogeneous focal mass (*arrows*) in the right lobe of the liver on axial ultrasonography images (*A*) associated with central vascularity on Doppler ultrasonography (*arrow*) (*B*). The mass (*arrow*) appears hyperintense on T2-weighted MR images (*C*) and hypointense on T1-weighted MR images (*D*). After injection of intravenous extracellular contrast material, the lesion (*arrow*) shows strong enhancement during the arterial phase (*E*) associated with subsequent gradual loss of enhancement during the portal venous (*F*) and delayed (*G*) phases where the lesion becomes isointense to the adjacent liver parenchyma. There is a T1-hypointense, T2-hyperintense central scar which does not enhance during the arterial phase and progressively enhances during the portal venous (*F*) and delayed phases (*G*).

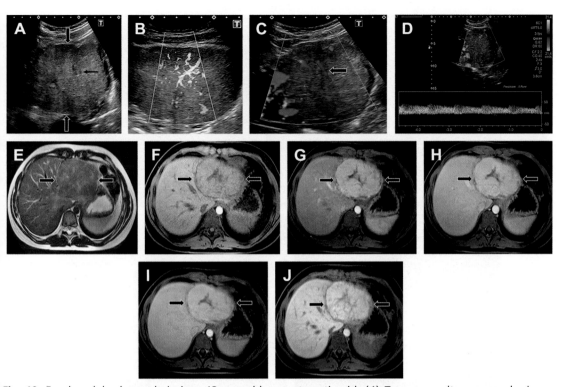

Fig. 10. Focal nodular hyperplasia in a 13-year-old asymptomatic girl. (*A*) Transverse ultrasonography image shows a large, heterogeneous, hyperechoic mass (*thick arrows*) with well-defined lobulated contours and hypoechoic central scar (*thin arrow*) involving the left lobe of the liver. (*B*) On color Doppler ultrasonography, there is dentritic vascularity in the mass. There is a prominent central feeding artery (*arrow*) on color Doppler ultrasonography image (*C*), which shows a low-resistance flow pattern (*D*). The lesion (*arrows*) is isointense on T2-weighted (*E*) and T1-weighted (*F*) MR images associated with a hypointense central scar on T1-weighted MR image. After intravenous Gd-EOB-DTPA injection, the lesion (*arrows*) shows avid enhancement during the arterial phase (*G*), and keeps the enhancement during the transient phases where the enhancement becomes similar to that of the liver (*H, I*). (*J*) There is persistent enhancement of the lesion (*arrows*) during the hepatobiliary phase (fifteenth minute). No enhancement is seen in the central scar with EOB-DTPA injection during the entire study unlike extracellular contrast agents.

hyperintense on T1-weighted sequences, and hyperintense on T2-weighted sequences, with moderate to avid enhancement. The enhancement may continue (inflammatory subtype) or may not continue (hepatocyte nuclear factor 1 alpha mutated type) during the portal venous phase and delayed phase.[9]

Nodular regenerative hyperplasia

Nodular regenerative hyperplasia of the liver is a benign proliferative entity characterized by multiple nodules varying from a few millimeters to several centimeters. There is typically no underlying cirrhotic liver disease or fibrosis. Nodular regenerative hyperplasia is associated with many clinical conditions, including lymphoproliferative disease, autoimmune disorders, collagen vascular disease, portal hypertension, biliary atresia, and Budd-Chiari syndrome.[52]

The imaging findings of nodular regenerative hyperplasia are nonspecific. On US, multiple hypoechoic and isoechoic nodules in varying sizes are seen on the background of homogeneous liver parenchyma (**Fig. 11**). On CT, small hepatic nodules may not be detected. They usually appear hypodense and do not enhance; however, isodense enhancement compared to the liver parenchyma in the portal venous phase may also be seen.[53,54] On MR imaging, the lesions appear hyperintense on T1-weighted MR images and isointense to hypointense on T2-weighted MR images. The enhancement pattern of hepatic nodular regenerative hyperplasia is variable.[9,54]

Malignant Hepatic Tumors in Older Children

Hepatocellular carcinoma

HCC is the second most common primary malignant tumor of the liver in childhood. It should be

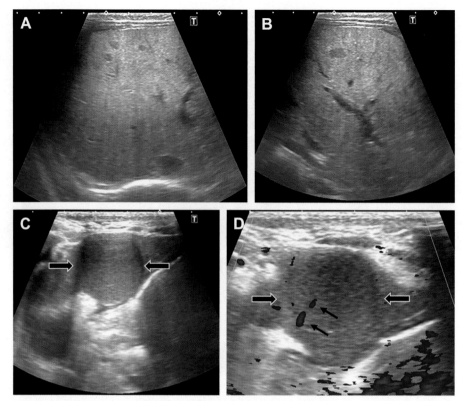

Fig. 11. Regenerative nodular hyperplasia in a 3-month-old boy who presented with bone marrow suppression, hepatosplenomegaly, and ascites. There are multiple isoechoic to hypoechoic nodular masses in varying sizes involving the liver diffusely on axial (*A*) and sagittal (*B*) ultrasonography images. The largest mass (*thick arrows*) appears as an ovoid mass with well-defined contours in the left lobe of the liver (*C*) and shows central vascularity (*thin arrows*) on color Doppler ultrasonography image (*D*).

differentiated from fibrolamellar carcinoma. HCC occurs much less frequently in children than in adults, with a prevalence of 0.5–1 cases per 1 million in Western countries.[1,25] HCC typically affects children over 10 years of age without any gender predilection. The age distribution is different from hepatoblastoma, which typically affects children less than 5 years of age. Predisposing factors include biliary atresia, cholestatic syndromes, hemochromatosis, hereditary tyrosinemia, glycogen storage disorders, Wilson's disease, and hepatitis B infection. Unlike in adults, cirrhosis is not a major predisposing factor. Serum alpha-fetoprotein levels are elevated in 55–65% of the cases.[55] Affected children usually present with an abdominal mass, constitutional symptoms, and abdominal pain.[17]

The appearance of HCC in children is similar to their adult counterpart. They may occur as a solitary mass, multifocal or diffusely infiltrative. HCC may appear homogeneous or heterogeneous depending on the presence of necrosis, hemorrhage, calcification, and fat. US findings are nonspecific; a heterogeneous mass with calcification may be seen (**Fig. 12**). On CT, the mass is usually hypodense or isodense with well-defined or ill-defined contours and may contain calcification (40%).[56] Early arterial enhancement and rapid wash-out is typical for HCC on dynamic CT and MR imaging studies. A capsule may be demonstrated during delayed phases. Vascular invasion including portal vein, hepatic veins, hepatic artery, and inferior vena cava may be demonstrated on CT.[57] On MR imaging, the appearance on T1-weighted imaging is variable; it may be hypointense, isointense, or hyperintense. Associated intratumoral fat and hemorrhage may be seen as focal areas of T1 hyperintensity. The lesion appears hyperintense on T2-weighted MR images and typically shows avid contrast enhancement during the arterial phase, with subsequent wash-out during the portal venous phase.[26,58]

Fibrolamellar carcinoma

Fibrolamellar carcinoma is a rare variant of HCC which primarily affects adolescents and young

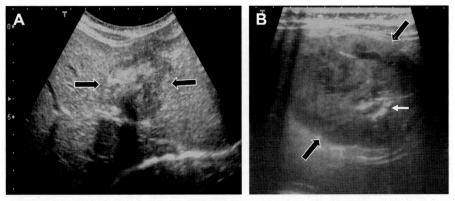

Fig. 12. Hepatocellular carcinoma in an 11-year-old boy with no known predisposing liver disease. A solid, heterogeneous mass (*black arrows*) with well-defined borders is seen at the junction of the right and left lobe of the liver on axial ultrasonography images by using a convex probe (*A*) and a linear probe (*B*). There is hyperechoic eccentric internal calcification (*white arrow*) with acoustic shadowing.

adults. The clinical, laboratory, and imaging features of fibrolamellar carcinoma are distinct from HCC. Unlike classic HCC, there is usually no predisposing factor such as cirrhosis or viral hepatitis in fibrolamellar carcinoma. The exact etiology is unknown.[25,59] Affected pediatric patients present with abdominal pain or palpable mass; however, rarely, gynecomastia and jaundice may be the presenting signs.[26] Serum alpha-fetoprotein levels are almost always within normal limits in patients with fibrolamellar carcinoma.

Unlike many other primary liver tumors, there is a left lobe predilection. There is usually a single, large mass with well-defined contours on imaging. On US, the lesion appears heterogeneous; associated calcification may be seen as hyperechoic foci with posterior acoustic shadowing. A central scar may be seen as a hyperechoic focus. On CT, there is usually a heterogeneous, hypodense mass with lobulated contours; calcification accompanies 35–68% of cases (**Fig. 13**).[60] The lesion enhances heterogeneously during the arterial phase and shows persistent enhancement during the portal venous and delayed phases close to liver parenchyma and becomes more homogeneous. This enhancement pattern is different than HCC where there is rapid wash-out during the venous phases; however, overlap of imaging features may occur between these two tumors. The lesion is usually isointense or hypointense on T1-weighted MR images and hyperintense on T2-weighted MR images, and shows avid contrast enhancement during the arterial phase with variable enhancement during the portal venous phase. The central scar is usually hypointense on both T1-weighted and

T2-weighted MR images and does not enhance unlike the scar of FNH (**Fig. 14**).[61]

Epithelioid hemangioendothelioma

Epithelioid hemangioendothelioma is an epithelial liver tumor classified under the category of malignant vascular tumors in the latest ISSVA classification.[14] Epithelioid hemangioendothelioma occurs almost exclusively in young adults, with a female predominance; children are only rarely affected. The most common clinical presentations are right upper quadrant pain, hepatomegaly, and weight loss; however, 25% of the affected patients are asymptomatic.[62]

On imaging, epithelioid hemangioendothelioma most often appears as multiple discrete nodules ranging from 0.5 cm to 12 cm, or as confluent masses with a tendency to coalesce. Peripheral lesions may cause flattening or retraction of the liver capsule in up to 69% of the cases. Compensatory hypertrophy of the unaffected liver may also be seen.[26]

On US, epithelioid hemangioendothelioma appears isoechoic or hypoechoic with or without a hypoechoic rim (**Fig. 15**). Association of hypoechoic rim may cause misinterpretation of the lesions as metastatic disease. On CEUS, most lesions show rimlike enhancement during the arterial phase with wash-out during the portal venous and delayed phases, which is a nonspecific sign of malignancy.[63]

On CT, epithelioid hemangioendothelioma demonstrate central hypodensity and nonenhancement due to presence of myxoid and hyalinized stroma or necrosis (**Fig. 16**). There is peripheral enhancement during the arterial phase corresponding to the hyperemia on pathology. During the portal

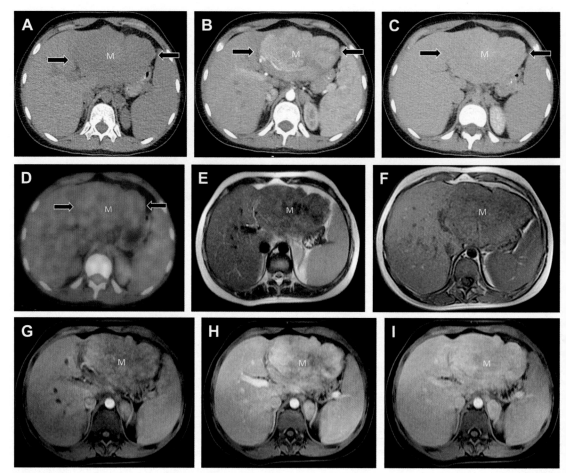

Fig. 13. Fibrolamellar carcinoma in a 15-year-old girl who presented with abdominal distension and pain. (*A*) There is a large hypoattenuating mass (M and *arrows*) occupying the left lobe of the liver with well-defined lobulated contours (*arrows*) on precontrast CT image. The mass (M and *arrows*) enhances heterogeneously during the arterial phase (*B*) and becomes isodense with the liver parenchyma during the delayed phase (*C*). (*D*) There is no FDG uptake on PET/CT image. The mass (M) is generally isointense with the liver parenchyma on T2-weighted MR images consisting of internal hypointense foci (*E*) and slightly hypointense on T1-weighted MR images (*F*). The mass (M) enhances heterogeneously during the arterial phase (*G*), shows progressive enhancement during the portal venous phase (*H*), and becomes isointense with the liver parenchyma during the delayed phase (*I*). There is no wash-out enhancement pattern. (*Courtesy of* Selim Doganay, MD, Turkey.)

venous and delayed phases, the lesion may show progressive centripetal enhancement; however, residual nonenhancing areas may persist. This central hypoenhancement and peripheral hyperenhancement may appear targetoid on CT. On MR imaging, the lesion appears hypointense on T1-weighted MR images and hyperintense on T2-weighted MR images. The central myxoid and hyalinized stroma may appear more hypointense on T1-weighted MR images and more hyperintense on T2-weighted MR images. The targetoid enhancement pattern is similar to that of CT.[64] Another characteristic finding of epithelioid hemangioendothelioma is the so-called lollipop sign, with

the hepatic or portal vein tapering toward the masses avascular core (**Fig. 17**).[65]

Metastatic Diseases of the Liver

Numerous malignancies may metastasize to the liver in children including neuroblastoma, Wilms tumor, rhabdomyosarcoma, germ cell tumors, neuroendocrine pancreatic tumors, pancreatoblastoma, gastrointestinal stromal tumor, and desmoplastic small round cell tumor.[4] The most common site of origin of liver metastases in children with solid tumors is neuroblastoma, followed by Wilms tumor. Involvement of liver is also

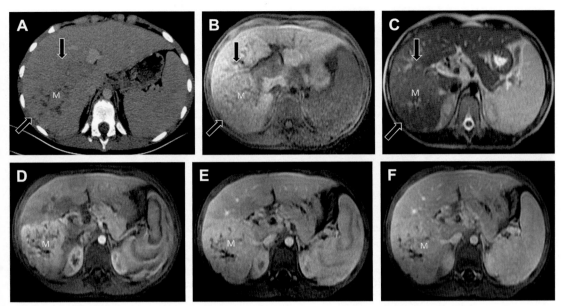

Fig. 14. Fibrolamellar carcinoma. (*A*) There is an isodense mass (M and *arrows*) involving segment 7 of the liver on the contrast-enhanced axial CT images during the portal venous phase consisting of multiple nonenhancing foci in keeping with scar tissue. The lesion (M and *arrows*) appears isointense on T1-weighted (*B*) and T2-weighted (*C*) MR images, enhances heterogeneously during the arterial phase (*D*), keeps the enhancement during the portal venous phase (*E*), and becomes isointense with the liver parenchyma during delayed phase (*F*). The central scar is hypointense to isointense on T1-weighted MR images, isointense to hyperintense on T2-weighted MR images, and does not enhance during the dynamic study.

encountered in 14% of the patients with non-Hodgkin lymphoma.[66,67]

The imaging findings of metastatic disease in liver are nonspecific. On US, there are usually multiple hypoechoic lesions (**Fig. 18**). On CT, the lesions generally appear hypodense compared to the surrounding liver parenchyma and enhances peripherally after contrast enhancement (**Fig. 19**). The metastatic lesions of neuroblastoma may involve the liver diffusely. On MR imaging, the lesions are typically hypointense on T1-weighted MR images, hyperintense on T2-weighted MR images, and may show peripheral ring enhancement similar to the CT.[67]

Primary Neoplasm of the Biliary Tree

Benign tumors involving the biliary tree and gallbladder are very uncommon in children. These neoplasms have a wide spectrum, including papillomatosis,[68] cystadenoma,[69] inflammatory myofibroblastic tumor,[70] yolk sac tumor,[71] and

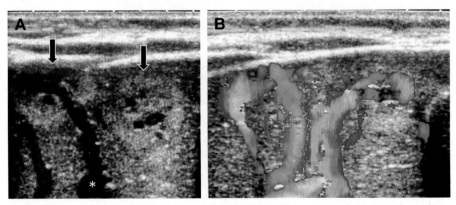

Fig. 15. Epithelioid hemangioendothelioma in an infant girl. (*A*) Ultrasonography image shows hyperechoic peripheral nodules (*arrows*). The lesion on the left is associated with a feeding vessel (*asterisk*) and demonstrates the typical the appearance of a "lollipop". (*B*) Color Doppler ultrasonography shows prominent feeding vessels.

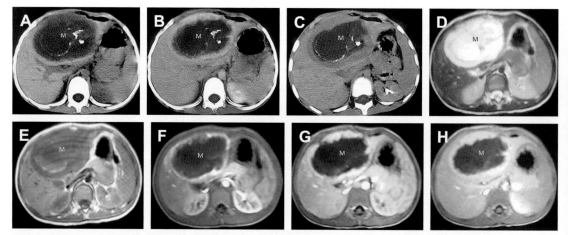

Fig. 16. Epithelioid hemangioendothelioma in a 12-year-old boy. (*A*) On noncontrast axial CT image, there is a large, markedly hypoattenuating mass (M) consisting of linear and coarse calcifications involving both right and left lobes of the liver. The periphery of the lesion (M) enhances during the portal venous phase (*B*) and shows wash-out during the delayed phase (*C*). The lesion (M) is markedly hyperintense on T2-weighted MR images (*D*) similar to fluid signal and hypointense on T1-weighted MR images (*E*). There is strong peripheral enhancement during the arterial phase (*F*) with subsequent partial centripetal fill-in during the portal venous (*G*) and delayed (*H*) phases. However, the large central stroma does not enhance. The calcifications in the mass appear hyperintense on T1-weighted MR images and hypointense on T2-weighted MR images.

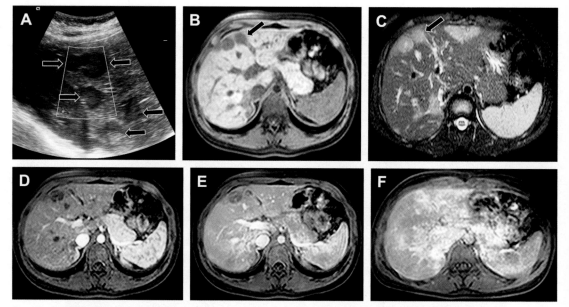

Fig. 17. Epithelioid hemangioendothelioma in a 17-year-old asymptomatic girl. (*A*) There are multiple nodular masses (*arrows*) in varying sizes scattered diffusely in the liver but predominantly involving the periphery of the liver on sagittal ultrasonography image. The lesions (*arrows*) are isoechoic to slightly hypoechoic centrally with the periphery being markedly hypoechoic. There is no flow on Doppler ultrasonography. The lesions (*arrows*) generally appear hypointense on T1-weighted (*B*) and hyperintense on T2-weighted (*C*) MR images, the center being more hypointense on T1-weighted MR images (*B*) and more hyperintense on T2-weighted images (*C*). The lesions do not show obvious enhancement during the arterial (*D*) and portal venous (*E*) phases. However, they enhance strongly during delayed phase while the contours of the lesions become ill-defined (*F*). One of the nodules abuts a branch of the portal vein to form the characteristic "lollipop sign" (*arrow*) on MR imaging (*B* and *C*).

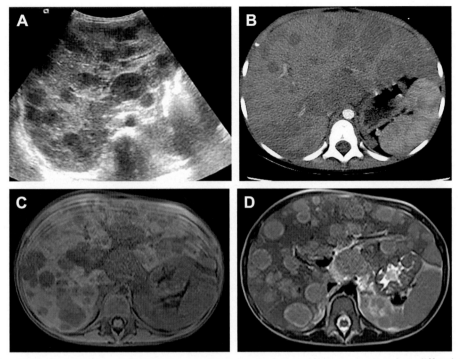

Fig. 18. Non-Hodgkin lymphoma. (*A*) There are multiple hypoechoic nodules in varying sizes diffusely involving the liver on axial ultrasonography image. (*B*) The nodules appear hypoattenuating on contrast-enhanced CT image. The lesions are hypointense on T1-weighted MR images (*C*) and slightly hyperintense on T2-weighted MR images compared with the adjacent liver parenchyma as the periphery of the lesions appear more hyperintense on T2-weighted MR images (*D*).

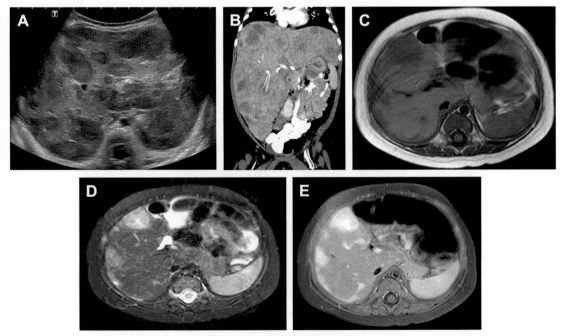

Fig. 19. Metastatic neuroblastoma in a 3-month-old girl. (*A*) There are multifocal lesions in the liver on axial ultrasonography image. The central portions of the lesions are isoechoic to slightly hypoechoic and the periphery is markedly hypoechoic. The liver is massively enlarged and the lesions enhance peripherally on coronal reformatted CT image (*B*). Follow-up MR imaging study after 6 months shows improvement. The lesions appear hypointense on T1-weighted MR images (*C*), hyperintense on T2-weighted MR images (*D*), and enhance homogeneously and avidly after gadolinium administration (*E*).

neuroendocrine tumor.[72] In contrast, malignant tumors of the biliary tree in children exclusively consist of rhabdomyosarcoma.[73–76] Unlike the adult population where benign and malignant primary tumors of the gallbladder are common, they are extremely rare in children. Primary tumors and tumorlike conditions of the gallbladder consist of adenomas, epithelial hyperplasia, gastric heterotopia, and cholesterol polyps.[1,77]

Rhabdomyosarcoma of the biliary tree typically presents at 3 years of age, with a range of 2–5 years. The affected child presents with jaundice, abdominal pain, nausea, vomiting, and/or fever. Jaundice is common at presentation and should alert for rhabdomyosarcoma since it is rarely seen in other malignant tumors. On laboratory analysis, increased conjugated bilirubin levels and normal alpha-fetoprotein levels in serum are typical.[24]

Biliary rhabdomyosarcoma typically shows an intraductal growth pattern. US usually demonstrates a hypoechoic intraductal mass causing biliary duct dilatation.[76] The mass infiltrates the biliary ducts and may show a grape-like or branching pattern. CT shows a heterogeneous mass with variable enhancement filling the biliary tree; however, when tumors reach a large size, the origin of the tumor may not be appreciated. On MR imaging, the lesion appears hypointense on T1-weighted MR images and hyperintense on T2-weighted MR images (**Fig. 20**). The enhancement pattern may vary from no enhancement to marked enhancement. MR cholangiography provides better anatomic delineation of the tumor by demonstrating the intraductal mass and associated biliary dilatation in a 3D fashion. The more commonly encountered congenital cysts of the biliary tree may resemble primary tumors of the biliary tree on imaging and may cause confusion.[72,73]

CONDITIONS THAT CAN MIMIC HEPATOBILIARY NEOPLASMS

Many nonneoplastic conditions may mimic hepatic tumors, including focal fatty infiltration (**Fig. 21**), hepatic infarction, infections, and peliosis hepatis.

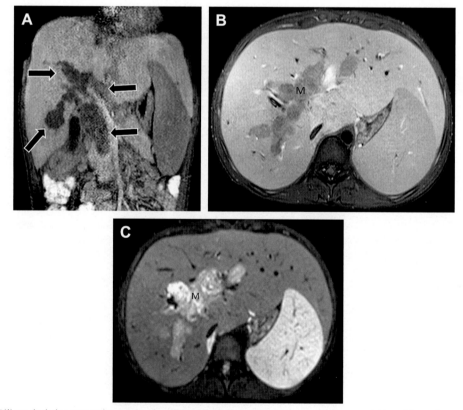

Fig. 20. Biliary rhabdomyosarcoma mixed with hepatocellular carcinoma in a 17-year-old boy. There is a nonenhancing intraductal mass (M and *arrows*) infiltrating the intrahepatic and extrahepatic bile ducts on coronal (*A*) and axial (*B*) postcontrast T1-weighted MR images. The mass appears heterogeneously hyperintense on diffusion-weighted MR images (b = 600 sec/mm2) (*C*). (*Reprint with permission from* Chavhan GB, Shelmerdine S, Jhaveri K, et al. Liver MR imaging in children: current concepts and technique. RadioGraphics 2016;36(5):1517–32.)

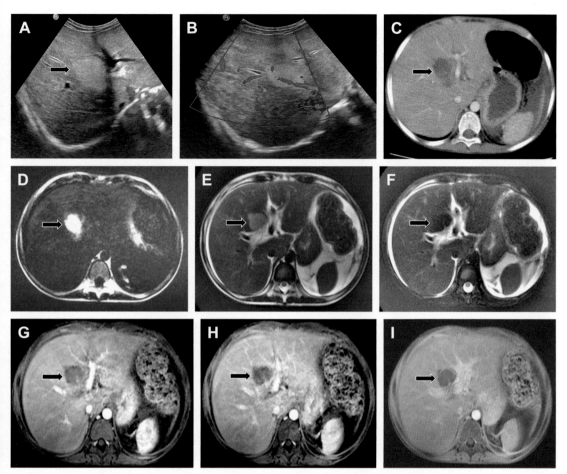

Fig. 21. Focal fatty infiltration in a 10-year-old girl with type I diabetes mellitus. (*A*) There is a hyperechoic focal lesion (*arrow*) with well-defined contours anterior to the right portal vein on axial ultrasonography images of the liver. (*B*) No vascularity of the mass is seen on color Doppler ultrasonography; however, the patent middle hepatic vein traverses the lesion without any associated mass effect or distortion. (*C*) The lesion (*arrow*) has a density of fat on axial CT image and does not enhance. The lesion (*arrow*) appears bright on fat-only LAVA MR images (*D*), slightly hyperintense on T2-weighted MR images (*E*), suppresses on T2-weighted fat-saturated MR images (*F*), and does not show contrast enhancement during the arterial (*G*), portal venous (*H*), and delayed phases (*I*).

Extrahepatic masses may also mimic a primary hepatic tumor especially when present with local extension into the liver.

SUMMARY

The treatment of children with hepatic tumors continues to evolve. Specifically, new advanced surgical techniques and transplantation options, more effective chemotherapy schemas, and increasing international collaboration between pediatric oncology groups have significantly improved morbidity and mortality rates. For instance, the overall survival in hepatoblastoma which is the most common primary hepatic tumor has increased from 30% to over 80%. As therapies grow more complex, state-of-the-art imaging of hepatobiliary tumors becomes

even more integral. There are many unique imaging features of these tumors that practicing radiologists should recognize in order to facilitate timely and accurate diagnosis. Finally, it is imperative for the radiologist to have a working knowledge of demographic, laboratory and clinical data in order to maximize diagnostic specificity and ultimately, improve outcomes.

REFERENCES

1. Birch JM. Epidemiology of pediatric liver tumors. In: Zimmermann A, Perilongo G, Malogolowkin M, et al, editors. Pediatric liver tumors. Pediatric oncology. 1st edition. Berlin; Heidelberg (Germany): Springer-Verlag; 2011. p. 15–26.
2. Rozell JM, Catanzano T, Polansky SM, et al. Primary liver tumors in pediatric patients: proper imaging

technique for diagnosis and staging. Semin Ultrasound CT MR 2014;35:382–93.

3. Lopez-Terrada D, Finegold MJ. Tumors of the liver. In: Suchy FJ, Sokol RJ, editors. Liver disease in children. 4th edition. Cambridge (United Kingdom): Cambridge University Press; 2014. p. 728–9.

4. Fernandez-Pineda I, Sandoval JA, Davidoff AM. Hepatic metastatic disease in pediatric and adolescent solid tumors. World J Hepatol 2015;7:1807–17.

5. Darge K, Papadopoulou F, Ntoulia A, et al. Safety of contrast-enhanced ultrasound in children for noncardiac applications: a review by the Society for Pediatric Radiology (SPR) and the International Contrast Ultrasound Society (ICUS). Pediatr Radiol 2013;43:1063–73.

6. Felsted AE, Shi Y, Masand PM, et al. Intraoperative ultrasound for liver tumor resection in children. J Surg Res 2015;198:418–23.

7. Frush DP. MDCT in children: scan techniques and contrast issues. In: Kalra MK, Sanjay S, Rubin GD, editors. Multidetector CT: from protocols to practice. 1st edition. Heidelberg (Germany): Springer-Verlag; 2008. p. 331–51.

8. Nievelstein RA, van Dam IM, van der Molen AJ. Multidetector CT in children: current concepts and dose reduction strategies. Pediatr Radiol 2010;40: 1324–44.

9. Pugmire BS, Towbin AJ. Magnetic resonance imaging of primary pediatric liver tumors. Pediatr Radiol 2016;46:764–77.

10. Chavhan GB, Mann E, Kamath BM, et al. Gadobenate-dimeglumine-enhanced magnetic resonance imaging for hepatic lesions in children. Pediatr Radiol 2014;44:1266–74.

11. Mitchell CL, Vasanawala SS. An approach to pediatric liver MRI. Am J Roentgenol 2011;196:W519–26.

12. Seale MK, Catalano OA, Saini S, et al. Hepatobiliary-specific MR contrast agents: role in imaging the liver and biliary tree. Radiographics 2009;29:1725–48.

13. Kolbe AB, Podberesky DJ, Zhang B, et al. The impact of hepatocyte phase imaging from infancy to young adulthood in patients with a known or suspected liver lesion. Pediatr Radiol 2015;45:354–65.

14. ISSVA classification of vascular anomalies ©2014 International Society for the Study of Vascular Anomalies. 2014. Available at: issva.org/classification. Accessed March 25, 2017.

15. Horii KA, Drolet BA, Frieden IJ, et al. Prospective study of the frequency of hepatic hemangiomas in infants with multiple cutaneous infantile hemangiomas. Pediatr Dermatol 2011;28:245–53.

16. Chang LC, Haggstrom AN, Drolet BA, et al. Growth characteristics of infantile hemangiomas: implications for management. Pediatrics 2008;122:360.

17. Brugières L. Clinical presentation and diagnosis. In: Zimmermann A, Perilongo G, Malogolowkin M, et al, editors. Pediatric liver tumors. Pediatric oncology.

1st edition. Berlin; Heidelberg (Germany): Springer-Verlag; 2011. p. 59–64.

18. Christison-Lagay ER, Burrows PE, Alomari A, et al. Hepatic hemangiomas: subtype classification and development of a clinical practice algorithm and registry. J Pediatr Surg 2007;42:62–7.

19. Kassarjian A, Zurakowski D, Dubois J, et al. Infantile hepatic hemangiomas: clinical and imaging findings and their correlation with therapy. Am J Roentgenol 2004;182:785–95.

20. Chung EM, Cube R, Lewis RB, et al. From the archives of the AFIP: pediatric liver masses: radiologic-pathologic correlation part 1. Benign tumors. Radiographics 2010;30:801–26.

21. Nasseri E, Piram M, McCuaig CC, et al. Partially involuting congenital hemangiomas: a report of 8 cases and review of the literature. J Am Acad Dermatol 2014;70:75.

22. Gorincour G, Kokta V, Rypens F, et al. Imaging characteristics of two subtypes of congenital hemangiomas: rapidly involuting congenital hemangiomas and non-involuting congenital hemangiomas. Pediatr Radiol 2005;35:1178–85.

23. Stringer MD, Alizai NK. Mesenchymal hamartoma of the liver: a systematic review. J Pediatr Surg 2005; 40:1681–90.

24. von Schweinitz D. Neonatal liver tumours. Semin Neonatol 2003;8:403–10.

25. Meyers RL. Tumors of the liver in children. Surg Oncol 2007;16:195–203.

26. Chung EM, Lattin GE Jr, Cube R, et al. From the archives of the AFIP: pediatric liver masses: radiologic-pathologic correlation. Part 2. Malignant tumors. Radiographics 2011;31:483–507.

27. Shelmerdine SC, Roebuck DJ, Towbin AJ, et al. MRI of paediatric liver tumours: How we review and report. Cancer Imaging 2016;16:21.

28. Meyers RL, Tiao G, de Ville de Goyet J, et al. Hepatoblastoma state of the art: pre-treatment extent of disease, surgical resection guidelines and the role of liver transplantation. Curr Opin Pediatr 2014;26:29–36.

29. Roebuck DJ, Olsen Ø, Pariente D. Radiological staging in children with hepatoblastoma. Pediatr Radiol 2006;36:176–82.

30. Abe T, Oguma E, Nozawa K, et al. Malignant rhabdoid tumor of the liver: a case report with US and CT manifestation. Jpn J Radiol 2009;27:462–5.

31. Martelli MG, Liu C. Malignant rhabdoid tumour of the liver in a seven-month-old female infant: a case report and literature review. Afr J Paediatr Surg 2013;10:50–4.

32. Yuri T, Danbara N, Shikata N, et al. Malignant rhabdoid tumor of the liver: case report and literature review. Pathol Int 2004;54:623–9.

33. Putra J, Ornvold K. Undifferentiated embryonal sarcoma of the liver: a concise review. Arch Pathol Lab Med 2015;139:269–73.

34. Adeyiga AO, Lee EY, Eisenberg RL. Focal hepatic masses in pediatric patients. Am J Roentgenol 2012;199:W422–40.

35. Plant AS, Busuttil RW, Rana A, et al. A single-institution retrospective cases series of childhood undifferentiated embryonal liver sarcoma (UELS): success of combined therapy and the use of orthotopic liver transplant. J Pediatr Hematol Oncol 2013;35:451–5.

36. Geramizadeh B, Safari A, Bahador A, et al. Hepatic angiosarcoma of childhood: a case report and review of literature. J Pediatr Surg 2011;46:e9–11.

37. Kirchner SB, Heller RM, Kasselberg AG, et al. Infantile hepatic hemangioendothelioma with subsequent malignant degeneration. Pediatr Radiol 1981;11:42–5.

38. Ackermann O, Fabre M, Franchi S, et al. Widening spectrum of liver angiosarcoma in children. J Pediatr Gastroenterol Nutr 2011;6:615–9.

39. Wang L, Lv K, Chang XY, et al. Contrast-enhanced ultrasound study of primary hepatic angiosarcoma: a pitfall of non-enhancement. Eur J Radiol 2012;81:2054–9.

40. Rademaker J, Widjaja A, Galanski M. Hepatic hemangiosarcoma: imaging findings and differential diagnosis. Eur Radiol 2000;10:129–33.

41. Bouyn CI, Leclere J, Raimondo G, et al. Hepatic focal nodular hyperplasia in children previously treated for a solid tumor. Incidence, risk factors, and outcome. Cancer 2003;97:3107–13.

42. Bartolotta TV, Midiri M, Scialpi M, et al. Focal nodular hyperplasia in normal and fatty liver: a qualitative and quantitative evaluation with contrast-enhanced ultrasound. Eur Radiol 2004;14:583–91.

43. Wu S, Tu R, Liu G, et al. The frequency and clinical significance of the halo sign in focal nodular hyperplasia of the liver. Med Ultrason 2012;14:278–82.

44. Roche V, Pigneur F, Tselikas L, et al. Differentiation of focal nodular hyperplasia from hepatocellular adenomas with low-mechanical-index contrast-enhanced sonography (CEUS): effect of size on diagnostic confidence. Eur Radiol 2015;25:186–95.

45. Bertin C, Egels S, Wagner M, et al. Contrast-enhanced ultrasound of focal nodular hyperplasia: a matter of size. Eur Radiol 2014;24:2561–71.

46. Ferlicot S, Kobeiter H, Tran Van Nhieu J, et al. MRI of atypical focal nodular hyperplasia of the liver: radiology-pathology correlation. Am J Roentgenol 2004;182:1227–31.

47. Sutherland T, Seale M, Yap K. Part 1: MRI features of focal nodular hyperplasia with an emphasis on hepatobiliary contrast agents. J Med Imaging Radiat Oncol 2014;58:50–5.

48. Towbin AJ, Luo GG, Yin H, et al. Focal nodular hyperplasia in children, adolescents, and young adults. Pediatr Radiol 2011;41:341–9.

49. Applegate KE, Ghei M, Perez-Atayde AR. Prenatal detection of a solitary liver adenoma. Pediatr Radiol 1999;29:92–4.

50. Morris MW, Berch B, Westmoreland T, et al. Resection of a giant hepatic adenoma in an eight-year-old girl. Am Surg 2013;79:889–90.

51. Vaithianathan R, Philipchandran, Selvambigai G, et al. Spontaneous hepatocellular adenoma in paediatric age group - case report. J Clin Diagn Res 2013;7:2962–3.

52. Trenschel GM, Schubert A, Dries V, et al. Nodular regenerative hyperplasia of the liver: case report of a 13-year-old girl and review of the literature. Pediatr Radiol 2000;30:64–8.

53. Yoon HJ, Jeon TY, Yoo SY, et al. Hepatic tumours in children with biliary atresia: single-centre experience in 13 cases and review of the literature. Clin Radiol 2014;69:113–9.

54. Wang HM, Lo GH, Hsu PI, et al. Nodular regenerative hyperplasia of the liver. J Chin Med Assoc 2008;71:523–7.

55. Murawski M, Weeda VB, Maibach R, et al. Hepatocellular carcinoma in children: does modified platinum- and doxorubicin-based chemotherapy increase tumor resectability and change outcome: lessons learned from the SIOPEL 2 and 3 studies. J Clin Oncol 2016;34:1050–6.

56. Jha P, Chawla SC, Tavri S, et al. Pediatric liver tumors–a pictorial review. Eur Radiol 2009;19:209–19.

57. Karahan OI, Yikilmaz A, Isin S, et al. Characterization of hepatocellular carcinomas with triphasic CT and correlation with histopathologic findings. Acta Radiol 2003;44:566–71.

58. Karahan OI, Yikilmaz A, Artis T, et al. Contrast-enhanced dynamic magnetic resonance imaging findings of hepatocellular carcinoma and their correlation with histopathologic findings. Eur J Radiol 2006;57:445–52.

59. Torbenson M. Fibrolamellar carcinoma: 2012 update. Scientifica (Cairo) 2012;2012:743790.

60. Ganeshan D, Szklaruk J, Kundra V, et al. Imaging features of fibrolamellar hepatocellular carcinoma. Am J Roentgenol 2014;202:544–52.

61. Smith MT, Blatt ER, Jedlicka P, et al. Best cases from the AFIP: fibrolamellar hepatocellular carcinoma. Radiographics 2008;28:609–13.

62. Mehrabi A, Kashfi A, Fonouni H, et al. Primary malignant hepatic epithelioid hemangioendothelioma: a comprehensive review of the literature with emphasis on the surgical therapy. Cancer 2006;107:2108–21.

63. Dong Y, Wang WP, Cantisani V, et al. Contrast-enhanced ultrasound of histologically proven hepatic epithelioid hemangioendothelioma. World J Gastroenterol 2016;22:4741–9.

64. Leonardou P, Semelka RC, Mastropasqua M, et al. Epithelioid hemangioendothelioma of the liver. MR imaging findings. Magn Reson Imaging 2002;20:631–3.

65. Alomari AI. The lollipop sign: a new cross-sectional sign of hepatic epithelioid hemangioendothelioma. Eur J Radiol 2006;59:460–4.

66. Das CJ, Dhingra S, Gupta AK, et al. Imaging of paediatric liver tumours with pathological correlation. Clin Radiol 2009;64:1015–25.

67. Biko DM, Anupindi SA, Hernandez A, et al. Childhood Burkitt lymphoma: abdominal and pelvic imaging findings. Am J Roentgenol 2009;192:1304–15.

68. Singh A, Sharma N, Panda SS, et al. Benign papillomatosis of common bile duct in children: a rare case report. J Indian Assoc Pediatr Surg 2014;19:44–5.

69. Wood JA, McLeary MS, Thomas RD, et al. Biliary cystadenoma in a child: CT and MR appearances. Pediatr Radiol 1998;28:922.

70. D'Cunha A, Jehangir S, Thomas R. Inflammatory myofibroblastic tumor of common bile duct in a girl. APSP J Case Rep 2016;7:28.

71. Munghate GS, Agarwala S, Bhatnagar V. Primary yolk sac tumor of the common bile duct. J Pediatr Surg 2011;46:1271–3.

72. Tonnhofer U, Balassy C, Reck CA, et al. Neuroendocrine tumor of the common hepatic duct, mimicking a choledochal cyst in a 6-year-old child. J Pediatr Surg 2009;44:E23–5.

73. Nemade B, Talapatra K, Shet T, et al. Embryonal rhabdomyosarcoma of the biliary tree mimicking a choledochal cyst. J Cancer Res Ther 2007;3:40–2.

74. Kebudi R, Görgun O, Ayan I, et al. Rhabdomyosarcoma of the biliary tree. Pediatr Int 2003;45: 469–71.

75. Perera MT, McKiernan PJ, Brundler MA, et al. Embryonal rhabdomyosarcoma of the ampulla of Vater in early childhood: report of a case and review of literature. J Pediatr Surg 2009;44:e9–11.

76. Kirli EA, Parlak E, Oguz B, et al. Rhabdomyosarcoma of the common bile duct: an unusual cause of obstructive jaundice in a child. Turk J Pediatr 2012;54:654–7.

77. Stringer MD, Ceylan H, Ward K, et al. Gallbladder polyps in children–classification and management. J Pediatr Surg 2003;38:1680–4.

Pediatric Urinary System Neoplasms
An Overview and Update

Michael George, MD, MFA[a],*, Jeannette M. Perez-Rosello, MD[a],
Ali Yikilmaz, MD[b], Edward Y. Lee, MD, MPH[a]

KEYWORDS

- Pediatric • Neoplasms • Urinary system

KEY POINTS

- Pediatric urinary system neoplasms may be stratified by the age of the child. In the neonatal period, the most common tumor is mesoblastic nephroma; in the first decade, Wilms tumor; and in the second decade, Wilms tumor and renal cell carcinoma occur with equal frequency.
- Wilms tumor is by far the most common renal malignancy of childhood, but many of the neoplasms formerly termed *variant Wilms* represent distinct entities.
- Pediatric and adult renal cell carcinoma differ substantially in their subtype, behavior, and association with cancer syndromes.
- Common mimics of pediatric urinary system neoplasms include focal infection, localized cystic renal disease, abscess, and renal infarction.
- Evolving treatment paradigms emphasize nephron- or bladder-conserving surgery, neoadjuvant chemotherapy, and possibly radiotherapy. With these changes, the role of the imaging shifts from presurgical planning to diagnosis that directs management before tissue confirmation.

INTRODUCTION

The classification and therapies of pediatric urinary system neoplasms are constantly evolving. Whereas previously many renal neoplasms were considered variants of Wilms tumor, increasingly sophisticated histopathologic investigation has refined and improved our understanding of these varied renal neoplasms. The clinical presentation of malignant renal masses is often nonspecific, overlapping with benign or even non-neoplastic causes. Because biopsy of renal lesions is rarely undertaken in the pediatric population due to of the risk of upstaging a malignancy, the presurgical distinction of a malignant versus benign lesion is of critical importance. Additionally, given the increasing use of neoadjuvant chemotherapy as advocated by the International Society of Pediatric Oncology, diagnostic radiology is called to make presumptive diagnoses that guide treatment.

The goal of this article is to provide an up-to-date review on neoplasms involving the urinary system, including the kidneys and bladder, as well as their mimics, with an emphasis on characteristic imaging findings and differential diagnostic considerations. Such improved understanding has a great potential to reach a timely and accurate diagnosis that, in turn, can lead to optimal pediatric patient care.

[a] Department of Radiology, Boston Children's Hospital, Harvard Medical School, 300 Longwood Avenue, Boston, MA 02115, USA; [b] Department of Radiology, Goztepe Research and Training Hospital, Istanbul Medeniyet University Medical School, Kadikoy, Istanbul 34722, Turkey
* Corresponding author.
E-mail address: Michael.George@childrens.harvard.edu

Radiol Clin N Am 55 (2017) 767–784
http://dx.doi.org/10.1016/j.rcl.2017.02.004

radiologic.theclinics.com

SPECTRUM OF RENAL NEOPLASM AND MIMICS
Benign Renal Neoplasms

Congenital mesoblastic nephroma

Congenital mesoblastic nephroma (CMN) is a renal tumor of newborns and infants. Although CMN is the most common renal tumor of the neonatal period, it remains rare overall, accounting for 3% to 6% of pediatric renal neoplasms.[1] Nearly 90% of affected pediatric patients present before 1 year of age,[2] and they may be diagnosed as early as the second trimester.[3] A slight (1.5:1.0) male predominance has been reported.[4] Although CMN is increasingly diagnosed in utero, it most frequently presents as a painless abdominal mass postnatally. There is an increased incidence (71%) of perinatal complications, including preterm delivery, hydrops, and polyhydramnios, with several neonates exhibiting hypertension.[5]

Two subtypes of CMN are currently described, classic and cellular, with substantial histologic, imaging, and prognostic distinctions. On gross inspection, the classic type is solid and unencapsulated, sometimes infiltrating the renal hilum. In contrast to the cellular subtype, the classic type is larger and may demonstrate necrosis, hemorrhage, or cystic changes.[1] Histologically, the classic CMN is composed of interlocking fibroblastic and myofibroblastic cells, whereas the cellular variant shows dense cellular proliferation, reminiscent of round blue cell tumors.[6] Aggressive behavior (5%–10%) occurs exclusively in the cellular variant,[7] potentially with metastases to the lung, liver, bone, or brain. Treatment is complete (or radical) nephrectomy, with chemotherapy reserved for partial nephrectomy.

The imaging features of CMN depend on the subtype. Classic CMNs appear as solid, homogenous soft tissue masses, frequently involving the renal sinus.[8] Ultrasound (US) may demonstrate alternating hyperechoic and hypoechoic rings as a consequence of vascular entrapment,[9] whereas prominent anechoic fluid may be seen in the cellular subtype (Fig. 1A). Computed tomography (CT) frequently shows an epicenter in the renal hilum (see Fig. 1B). On MR imaging, enhancement is typically peripheral,[10] with diffusion restriction reflecting increased cellularity. Alternatively, the cellular variant may be marked by more central and punctate enhancement, with areas of cystic change and hemorrhage. Locally aggressive features, such as vessel encasement and organ invasion, may be observed.[5] Differential considerations include Wilms tumor, clear cell sarcoma, and rhabdoid tumor, which are discussed in the later sections of this article.

Most recently, cytogenetic analysis has led to a deeper understanding of CMN. It has been shown that the chromosomal abnormalities of the cellular subtype (ETV6-NTRK3 gene fusion) are identical to those in infantile fibrosarcoma, whereas the more benign classic subtype is thought to represent a variant of infantile fibromatosis.[6]

Ossifying renal tumors of infancy

Ossifying renal tumors of infancy (ORTI) are very rare benign neoplasms of infancy and early childhood, with only 17 cases reported in the literature.[11] The tumor presents between 6 days and 30 months of age, mostly in boys (75%),[12] with macroscopic hematuria. Thus far, only one case has presented as a palpable mass.[13]

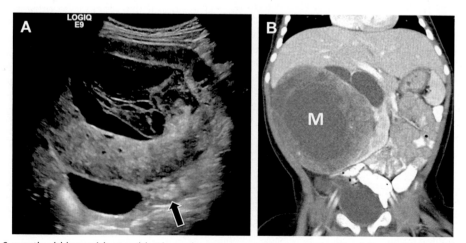

Fig. 1. A 6-month-old boy with mesoblastic nephroma, presenting as a palpable abdominal mass. (A) Longitudinal US and (B) coronal enhanced soft tissue window CT images show a complex solid and cystic mass (M) originating from the right kidney. The US image additionally shows medullary nephrocalcinosis (arrow).

On gross inspection, ORTI are generally small (between 2–3 cm) and solid, most commonly found in the upper pole (69%) of the left kidney (75%).[2] They are typically attached to the renal papilla, from which they grow into the calyx, often resulting in local caliectasis. Histologically, they demonstrate eosinophilic osteoid matrix surrounding a core of osteoid and spindle cells. The pathogenesis of the tumor is uncertain, but it may arise from nephrogenic rests or urothelial cells.[8]

Imaging studies demonstrate a calcified mass, typically causing local hydronephrosis, with an appearance similar to a staghorn calculus. The mass is strongly echogenic on US, with acoustic shadowing and intratumoral blood flow on color Doppler.[11] The mass can be distinguished from calculus on CT and MR imaging by variable contrast enhancement. Differential considerations of a calcified mass in this age group include Wilms tumor, nephrogenic rests, renal cell carcinoma, calcified hematoma, and post-tubercular calcification. Because the tumor may be enucleated without the need for hemi-nephrectomy,[14] presurgical diagnosis may reduce morbidity.

Recently, Seixas-Mikelus and colleagues[15] reported a case of ORTI coincident with granulosa cell tumor of the testis; but it is unclear whether this represents a reproducible association. No cases of recurrence or metastasis have been described.

Angiomyolipoma

Renal angiomyolipoma (AML) is a benign mesenchymal tumor representing less than 3% of renal tumors in the pediatric population.[16] Although they may be sporadic in adults, AML is almost invariably syndromic in children. AML occurs in 40% to 80% of patients with tuberous sclerosis complex (TSC)[17] and is also associated with neurofibromatosis, von Hippel-Lindau syndrome, and Sturge-Weber syndrome. In the setting of TSC, 80% of AMLs are diagnosed before 10 years of age, usually on surveillance imaging.[18] Although typically asymptomatic, lesions greater than 4 cm[19] may present with spontaneous hemorrhage leading to abdominal pain, hematuria, and even hemodynamic instability.[20]

AMLs are highly cellular tumors composed of varying elements of smooth muscle, vascular elements, and bulk fat, although tumors associated with TSC are usually lipid poor.[21] The imaging characteristics of AML vary according to the proportion of these elements. The presence of bulk fat on CT has been said to be pathognomic for AML, although it can also be seen in clear-cell renal cell carcinoma (RCC) and Wilms tumor.[22] On US, AMLs (and occasionally RCCs) are hyperechoic to renal cortex (**Fig. 2**A),[23] usually with a prominent vascular component (see **Fig. 2**B). Although acoustic shadowing is more commonly seen in AML,[24] RCC may be distinguished by intratumoral cysts.[25] MR imaging is of special importance in distinguishing fat-containing lesions. On out-of-phase imaging, the presence of intralesional or perilesional India-ink artifact indicates the presence of bulk fat and is strongly suggestive of AML,[26] especially in the absence of ossification. Rarely, AMLs show local aggressive behavior. Invasion of the inferior vena cava (IVC) and malignant transformation have been described.[8]

Most recently, there have been advances in the understanding, treatment, and imaging of AMLs. We now recognize that mutations in TSC genes alter the mammalian target of rapamycin (mTOR) signaling pathway, a central regulator of cell metabolism and proliferation with important roles in insulin-resistance and oncogenesis. Suppression of mTOR signaling with sirolimus causes AML to regress.[27] Additionally, researchers have recently

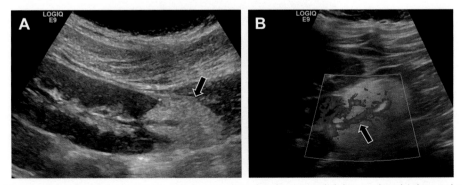

Fig. 2. A 12-year-old girl with a chromosomal abnormality, developmental delay, and multiple renal angiomyolipomas. (*A*) Prone, longitudinal US of the right kidney shows a 4 cm hyperechoic and predominantly exophytic lesion (*arrow*). (*B*) The supine, power Doppler US image of the lesion shows an enlarged feeding artery (*arrow*).

suggested that lipid-poor AML may be distinguished from RCC using wash-out kinetics on contrast-enhanced CT.[28]

Multilocular cystic renal tumors

Multilocular cystic renal tumors (MCRTs) were classically described as a spectrum of septated, cystic neoplasms ranging from the benign cystic nephroma (CN) to the more intermediate-risk cystic partially differentiated nephroblastoma (CPDN).[29] These rare tumors were thought to have a bimodal age and sex distribution,[30] occurring in young boys (3 months to 4 years) and middle-aged women,[8] although recent histopathology suggests that adult MCRTs represent a distinct clinical entity.[31] In children, most MCRTs present as a painless intra-abdominal mass, although they may less frequently present with hematuria or urinary tract infection.[32]

On gross inspection, MCRTs are well-circumscribed masses composed of cysts of varying sizes, surrounded by a thick fibrous capsule. Histopathologically, the cysts of MCRTs are lined by flattened epithelium, with eosinophilic cuboidal cells protruding into the lumen, giving them a hobnail appearance.[5]

Imaging studies demonstrate a multilocular, cystic mass with hair-like septa and no solid component,[33] features easily distinguished on US (Fig. 3A). Peripheral calcifications may be present, although only 5% are evident on radiographs.[4] A more typical plain film appearance is nonspecific mass effect on bowel loops (see Fig. 3B). The fibrous capsule typically demonstrates faint enhancement (see Fig. 3C); nodular enhancement of the cyst wall is uncommon (18%).[34] On MR imaging, the cystic component typically exhibits variable T1 hyperintensity due

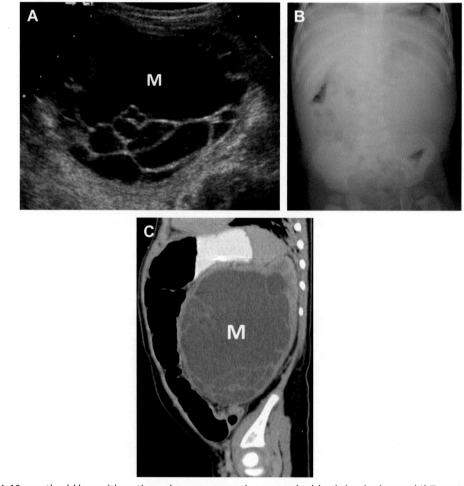

Fig. 3. A 10-month-old boy with cystic nephroma, presenting as a palpable abdominal mass. (*A*) Transverse US and (*B*) upright radiograph of the abdomen shows displacement of the bowel by a left abdominal mass (M). (*C*) Sagittal enhanced soft tissue window CT image shows a multilocular cystic mass (M) originating from the left kidney.

to protein and blood content. Rarely, the densely packed septa of the cysts may mimic a solid mass on CT.[5] Differential considerations for MCRT include cystic mesoblastic nephroma (if in the perinatal period), cystic Wilms tumor, and segmental multicystic dysplastic kidney, the latter of which may be suggested by an ectopic ureter. Because the imaging and clinical presentation of MCRT is nonspecific, treatment is surgical, with full or partial nephrectomy.

Most recently, the classification of MCRT has changed. Under the old schema, CPDN was distinguished from pediatric CN by the presence of blastema cells; the World Health Organization now recommends all MCRTs be classified as CPDN.[35] Additionally, a significant association with familial pleuropulmonary blastoma has been described, with the common pathway of the DICER1 mutation.[36]

Malignant Renal Neoplasms

Wilms tumor

Wilms tumor (nephroblastoma) is a malignant neoplasm arising from mesodermal precursors in the renal parenchyma. It is by far the most common renal neoplasm of childhood, accounting for 87% of renal masses.[37] The peak incidence of Wilms tumor is between 3 and 4 years of age,[38] and it is exceptionally rare in neonates (0.16%).[30] Most cases present as a painless abdominal mass, although secondary hypertension may also occur in a quarter of cases, due to renin production.[2] Bilateral nephroblastoma occurs in 4% to 13% of cases and present slightly earlier (mean age 33 months) than unilateral tumors, suggesting a genetic predisposition.[1]

On gross inspection, Wilms tumors are well-circumscribed or macrolobulated masses, frequently with central necrosis. Histologically, nephroblastomas are composed of variable amounts blastema, stroma, and epithelium, although not all elements may be present. The presence of anaplastic elements (10%) suggests resistance to chemotherapy and is the single most important indicator of poor prognosis.[39] Although most Wilms tumors are sporadic, 2 loci on chromosome 11 (WT1 and WT2) have been implicated with nephroblastoma in association with other syndromes, including WAGR (Wilms tumor, aniridia, genitourinary anomalies, and intellectual disability), Denys-Drash (congenital nephropathy, Wilms tumor, and intersex disorders), Beckwith-Wiedemann syndrome (BWS), and hemihypertrophy.[8]

Imaging demonstrates solid masses centered in the kidney, possibly with a claw of surrounding renal tissue (**Fig. 4**). Nephroblastoma tends to displace rather than encase surrounding structures and commonly invades the renal vein (**Fig. 5**A) and the IVC (see **Fig. 5**B). Metastases are found on presentation in 11% of the cases, most commonly to the lungs (85%) (see **Fig. 5**C), liver (20%), and bone (infrequent).[2] On US, nephroblastoma has a heterogeneous appearance, with hypoechoic and hyperechoic regions corresponding with hemorrhage and necrosis. Shadowing calcifications are present in 9% of cases.[40] On CT, the tumors are heterogeneous and enhance less robustly than the surrounding kidney and calcifications are seen more frequently than on US (15%).[5] MR imaging demonstrates a lobulated, heterogeneous lesion that is T1 hypointense and T2 hyperintense to the renal parenchyma (**Fig. 6**).[8] The most important differential consideration of Wilms tumor is neuroblastoma, which is extrarenal in origin, more frequently calcifies (80%–90%), and encases adjacent structures.

Staging of Wilms tumor in the United States remains surgical, although preoperative imaging

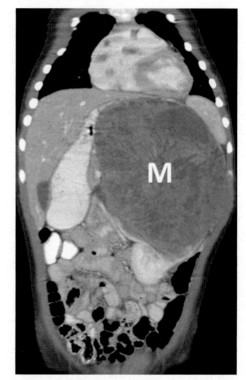

Fig. 4. A 5-year-old girl with Wilms tumor, presenting as a palpable abdominal mass. Coronal enhanced soft tissue window CT image shows a large, heterogeneous left renal mass (M) crossing midline and displacing vessels and other organs. Renal parenchyma is stretched around the mass in a claw sign indicating renal origin.

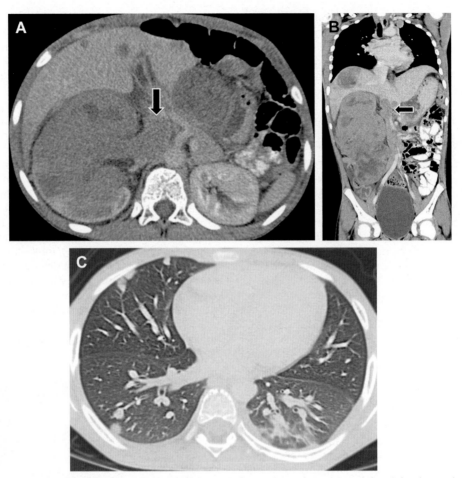

Fig. 5. An 8-year-old boy with Wilms tumor, presenting after 2 days of vomiting. (*A*) Axial enhanced soft tissue window CT image shows a right renal mass with invasion (*arrow*) of the right renal vein. (*B*) Coronal enhanced CT image shows invasion (*arrow*) of the IVC and multiple liver masses. (*C*) Axial lung window CT image shows multiple lung nodules consistent with pulmonary metastasis.

strongly influences treatment. Factors that may change surgical approach include bilaterality, invasion of the renal vein (4%–10%) or IVC, and tumor rupture, which may manifest by poorly defined tumor margins, perinephric fat stranding, retroperitoneal fluid, or ipsilateral pleural effusion.[41] The mainstay of treatment remains total nephrectomy, followed by chemotherapy and possibly therapeutic radiation. In the setting of bilateral disease, chemotherapy may precede nephron-sparing surgery to reduce the extent of disease and the possibility of tumor spillage.[7]

Most recently, collaboration between the Children's Oncology Group (COG) and the International Society of Pediatric Oncology (SIOP) has led to refined risk stratification by gene locus heterogeneity in combination with traditional staging and histologic grade.[42] This refined risk stratification has increased the overall survival of Wilms tumors to well more than the 90% benchmark set forth by the COG.

Nephroblastomatosis

Closely associated with Wilms tumor, nephroblastomatosis is defined by diffuse or multifocal persistence of nephrogenic rests. These rests are composed of metanephric blastema, the embryonic structure that gives rise to the nephron.[43] They are normally present until the 36th week of gestation and are found incidentally in 1% of infants.[38] They are also a precursor of Wilms tumor, found in 30% to 40% of cases after surgical resection, and in nearly all cases of bilateral nephroblastoma.[44] The lesions are asymptomatic, and most frequently encountered during surveillance imaging for tumor syndromes, including BWS, WAGR, Denys-Drash, and sporadic aniridia.

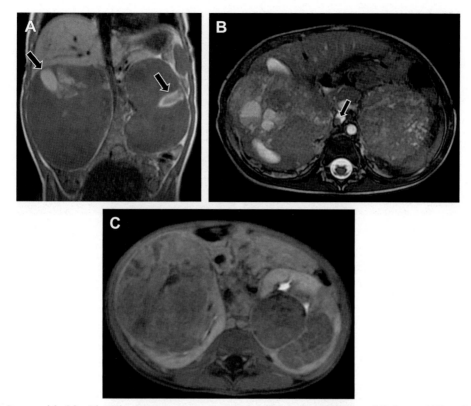

Fig. 6. A 3-year-old girl with Wilms tumor, presenting with a distended abdomen. (*A*) Coronal T1-weighted MR image shows bilateral renal masses with areas of hemorrhage (*arrows*). (*B*) Axial fast imaging employing steady-state acquisition MR image shows invasion (*arrow*) of tumor into the IVC. (*C*) Axial enhanced T1-weighted MR image with fat saturation shows heterogeneous enhancement of the renal masses.

At gross inspection, nephrogenic rests are tan nodules surrounded by normal renal parenchyma; when multiple, they may form a rind on the periphery of the kidney.[1] Rests may be perilobar, peripherally located or along a column of Bertin, or intralobar, found centrally. Although perilobar rests are more common, intralobar rests have a higher rate of malignant transformation. Histologically, rests are classified as dormant, sclerosing, hyperplastic, or neoplastic. Like Wilms tumor, nephrogenic rests are associated with WT1 and WT2 abnormities on chromosome 11, in addition to defects in the WTX domain of the X chromosome and the TP53 tumor suppressor gene on chromosome 17, which is associated with anaplasia.[45]

Imaging evaluation of nephroblastomatosis demonstrates homogenous round, ovoid, or irregular nodules, many of which are peripheral in location. On CT, the nephroblastomatosis nodules show low attenuation and poor enhancement when compared with surrounding parenchyma.[8] MR imaging typically shows T1 hypointensity and variable T2 hyperintensity (**Fig. 7**A, B) and poor enhancement (see **Fig. 7**C). US is the least sensitive modality, as the rests may appear hypoechoic, isoechoic, or hyperechoic; they may also diffusely enlarge the kidney, increasing its echogenicity and decreasing corticomedullary differentiation.[6] The primary differential consideration for nephroblastomatosis is lymphoma, which is rare in infants.

Treatment of nephroblastomatosis is currently somewhat controversial. Some investigators advocate treatment with chemotherapy until imaging resolution, whereas others recommend serial imaging with US at 3-month intervals until 8 years of age,[2] at which point the risk of Wilms tumor is equal to that of the general population. The frequency of follow-up allows for partial rather than full nephrectomy, which is of significance given the potential development of malignant transformation in multiple rests. Transformation is suggested by increasing heterogeneity, size, and sphericity.[3] Recently, an association has been made with the absence of tracheal cartilage, possibly mediated by Sonic Hedgehog signaling,[46] a protein essential in embryonic development.

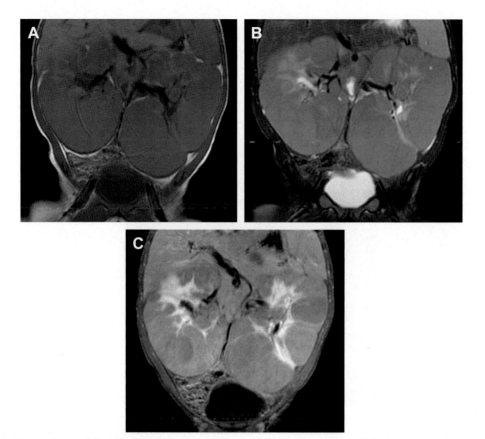

Fig. 7. A 14-month-old girl with nephroblastomatosis, presenting with a distended abdomen and poor growth. This child went on to develop bilateral Wilms tumor. Coronal T1-weighted (*A*) and T2-weighted (*B*) MR images show enlargement of the kidneys by a rind of multiple peripheral masses that are T1 and T2 hypointense. (*C*) Coronal postcontrast T1-weighted MR image shows decreased enhancement of the masses relative to the normal enhancing renal parenchyma.

Rhabdoid tumor of the kidney

Rhabdoid tumor (RT) of the kidney is a rare, exclusively pediatric neoplasm accounting for less than 2% of pediatric renal tumors.[8] Sixty percent of RTs occur before 1 year of age, and 80% occur before 2 years of age. A slight male predominance has been reported. These highly malignant renal tumors are most often (80%) metastatic at presentation, with regional symptoms including a palpable mass, pain, hematuria, and fever (50%). Hypercalcemia may be present because of elevated parathormone levels.[47] There is a well-described association (15%) with synchronous intracranial neoplasms, usually arising in the midline of the posterior fossa.[7]

The gross appearance of RT is nonspecific. The masses are typically large and centrally located in the renal hilum, with invasion of the collecting system. Vascular invasion, linear calcifications, and areas of hemorrhage are common. Histologically, RTs resemble skeletal muscle, with monomorphic

cells containing prominent eosinophilic nuclei and intracytoplasmic inclusions.[30] Despite aggressive treatment with both radical nephrectomy and chemotherapy, prognosis remains the worst of any pediatric renal tumor.

Imaging of RT usually shows a large, central, heterogeneous soft tissue mass with indistinct margins (**Fig. 8**).[1] Characteristic subcapsular fluid collections, representing hemorrhage or necrosis, occur in 71% of RTs. Additional typical findings of RT on CT include vascular invasion and tumor lobules, often outlined by curvilinear calcifications.[48] Differential considerations include Wilms tumor in young children and mesoblastic nephroma in infants.

In recent years, advances have been made in the understanding and treatment of RT. Molecular genetics have identified deletions in chromosome locus 22q11 (SMARCB1) likely related to epigenetic modification, which are also present in atypical teratoma RT.[2] The COG has now begun

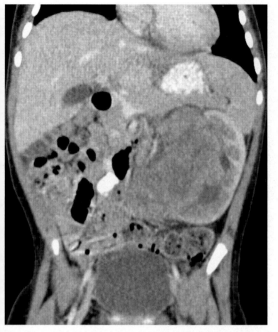

Fig. 8. A 22-month-old girl with rhabdoid tumor of the kidney, presenting with fever of unknown origin. Coronal enhanced soft tissue window CT image shows a heterogeneous left renal mass. There is a characteristic central location and invasion of the renal hilum. MR imaging of the brain was normal.

screening all RTs for SMARCB1 mutations in order to improve classification and clarify prognosis. Additionally, 2 reports have described the successful use of stem cell therapy and high-dose chemotherapy in the treatment of renal RT.[49]

Clear cell sarcoma of the kidney

Clear cell sarcoma of the kidney (CCSK) is a malignant mesenchymal tumor of the kidney unique to the pediatric population. Although rare, with an incidence of 10 to 20 cases per year, CCSK is the second most common malignant neoplasm of the kidney in the pediatric population. The average age at diagnosis is 3 years, with a 2:1 male predilection.[1] Most cases present with a palpable abdominal mass; hematuria, hypertension, and bone pain are less common.[50] Unlike Wilms tumor, CCSK does not seem to be associated with other syndromes.[51]

On gross inspection, CCSK is a well-circumscribed solid mass centered in the renal medulla.[7] Intratumoral cysts are a common finding, ranging in size between 0.5 and 5.0 cm,[52] as are hemorrhage and necrosis (70%). The histologic appearance is varied, with as many as 9 variants described, with the common findings of cords of round or spindle-shaped cells surrounded by a "chicken wire" of fibrovascular septa.[2] Cytogenetic abnormalities involving translocations in t(10;17) (q22;p13/p12) and deletion of 14q24q31 have been described.[45]

Imaging features of CCSK are nonspecific and frequently overlap with Wilms tumor. The mass appears heterogeneous, with varying degrees of necrosis. On US, small cysts may be present and may occasionally predominate, mimicking multi-locular CN.[4] The mass is hypoattenuating on CT (**Fig. 9**A), and on MR imaging it demonstrates low to intermediate T1 signal and pronounced T2 hyperintensity. Because of necrosis, it may enhance less robustly than the surrounding renal parenchyma.[4] Although the tumor may cross the midline, vascular invasion is rare. One important distinguishing factor of CCSK is a propensity for bony metastases (see **Fig. 9**B–D), present in 13% to 20% of cases.[19]

The prognosis of CCSK remains worse than that of Wilms tumor. Relapse occurs in 20% to 40% of cases and has been described as long as 3 years after diagnosis.[53] Treatment is radical nephrectomy and high-dose chemotherapy. Most recently, the COG has advocated the addition of central nervous system–targeting chemotherapy and radiotherapy in select tumors.[8]

Renal cell carcinoma

RCC is a rare malignant neoplasm in children, accounting for 1% to 2% of all pediatric renal tumors.[54] Although case reports exist of the tumors occurring in infancy, most pediatric RCCs are diagnosed in the second decade, during which Wilms tumor and RCC occur with equal frequency.[55] It is more frequent in girls than boys (58%) and slightly more common in non-Hispanic blacks.[56] RCC is frequently associated with von Hippel-Lindau (VHL). VHL should be excluded in any child diagnosed with RCC.[8] Additional associations are seen with TSC, sickle cell hemoglobinopathies, and transplant recipients.[57] Pediatric RCC may present with the classic triad of gross hematuria, flank pain, and a palpable mass.

On gross inspection, RCC is indistinguishable from other common pediatric tumors,[58] appearing as a solid mass with variable necrosis, hemorrhage, and cystic degeneration, although the lesions tend to be smaller in size[4] and more commonly (25%) calcify.[38] The histologic appearance and classification of pediatric RCC differs substantially from adult tumors. Clear-cell RCC is exceedingly rare in children, with the most common subtypes including the Xp11 translocation (20%–40%), papillary (30%), medullary, and oncocytic variants.[59] Translocation RCC, medullary RCC, and oncocytic RCC are associated with prior

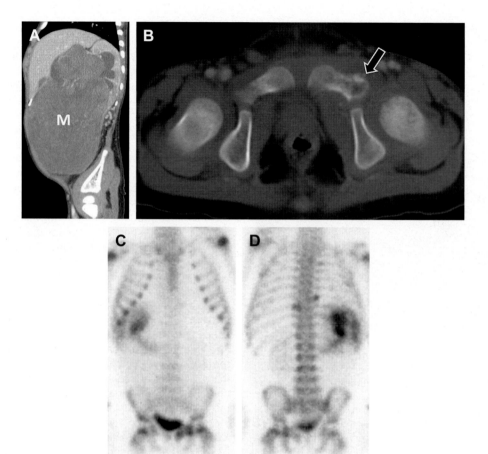

Fig. 9. A 2-year-old boy with clear cell sarcoma, presenting with a palpable abdominal mass. (*A*) Sagittal enhanced soft tissue window CT image shows a large, heterogeneous renal mass (M). (*B*) Axial bone window CT image shows a destructive lesion (*arrow*) in the left superior pubic ramus. (*C*) Anterior and (*D*) posterior Technetium-99m methylene diphosphonate scan images show radiotracer uptake in the left superior pubic ramus, right eighth vertebral transverse process, and left ninth vertebral transverse process consistent with metastatic lesions. There is increase radiotracer accumulation in the obstructed right collecting system.

chemotherapy,[59] sickle cell disease, and neuroblastoma,[60] respectively. All variants may metastasize to the liver, bone, lungs, and brain. Aggressive regional spread is common, particularly in the medullary subtype.

The imaging appearance of RCC is nonspecific. On US, RCC may appear hyperechoic, hypoechoic, or isoechoic to renal cortex, often with characteristic intratumoral cysts (**Fig. 10**). Cross-sectional imaging typically shows a heterogeneous mass that may be well or poorly circumscribed,[61] noncalcified, or harboring small calcifications (**Fig. 11**A). Contrast enhancement is typically poor,[62] particularly in the papillary variant. Important imaging findings for staging purposes include locoregional lymphadenopathy (see **Fig. 11**B) and vascular invasion (see **Fig. 11**C).

Stage of RCC at presentation remains the most important factor in mortality. Because of the insensitivity to chemotherapy and radiotherapy, the mainstay of therapy is radical nephrectomy.[63] Prognosis in RCC remains lower than in Wilms tumor, with an overall survival of 64%.[64]

Desmoplastic small round cell tumor

Desmoplastic small round cell tumor (DSRCT) is an exceeding rare, highly aggressive malignant neoplasm of childhood and young adulthood.[65] While DSRCT most commonly occur in the serosal surface of the abdomen, they have also arisen from the serosal surfaces of the pleural cavity, scrotum, and ovary.[66] There is a strong male (4:1) predilection.[67] Three case reports describe DSRCT isolated to the kidney[68,69]; in this setting, each patient presented with gross hematuria.

On gross inspection, DSRCTs are firm, lobulated masses. Histologically, they appear as nests of small round cells in a lattice of fibrous

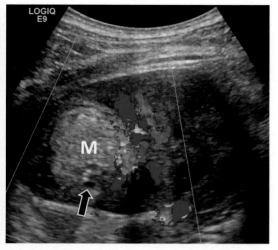

Fig. 10. A 15-year-old girl with renal cell carcinoma (RCC) presenting with gross hematuria. Longitudinal Doppler US image shows a hyperechoic mass (M) in the upper pole of the right kidney. The intratumoral cyst (*arrow*) is suggestive of RCC and would be atypical of angiomyolipoma.

connective tissue,[70] with a unique EWS-WT1 t(11;22)(p13;q12) translocation that has been implicated in their pathogenesis.[71]

Imaging of DSRCT demonstrates a heterogeneous, well-circumscribed mass with prominent punctate calcifications (**Fig. 12**).[72] On US, DSRCT tends to be hypoechoic, though renal DSRCTs have appeared slightly hyperechoic to renal cortex.[73] The lesions appear low attenuation and hypovascular on CT, with very little enhancement appreciable in the corticomedullary and nephrographic phases.[5]

Very recently, DSRCT has been described in association with sclerotic bony metastasis,[74] and other case reports have described a more indolent clinical course than previously recorded.[73]

Ewing sarcoma of the kidney

Extraosseous Ewing sarcoma (EOES) is a high-grade tumor of neuroectodermal origin, typically found in children and adolescents. Although most commonly originating from bone, they may rarely arise from the skin and viscera, including the kidney.[75] Although renal Ewing sarcoma can arise in children, it is most common in young adult men.[76] The lesions are typically asymptomatic until they present with symptoms of mass effect, at which point they range between 5.5 and 23.0 cm in size.[2]

Histopathologically, Ewing sarcoma belongs to the family of small, round blue cell tumors. It can be challenging to distinguish EOES from primitive neuroectodermal tumor (PNET), although Homer-Wright–type rosettes in pathology are only seen in PNET.

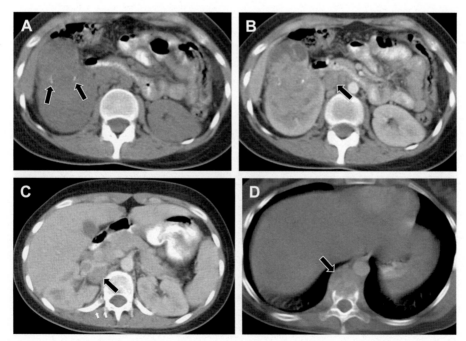

Fig. 11. A 16-year-old boy with renal cell carcinoma, presenting with abdominal pain. (*A*) Axial nonenhanced soft tissue window CT image shows calcifications (*arrows*) in a right renal mass. (*B, C*) Axial enhanced soft tissue window CT images show poor definition of the margins of the mass and perihilar adenopathy (*arrows*). (*D*) Axial bone window CT image shows osseous metastatic disease (*arrow*) of the T9 vertebral body.

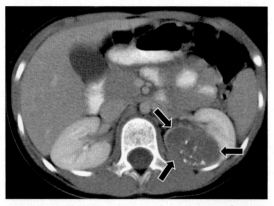

Fig. 12. A 6-year-old boy with desmoplastic small round blue cell tumor presenting with gross hematuria. Axial enhanced CT image of the left kidney shows punctate calcifications in the mass (*arrows*).

The imaging appearance of EOES is nonspecific and indistinguishable from RCC.[77] CT typically demonstrates a large, heterogeneous mass that replaces the kidney. Hemorrhage, necrosis, and calcification are common; invasion of the renal vein has been described.[75] Signal on T1-weighted MR imaging depends of the presence of blood products, which is variable, whereas T2 hyperintensity is typically present. Because the appearance is nonspecific, diagnosis is typically made following radical nephrectomy for presumed RCC.

Metastatic Renal Disease

Renal lymphoma
Lymphoma is the third most common malignancy of childhood; as many as 62% of children with lymphoma have renal involvement and most of these cases are appreciable by CT.[78,79] Because the kidney does not contain native lymphatic tissue, involvement of the kidney is secondary to disseminated disease; presentation typically reflects other symptoms of the diffuse disease process. Burkitt and T-cell lymphoblastic lymphoma have particular predilections for the kidney.[80]

As in the adult population, the imaging appearance of renal pediatric lymphoma is varied. It may present as solitary or multifocal masses of 1 to 3 cm, direct extension of retroperitoneal lymphadenopathy, diffuse infiltration, or perinephric disease.[81,82] When present, masses are hypoattenuating on CT (**Fig. 13**A), hypoechoic on US,[8] and fluorodeoxyglucose (FDG)-avid on PET (see **Fig. 13**B). The homogenous cellularity of the tumor results in increased through-transmission on US as well as T2 hyperintensity and restricted diffusion on MR imaging. Diagnostic certainty can be increased by coincident findings, such as

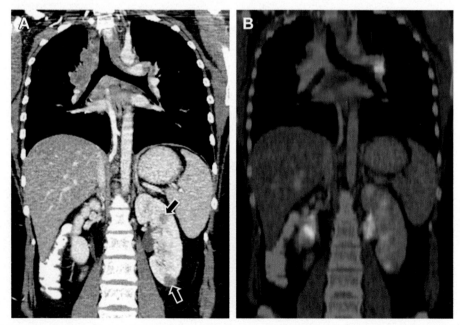

Fig. 13. A 16-year-old girl with large B-cell lymphoma. (*A*) Coronal enhanced soft tissue window CT image shows homogenous hypodense masses (*arrows*) in the left kidney and a heterogeneous mediastinal mass. (*B*) Coronal fluorodeoxyglucose (FDG)-PET image shows FDG uptake in the renal masses, mediastinal mass, and in a previously unseen liver lesion.

retroperitoneal lymphadenopathy, mediastinal mass, or splenomegaly.

Renal Neoplasm Mimics

Acute focal nephritis

Acute focal nephritis (AFN) is a common mimic of pediatric renal neoplasms in both its clinical presentation and imaging appearance. It is distinguished from acute pyelonephritis (APN) by its focality and more often leads to scarring and abscess formation. The most common clinical signs are fever and/or flank pain[83]; but these are also commonly present in Wilms tumor, RCC, and other renal masses of childhood; additionally, urinalysis with leukocyte esterase and leukocytosis may be insensitive (70%–90%) and nonspecific, respectively.[2] Although imaging in the setting of acute infection is not currently recommended,[84] it may be performed in the setting of treatment failure, suspected complication, or to assess for anatomic abnormalities.

Because AFN lies on a spectrum between diffuse APN and renal abscess, the imaging appearance is varied. On US, the most common appearance is a normal kidney,[85] although confirming focally decreased blood flow on power Doppler increases sensitivity.[86] When a textural abnormality is perceptible, it may appear masslike and is more commonly hyperechoic than hypoechoic.[87] On contrast-enhanced CT, AFN progresses from wedgelike to masslike regions of decreased enhancement (**Fig. 14**) and finally abscess; the radiographic progression may correlate with clinical severity.[1] More recently, MR imaging has been used to confirm pyelonephritis by identifying restricted diffusion in children with renal insufficiency.[88]

Renal infarction

Renal infarction stems from interruption of the vascular supply to the kidney and in children most commonly stems from vasculitis, dissection (especially in the setting of fibromuscular dysplasia or prior catheterization), or thromboembolism. The distribution and scope of the insult depends on the variable vascular supply of the kidney and level of interruption.[89] The clinical presentation may mimic that of renal masses, with flank pain, fever, hematuria, proteinuria, or hypertension secondary to renin release.[90]

On US, acute infarct may not have a textural correlate; but decreased flow should be present on Doppler interrogation.[91] CT typically shows wedgelike, round or global nonenhancement, depending on the level of occlusion.[3] One potentially distinguishing feature of infarct is the cortical rim sign, in which the nonenhanced infarct is

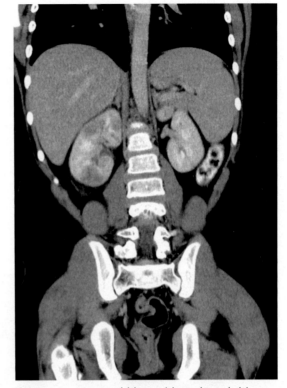

Fig. 14. An 11-year-old boy with pyelonephritis, presenting with severe pain and fever. The patient has past medical history of vesicoureteric reflux and urinary tract infections. Coronal enhanced soft tissue window CT image shows multiple masslike regions of nonenhancement in the right kidney.

bordered by 1 to 3 mm of enhancing peripheral cortex. This sign is thought to stem from the independent supply of the capsular perforating arteries and is variably present depending on the level of occlusion.[92] It may also be seen in venous infarction and acute tubular necrosis.[93] Renal infarct may also be diagnosed by the absence of Doppler flow in the renal arteries or abrupt cutoff of contrast as seen on contrast-enhanced CT.

SPECTRUM OF BLADDER NEOPLASM AND MIMICS
Bladder Neoplasms

Rhabdomyosarcoma

Rhabdomyosarcoma is a malignant neoplasm arising from primitive muscles cells. Although rare overall, accounting for 3.5% of childhood cancers, it the most common lower urogenital neoplasm of childhood. The mean presenting age is 4 years,[2] although a second peak in late adolescence has also been noted in paratesticular tumors.[94] Boys are more often affected than girls (3:1).[1] Common presenting signs include gross hematuria, difficulty voiding, urinary retention, and urgency.[95] Associations exist with Li-Fraumeni, pleuropulmonary blastoma (with DICER1 mutation), neurofibromatosis type 1, and BWS.[96]

On gross inspection, rhabdomyosarcomas are poorly infiltrating masses of the bladder wall, often necessitating a wide surgical margin. If intraluminal extension is present, the tumor may have a polypoid or grapelike appearance (sarcoma botryoides). Histologically, the lesions are composed of malignant spindle cells invested with loose, myoid stroma.[1] Embryonal, alveolar, and pleomorphic subtypes have been described, with embryonal subtype representing 90% of bladder tumors.[97]

Imaging often demonstrates bladder obstruction, with mural or intraluminal masses. Infiltration into the prostate is common. US may demonstrate a fungating intraluminal mass (**Fig. 15A**), whereas fluoroscopic cystogram will show a fixed polypoid mural-based filling defect (see **Fig. 15**B, C). On MR imaging, rhabdomyosarcoma show T1 lengthening and high signal on T2-weighted MR imaging sequences, with heterogeneous enhancement (see **Fig. 15**D).[6] CT shows local osseous destruction in up to 20% of cases.[98]

Optimal management of pediatric bladder rhabdomyosarcoma is controversial. Whereas the COG advises early radiotherapy to improve event-free survival, the SIOP emphasizes subtotal surgery followed by chemotherapy. Both approaches stress the goal of organ sparing, as opposed to the traditional approach of radical cystectomy. This information suggests that

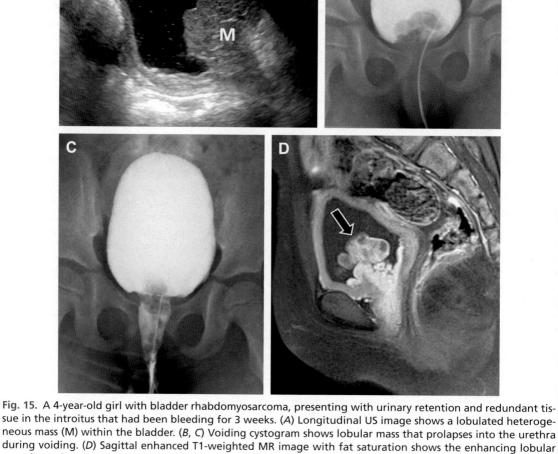

Fig. 15. A 4-year-old girl with bladder rhabdomyosarcoma, presenting with urinary retention and redundant tissue in the introitus that had been bleeding for 3 weeks. (*A*) Longitudinal US image shows a lobulated heterogeneous mass (M) within the bladder. (*B, C*) Voiding cystogram shows lobular mass that prolapses into the urethra during voiding. (*D*) Sagittal enhanced T1-weighted MR image with fat saturation shows the enhancing lobular mass (*arrow*).

high-resolution multi-parametric MR imaging, well described in the adult literature,[99] may be of benefit given the goal of tissue conservation.

Fibroepithelial Polyps

Fibroepithelial polyps (FEPs) are rare, benign mesodermal tumors typically seen in infants and children.[100] They may appear anywhere from the ureter to the urethra and may be isolated or multiple. These pedunculated tumors are composed of fibrovascular stroma covered by normal epithelium[101] and tend to present with episodic flank pain due to intermittent ureteropelvic junction (UPJ) obstruction. Up to 5% of UPJ obstructions may be caused by FEPs.[102] The radiologic appearance is variable, depending on whether the lesion is stalklike or polypoid; but overall preoperative detection rates are poor, ranging between 0% and 27% on fluoroscopic excretory urography and 21% for MR urography.[102]

Bladder Neoplasm Mimics

Debris and clot may both have a masslike appearance, although they may readily be distinguished from neoplasm by their mobility and lack of flow on color Doppler US or enhancement on cross-sectional imaging studies. Cystitis may provide a more challenging diagnostic dilemma, as it may occasionally present with focal rather than diffuse wall thickening in the setting of hematuria.[103]

SUMMARY

Advances in the histopathologic classification of pediatric urinary system tumors have led to increasingly successful and complex treatment algorithms for these important tumors. As these treatments moved away from radical nephrectomy and cystectomy in favor of organ-sparing surgery and neoadjuvant chemotherapy, the role of the radiologist has also changed. In the new paradigm described by the International Society of Pediatric Oncology, which is now being adopted in the United States, the radiologist is not interpreting studies solely to aid in preoperative planning but making diagnoses that direct management before tissue confirmation. Knowledge of the clinical and imaging features of these pediatric urinary system lesions is crucial to this endeavor.

REFERENCES

1. Chung E, Graeber A, Conran R. Renal tumors of childhood: radiologic-pathology correlation part 1. Radiographics 2016;36:499–522.
2. Murphy WM, Grignon DJ, Perlman EJ. Kidney tumors in children. In: Prichard-Jones K, Dome J, editors. Tumors of the kidney, bladder, and related urinary structures. Washington, DC: American Registry of Pathology; 2004. p. 1–99.
3. Chen WY, Lin CN, Chao CS, et al. Prenatal diagnosis of congenital mesoblastic nephroma in mid-second trimester by sonography and magnetic resonance imaging. Prenat Diagn 2003;23:927–31.
4. Powis M. Neonatal renal tumours. Early Hum Dev 2010;86:607–12.
5. Bayindir P, Guillerman RP, Hicks MJ, et al. Cellular mesoblastic nephroma (infantile renal fibrosarcoma): institutional review of the clinical, diagnostic imaging, and pathologic features of a distinctive neoplasm of infancy. Pediatr Radiol 2009;39:1066–74.
6. Vujanić GM. Renal tumours of childhood: an overview. Diagn Histopathol 2009;15:501–9.
7. Husain AN, Pysher TJ. The kidney and lower urinary tract. In: Stocker JT, Dehner LP, Husain AN, editors. Stocker and Dehner's pediatric pathology. 3rd edition. Philadelphia: Lippincott Williams & Wilkins; 2011. p. 779–836.
8. Lowe LH, Isuani BH, Heller RM, et al. Wilms tumor and beyond. Radiographics 2000;20:1585–603.
9. Chaudry G, Perez-Atayde AR, Ngan BY, et al. Imaging of congenital mesoblastic nephroma with pathological correlation. Pediatr Radiol 2009;39:1080–6.
10. Kirks DR, Kaufman RA. Function within mesoblastic nephroma: imaging-pathologic correlation. Pediatr Radiol 1989;19:136–9.
11. Lee SH, Choi YH, Kim WS, et al. Ossifying renal tumor of infancy: findings at ultrasound, CT and MRI. Pediatr Radiol 2014;44:625–8.
12. Flannigan RK, Heran MK, Oviedo A, et al. Case report and literature review of a rare diagnosis of ossifying renal tumour of infancy. Can Urol Assoc J 2014;8(3–4):E184–7.
13. Vazquez JL, Barnewolt CE, Shamberger RC, et al. Ossifying renal tumor of infancy presenting as a palpable abdominal mass. Pediatr Radiol 1998;28:454–7.
14. Steffens J, Kraus J, Misho B, et al. Ossifying renal tumor of infancy. J Urol 1993;149:1080–1.
15. Seixas-Mikelus SA, Khan A, Williot PE, et al. Three-month-old boy with juvenile granulosa cell tumor of testis and ossifying renal tumor of infancy. Urology 2009;74:311–3.
16. Xi S, Chen H, Wu X, et al. Malignant renal angiomyolipoma with metastases in a child. Int J Surg Pathol 2014;22:160–6.
17. Hennigar RA, Beckwith JB. Nephrogenic adenofibroma: a novel kidney tumor of young people. Am J Surg Pathol 1992;16:325–34.
18. Ewalt DH, Sheffield E, Sparagana SP, et al. Renal lesion growth in children with tuberous sclerosis complex. J Urol 1998;160:141–5.

19. Geller E, Smergel EM, Lowry PA. Renal neoplasms of childhood. Radiol Clin North Am 1997; 35:1391–413.

20. Lemaitre L, Robert Y, Dubrulle F, et al. Renal angiomyolipoma: growth followed up with CT and/or US. Radiology 1995;197:598–602.

21. Pargaonkar V, Nadkarni N, Thiele E, et al. Lipid poor renal lesions in tuberous sclerosis complex. Conference paper, presented at 98th Scientific Assembly and Annual Meeting, Radiological Society of North America, Chicago, November 25–30, 2012.

22. Milner J, McNeil B, Alioto J, et al. Fat poor renal angiomyolipoma: patient, computerized tomography and histological findings. J Urol 2006;176:905–9.

23. Siegel CL, Middleton WD, Teefey SA, et al. Angiomyolipoma and renal cell carcinoma: US differentiation. Radiology 1996;198:789–93.

24. Malhi H, Grant EG, Duddalwar V. Contrast-enhanced ultrasound of the liver and kidney. Radiol Clin North Am 2014;52:1177–90.

25. Yamashita Y, Ueno S, Makita O, et al. Hyperechoic renal tumors: anechoic rim and intramural cysts in US differentiation of renal cell carcinoma from angiomyolipoma. Radiology 1993;188:179–82.

26. Israel GM, Hindman N, Hecht E, et al. The use of opposed-phase chemical shift MRI in the diagnosis of renal angiomyolipomas. AJR Am J Roentgenol 2005;18:1868–72.

27. Bissler JJ, McCormack FX, Young LR. Sirolimus of angiomyolipoma in tuberous sclerosis complex or lymphangioleiomyomatosis. N Engl J Med 2008; 358:140–51.

28. Xie P, Yang Z, Yuan Z. Lipid-poor renal angiomyolipoma: differentiation from clear cell renal cell carcinoma using wash-in and washout characteristics on contrast-enhanced computed tomography. Oncol Lett 2016;11:2327–31.

29. Joshi VV, Beckwith JB. Multilocular cyst of the kidney (cystic nephroma) and cystic, partially differentiated nephroblastoma: terminology and criteria for diagnosis. Cancer 1989;64:466–79.

30. Charles AK, Vujani GM, Berry PJ. Renal tumours of childhood. Histopathology 1998;32:293–309.

31. Antic T, Perry KT, Harrison K, et al. Mixed epithelial and stromal tumor of the kidney and cystic nephroma share overlapping features: reappraisal of 15 lesions. Arch Pathol Lab Med 2006;130:80–5.

32. Madewell JE, Goldman SM, Davis CJ Jr, et al. Multilocular cystic nephroma: a radiographic-pathologic correlation of 58 patients. Radiology 1983;146:309–21.

33. Freire M, Remer EM. Clinical and radiology features of cystic renal masses. AJR Am J Roentgenol 2009;192:1367–72.

34. Lane BR, Campbell SC, Remer EM, et al. Adult cystic nephroma and mixed epithelial and stromal tumor of the kidney: clinical, radiographic, and pathologic characteristics. Urology 2008;71:1142–8.

35. Eble JN. Cystic partially differentiated nephroblastoma. In: Eble JN, Sauter G, Epstein JI, et al, editors. Tumours of the urinary system and male genital organs. Geneva (Switzerland): World Health Organization; 2004. p. 55.

36. Hill DA, Ivanovich J, Priest JR, et al. DICER1 mutations in familial pleuropulmonary blastoma. Science 2009;325(5943):965.

37. Julian JC, Merguerian PA, Shortliffe LMD. Pediatric genitourinary tumors. Curr Opin Oncol 1995;7: 265–74.

38. Lonergan GJ, Martinez-Leon MI, Agrons GA, et al. Nephrogenic rests, nephroblastomatosis, and associated lesions of the kidney. Radiographics 1998;18:947–68.

39. National Cancer Institute at the National Institutes of Health. Wilms tumor and other childhood kidney tumors treatment (PDQ).

40. Brisse HJ, Smets AM, Kaste SC, et al. Imaging in unilateral Wilms tumour. Pediatr Radiol 2008;38: 18–29.

41. Khanna G, Naranjo A, Hoffer F, et al. Detection of preoperative Wilms tumor rupture with CT: a report from the Children's Oncology Group. Radiology 2013;266:610–7.

42. Dome JS, Graf N, Geller GI, et al. Advances in Wilms tumor treatment and biology: progress through international collaboration. J Clin Oncol 2015;33:1–11.

43. Glassberg KI. Normal and abnormal development of the kidney: a clinician's interpretation of current knowledge. J Urol 2002;167:2339–50.

44. White KS, Grossman H. Wilms' and associated renal tumors of childhood. Pediatr Radiol 1991;21:81–8.

45. Royer-Pokora B. Genetics of pediatric renal tumors. Pediatr Nephrol 2013;28:13–23.

46. Rodriguez MM, Correa-Medina M, Whittington EE. Bilateral renal dysplasia, nephroblastomatosis, and bronchial stenosis: a new syndrome? Fetal Pediatr Pathol 2015;34:190–6.

47. Amar AM, Tomlinson G, Green DM, et al. Clinical presentation of rhabdoid tumors of the kidney. J Pediatr Hematol Oncol 2001;23:105–8.

48. Chung CJ, Lorenzo R, Rayder S, et al. Rhabdoid tumors of the kidney in children: CT findings. AJR Am J Roentgenol 1995;164:697–700.

49. Koga Y, Matsuzaki A, Suminoe A, et al. Long-term survival after autologous peripheral blood stem cell transplantation in two patients with malignant rhabdoid tumor of the kidney. Pediatr Blood Cancer 2009;52:888–90.

50. Argani P, Perlman EJ, Breslow NE, et al. Clear cell sarcoma of the kidney: a review of 351 cases from the National Wilms Tumor Study Group Pathology Center. Am J Surg Pathol 2000;2:4–18.

51. Sotelo-Avila F, Gonzalez-Crussi S, Sadowinski WM, et al. Clear cell sarcoma of the kidney: a

clinicopathologic study of 21 patients with long-term follow-up evaluation. Hum Pathol 1986;16:1219–30.

52. Glass RB, Davidson AJ, Fernbach SK. Clear cell sarcoma of the kidney: CT, sonographic, and pathologic correlation. Radiology 1991;180:715–7.

53. Gooskens SL, Furtwängler R, Vujanic GM, et al. Clear cell sarcoma of the kidney: a review. Eur J Cancer 2012;48:221926.

54. Pastore G, Znaor A, Spreafico F, et al. Malignant renal tumours incidence and survival in European children (1978–1997); report from the ACCIS project. Eur J Cancer 2006;42:2103–14.

55. Hartman DS, Davis CJ Jr, Madewell JE, et al. Primary malignant renal tumors in the second decade of life: Wilms tumor versus renal cell carcinoma. J Urol 1982;127:888–91.

56. Silberstein J, Grabowski J, Saltzstein SL. Renal cell carcinoma in the pediatric population: results from the California Cancer Registry. Pediatr Blood Cancer 2009;52:237–41.

57. Greco AJ, Baluarte JH, Meyers KE, et al. Chromophobe renal cell carcinoma in a pediatric living-related kidney transplant recipient. Am J Kidney Dis 2005;45(6):e105–8.

58. Perlman EJ. Pediatric renal cell carcinoma. Surg Pathol Clin 2010;3:641–51.

59. Eble JN, Sauter G, Epstein JI, et al. World Health Organization classification of tumours; pathology and genetics of tumours of the urinary system and male genital organs. Lyon (France): IARC-Press; 2004.

60. Medeiros LJ, Palmedo G, Krigman HR, et al. Oncocytoid renal cell carcinoma after neuroblastoma: a report of four cases of a distinct clinicopathologic entity. Am J Surg Pathol 1999;23:772–80.

61. Lee EY. CT imaging of mass-like renal lesions in children. Pediatr Radiol 2007;37:896–907.

62. Siegel MJ. Pediatric body CT. Philadelphia: Lippincott Williams & Wilkins; 1999. p. 226–52.

63. Sausville JE, Hernandez DJ, Argani P. Pediatric renal cell carcinoma. J Pediatr Urol 2009;5:308–14.

64. Leuschner I, Harms D, Schmidt D. Renal cell carcinoma in children: histology, immunohistochemistry, and follow-up of 10 cases. Med Pediatr Oncol 1991;19:33–41.

65. Gerald WL, Rosai J. Desmoplastic small cell tumor with divergent differentiation. Pediatr Pathol 1989;9:177–83.

66. Baltogiannis N, Mavridis G, Keramidas D. Intraabdominal desmoplastic small round cell tumor: report of two cases in paediatric patients. Eur J Pediatr Surg 2002;12:333–6.

67. Ordonez NG. Desmoplastic small round cell tumor: a histopathologic study of 39 cases with emphasis on unusual histological patterns. Am J Surg Pathol 1998;22:1303–13.

68. Eaton SH, Cendron MA. Primary desmoplastic small round cell tumor of the kidney in a 7-year-old girl. J Pediatr Urol 2006;2:52–4.

69. Egloff AM, Lee EY, Dillon JE, et al. Desmoplastic small round cell tumor of the kidney in a pediatric patient: sonographic and multiphase CT findings. AJR Am J Roentgenol 2005;185:1347–9.

70. Su MC, Jeng YM, Chu YCH. Desmoplastic small round cell tumor of the kidney. Am J Surg Pathol 2004;28:1379–83.

71. Crapanzano JP, Cardillo M, Lin O, et al. Cytology of desmoplastic small round cell tumor. Cancer 2002;96:21–31.

72. Kim JH, Goo HW, Yoon CH. Intra-abdominal desmoplastic small round cell tumor: multiphase CT findings in two children. Pediatr Radiol 2003;33:418–21.

73. Eklund MJ, Cundiff C, Shehata BM, et al. Desmoplastic small round cell tumor of the kidney with unusual imaging features. Clin Imaging 2015;39:904–7.

74. Walton WJ, Flores RR. Desmoplastic small round cell tumor of the kidney: AIRP best cases in radiologic-pathologic correlation. Radiographics 2016;36:1533–8.

75. Ellinger J, Bastian PJ, Hauser S, et al. Primitive neuroectodermal tumor: rare, highly aggressive differential diagnosis in urologic malignancies. Urology 2006;68:257–62.

76. Lalwani N, Prasad SR, Vikram R, et al. Pediatric and adult primary sarcomas of the kidney: a cross-sectional imaging review. Acta Radiol 2011;52:448–57.

77. Ekram T, Elsayes KM, Cohan RH, et al. Computed tomography and magnetic resonance features of renal Ewing sarcoma. Acta Radiol 2008;49:1085–90.

78. Reznek RH, Mootoosamy I, Webb JAW, et al. CT in renal and perirenal lymphoma: a further look. Clin Radiol 1990;42:233–8.

79. Cohan RH, Dunnick NR, Leder RA, et al. Computed tomography of renal lymphoma. J Comput Assist Tomogr 1990;14:933–8.

80. Abramson SJ, Price AP. Imaging of pediatric lymphomas. Radiol Clin North Am 2008;46:313–38.

81. Sheth S, Ali S, Fishman E. Imaging of renal lymphoma: patterns of disease with pathologic correlation. Radiographics 2006;26:1151–68.

82. Huang JJ, Sung JM, Chen KW, et al. Acute bacterial nephritis: a clinicoradiologic correlation based on computed tomography. Am J Med 1992;93:289–98.

83. Raszka WV, Khan O. Pyelonephritis. Pediatr Rev 2005;66:364–70.

84. Hoberman A, Charron M, Hickey RW, et al. Imaging studies after a first febrile urinary tract infection in young children. N Engl J Med 2003;348:195–202.

85. Thurston W, Wilson SR. The urinary tract. In: Ruck CM, Wilson SR, Charboneau JW, editors. Diagnostic ultrasound. 2nd edition. St Louis (MO): Mosby; 1998. p. 329–97.

86. Dacher JN, Pfister C, Monroc M, et al. Power Doppler sonographic pattern of acute pyelonephritis in children: comparison with CT. AJR Am J Roentgenol 1996;166:1451–5.

87. Farmer KD, Gellett LR, Dubbins PA. The sonographic appearance of acute focal pyelonephritis: 8 years experience. Clin Radiol 2002;57:483–7.

88. Vivier PH, Beurdeley SA, Lim RP, et al. MRI and suspected acute pyelonephritis in children: comparison of diffusion-weighted imaging with gadolinium-enhanced T1-weighted imaging. Eur Radiol 2014;24:19–25.

89. Bluth EI, Arger PH, Benson CB, et al, editors. Ultrasound, a practical approach to clinical problems. New York: Thieme; 2008.

90. Jennette JC, Olson JL, Schwartz M, et al, editors. Heptinstall's pathology of the kidney. New York: Lippincott Williams and Wilkins; 2006.

91. Son J, Lee EY, Restrepo R, et al. Focal renal lesions in pediatric patients. AJR Am J Roentgenol 2012; 199:W668–82.

92. Dyer RB, Chen MY, Zagoria RJ. Classic signs in uroradiology. Radiographics 2004;24(suppl 1): S247–80.

93. Hann L, Pfister RC. Renal subcapsular rim sign: new etiologies and pathogenesis. Am J Roentgenol 1982;138:51–4.

94. Agrons GA, Wagner BJ, Lonergan GJ, et al. Genitourinary rhabdomyosarcoma in children: radiologic-pathologic correlation. Radiographics 1997;17:919–37.

95. Wu HY. The surgical management of paediatric bladder and prostate rhabdomyosarcoma. Arab J Urol 2013;11:40–6.

96. Gurney JG, Young JL Jr, Roffers SD, et al. Soft tissue sarcomas. In: Ries LA, Smith MA, Gurney JG, et al, editors. Cancer incidence and survival among children and adolescents: United States SEER Program 1975-1995. Bethesda (MD): National Cancer Institute, SEER Program; 1999. p. 111–23. NIH Pub.No. 99-4649.

97. Wong-You JJ, Woodward PJ, Manning MA, et al. Neoplasms of the urinary bladder: radiologic-pathologic correlation. Radiographics 2006;26:553–80.

98. Schepper AM. Imaging of soft tissue tumors. Berlin (Germany): Springer Verlag; 2006.

99. Verma S, Rajesh A, Prasad R, et al. Urinary bladder cancer: the role of MR imaging. Radiographics 2012;32:371–87.

100. Liddell RM, Weinberger E, Schofield DE, et al. Fibroepithelial polyp of the ureter in a child. AJR Am J Roentgenol 1991;157:1273–4.

101. Debruyne FMJ, Moonen WA, Daenekindt AA, et al. Fibroepithelial polyp of the ureter. Urology 1980;16: 355–9.

102. Li R, Lightfoot M, Alsyouf M, et al. Diagnosis and management of fibroepithelial polyps in children: a new treatment regimen. J Pediatr Urol 2015;11:22.e1-6.

103. Shinagare AB, Sadow CA, Sahni A, et al. Urinary bladder: normal appearance and mimics of malignancy at CT urography. Cancer Imaging 2011;11: 100–8.

Musculoskeletal Traumatic Injuries in Children
Characteristic Imaging Findings and Mimickers

Victor M. Ho-Fung, MD[a],*, Matthew A. Zapala, MD, PhD[b],
Edward Y. Lee, MD, MPH[c,d]

KEYWORDS

- Salter-Harris classification • Greenstick fracture • Bone bridge • Bone growth disturbance
- Pediatric musculoskeletal injury

KEY POINTS

- In the skeletally immature, the physis is more fragile and prone to injury than the ligamentous structures.
- Young children demonstrate greater fracture healing capacity due to the higher biologic activity and osteogenic potential of their periosteum compared with adults.
- Premature physeal closure in children is most often posttraumatic.
- Most acute traumatic bone injuries can be diagnosed with conventional radiographs.
- MR imaging is an excellent tool for differentiation of chronic repetitive trauma versus an acute musculoskeletal injury related to sports participation.

INTRODUCTION

Nearly one-third of emergency department visits in children and adolescents in the United States are related to traumatic injuries.[1] There is increased participation of children and adolescents in sports with a concomitant increased risk of traumatic injuries.[2] Diagnostic imaging of musculoskeletal traumatic injuries in children is crucial for the management of acute and long-term complications. This review article discusses currently available imaging modalities and techniques, physiology of normal bone growth, injury patterns, healing, and complications relevant to the imaging evaluation of musculoskeletal traumatic injuries in children with particular emphasis on the long bones. In addition, mimickers of musculoskeletal traumatic injuries in the pediatric population are reviewed.

All authors certify that there is no actual or potential conflict of interest in relation to this article.
[a] Department of Radiology, Children's Hospital of Philadelphia, Perelman School of Medicine, University of Pennsylvania, 3401 Civic Center Boulevard, Philadelphia, PA 19104, USA; [b] Pediatric Radiology Section, Department of Radiology and Biomedical Imaging, Benioff Children's Hospital, University of California, San Francisco, 1975 Fourth Street, San Francisco, CA 94158, USA; [c] Division of Thoracic Imaging, Department of Radiology, Boston Children's Hospital, Harvard Medical School, 300 Longwood Avenue, Boston, MA 02115, USA; [d] Department of Medicine, Boston Children's Hospital, Harvard Medical School, 300 Longwood Avenue, Boston, MA 02115, USA
* Corresponding author.
E-mail address: hov@email.chop.edu

0033-8389/17/© 2017 Elsevier Inc. All rights reserved.

IMAGING MODALITIES AND TECHNIQUES
Radiography

Conventional radiography remains the main imaging tool for assessment of traumatic injuries in children and adults. Most acute traumatic bone injuries can be diagnosed with conventional radiographs. Attention to appropriate positioning and technique is essential for accurate diagnosis of subtle fractures and assessment of joint derangement. The routine use of comparison radiographs remains a controversial topic. In the opinion of the authors, obtaining routine comparison radiographs of the contralateral joint in young children is not always necessary and can increase unnecessary ionizing radiation exposure.[3,4] A more reasonable approach is the evaluation of the initial images and deciding if additional comparison images of the contralateral joint are truly necessary. This approach is in line with the principle of as low as reasonably achievable (ALARA) in the judicious use of ionizing radiation in pediatric patients.

Ultrasound

The application of ultrasound evaluation of musculoskeletal injuries in young patients and adolescents for a variety of specific traumatic injuries is currently growing.[5] The assessment of soft tissue injuries using dynamic maneuvers with reproducibility of symptoms, availability of the contralateral extremity for comparison, lack of radiation exposure, and avoidance of general anesthesia are main attractive features of ultrasound.[6] However, as in all imaging modalities with novel applications, more experience and better normative data of the sonographic appearance of the growing skeleton is needed before expanding the indications of ultrasound in pediatric traumatic injuries.

Computed Tomography

Computed tomography (CT) utilization has been under a substantial amount of scrutiny in recent years due to the inherent risk of ionizing radiation in patients, particularly young children.[7] However, CT 3-dimensional reconstructions play an important role in the evaluation of polytraumatized patients and the assessment of complex fractures requiring emergent surgical planning, such as transitional fractures of the distal tibia, complex pelvic fractures, and unstable vertebral spine fractures.[8,9] Up-to-date reference resources are available from the Image Gently Alliance for the appropriateness criteria and radiation dose optimization when imaging children.[10]

MR Imaging

MR imaging is an excellent tool for the assessment of the bone marrow, cartilaginous components of the growing skeleton, and soft tissues.[11,12] MR imaging allows for superior tissue resolution combined with multiplanar evaluation. Several important indications for the use of MR imaging in children include radiographically occult fractures in pediatric patients with persistent pain, assessment of potential internal derangement, and complications of prior trauma, such as premature physeal closure and growth abnormalities of the developing skeleton. In addition, MR imaging is an excellent tool for differentiation of chronic repetitive trauma versus an acute injury related to sports participation. However, availability in the acute traumatic setting, cost-efficiency, and potential sedation or general anesthesia in young children are important considerations for the use of MR imaging in the assessment of musculoskeletal traumatic injuries.

NORMAL BONE GROWTH OF THE PEDIATRIC SKELETON

Longitudinal growth of the long bones is based on endochondral ossification, in which bone formation depends on a sequential transformation from a cartilaginous precursor. The physis or growth plate is a thin disk structure located between epiphyseal cartilage and the metaphysis that provides this cartilaginous precursor. The presence of the growth plate in children allows for a unique subset of fractures not present in adults. In addition, disruption of the rich vascular supply of the metaphysis can derange the normal apoptosis of chondrocytes in the hypertrophic zone of the physis and prevent normal mineralization leading to growth disturbances[13] (Fig. 1).

FRACTURE HEALING IN TRAUMATIC INJURIES IN CHILDREN

Fracture healing is a complex sequential process. Acutely, an immediate inflammatory phase occurs with hematoma formation at the end of the fracture fragments. This is followed by a reparative phase in which initial callous is predominantly immature woven bone. Finally, a remodeling phase occurs in which woven bone matures into lamellar bone and the shape of the bone returns to its initial configuration.[14] Periosteal membranous ossification plays a key role in fracture healing because undifferentiated cells in the periosteum differentiate into osteoblasts capable of forming bone

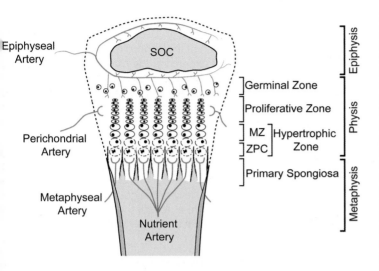

Fig. 1. Normal components of the immature skeleton and endochondral ossification. The epiphyses is the articulating end of a long bone, composed of hyaline cartilage with progressive development of a secondary ossification center (SOC). The physeal cartilage is highly cellular with a distinct columnar arrangement parallel to the long axis of the bones. The chondrocytes originate in the germinal zone near the epiphysis, then advance toward the metaphysis with sequential proliferation, undergo hypertrophy at the maturation zone (MZ), and finally apoptosis with mineralization of the matrix in the zone of provisional calcification (ZPC). The primary spongiosa in the metaphy-

sis is the newest bone formed in the skeleton. There is a rich vascular supply to the metaphysis from nutrient and metaphyseal arteries, rendering this region vulnerable to blood borne diseases and infection. The epiphysis vascular supply through the epiphyseal artery does not form a capillary bed but instead courses through canals in the cartilage, which play a critical role in the formation of the SOC. The perfusion to the epiphysis is fragile and scant, which predisposes the region to avascular necrosis.

without a cartilaginous model. Young children demonstrate greater fracture healing capacity due to the higher biologic activity and osteogenic potential of their periosteum compared with adults (Fig. 2). The periosteum in children is also thicker, more vascular, and less frequently disrupted around the entire circumference of the bone, allowing for greater fracture stability.[15,16]

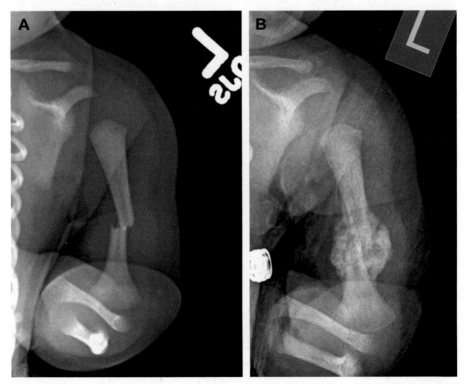

Fig. 2. Newborn infant boy with left arm swelling after difficult breech delivery. (*A*) Initial frontal radiograph of the left humerus demonstrates transverse acute midshaft fracture. (*B*) Follow-up radiograph obtained at 21 days of age demonstrates extensive callous formation and periosteal reaction consistent with interval healing.

CLASSIFICATION OF ACUTE PEDIATRIC FRACTURES
Long Bone Fractures

Pediatric fractures in the long bones can be classified into (1) plastic deformations, (2) greenstick fractures, (3) buckle fractures, (4) physeal fractures, and (5) complete fractures. The first 4 categories are unique to the pediatric skeleton due to anatomic and biomechanical differences from the adult skeleton. The mechanical properties of bone depend on its material composition and its complex architecture.[17] The pediatric bone is less stiff than adult bone and is, therefore, able to absorb more energy before fracturing resulting in a greater capacity to undergo plastic deformation.[18]

Plastic deformation

Plastic deformation is most commonly seen in the forearm, particularly the ulna.[19] The radius and ulna in normal children are often slightly bowed. Longitudinal compressive forces to the ends of long curved tubular bones would cause variable degrees of deformity, depending on the magnitude and duration of the applied force.[20,21] Intermediate forces not exceeding the maximal strength of the bones can result in radiographically occult microfractures and plastic deformation with increased bowing. Radiographs most often demonstrate bowing in 1 bone and fracture in the other (Fig. 3A). It is important to recognize that radiographs performed in the first few weeks following acute plastic deformation usually demonstrate absence of or a small amount of new bone formation.[21] If the deformity occurs in children younger than 4 years of age, or if the deformity is less than 20°, the angulation usually corrects with growth.[17]

Greenstick fracture

Greenstick fractures typically occur in long bones, particularly in the radius and ulna. The increased capacity of plastic deformation, lower mineral content, and the increased porosity of bone in children can prolong the time and energy absorption and allow incomplete propagation of the fracture line

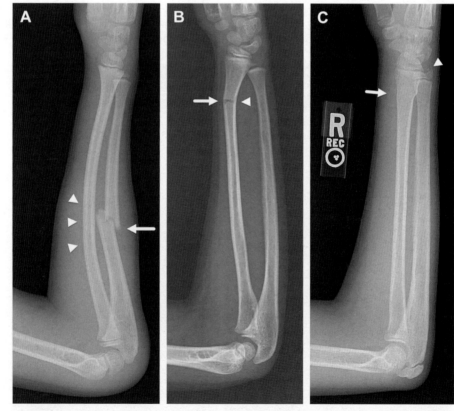

Fig. 3. Long bone fractures in children. (A) Lateral radiograph of the forearm shows plastic deformation of the radius (*arrowheads*) and transverse fracture of the ulnar midshaft (*arrow*). (B) Lateral radiograph of the forearm shows greenstick fracture of the distal radial shaft with cortical disruption at the radial side (*arrow*) and plastic bowing of the ulnar side (*arrowhead*). (C) Lateral radiograph of the forearm shows buckle fracture of the distal radius metadiaphysis (*arrow*) and ulnar styloid avulsion fracture (*arrowhead*).

through the bone.[15,18] This results in plastic deformity in the compression side of the bone with formation of the fracture line along the tension side and a greenstick type fracture (see **Fig. 3**B).

Buckle fracture
Buckle fractures are common. They result from compression failure of the bone at the junction of the metaphysis and diaphysis. Porosity in the metaphysis is larger relative to the denser bone of the diaphysis, causing buckling of the cortex

at this location with compressive forces (see **Fig. 3**C). Historically, when a buckle fracture is noted circumferentially along the metaphyseal region, it is called a torus fracture, because of its similarity to the raised band around the base of a classical Greek column.[15] These fractures occur more commonly in the distal radius and ulna, proximal radius, distal tibia and fibula, and small bones of the hand and feet.[22] Buckle fractures can be subtle and a high level of suspicion for these fractures should be present when noting subtle

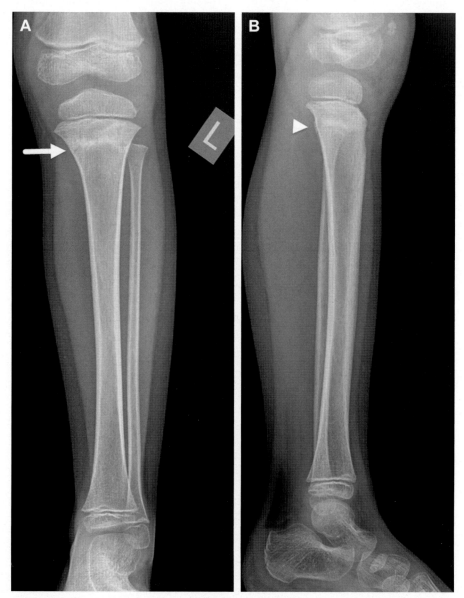

Fig. 4. Buckle fracture of the proximal tibia associated to trampoline injury in a 5-year-old boy. (A) Frontal and (B) lateral radiographs obtained 4 weeks after initial injury demonstrate subtle buckling of the proximal tibial cortex with dense transverse sclerotic line (*arrow*) and posterior periosteal reaction (*arrowhead*) in keeping with healing changes. The initial radiographs were interpreted as normal (not shown).

increased angulation or small convexity at the junction of the metaphysis and diaphysis in young children. Usually these fractures are stable and can be simply splinted or casted with good result.

In the proximal tibia, a buckle fracture can be seen associated with acute trampoline injuries in young children (aged 2–5 years; **Fig. 4**). The mechanism is likely related to differences in weight when jumping together with a heavier individual and increased impaction forces in the proximal tibia of the young children during landing on the trampoline mat.[23] Other investigators have described similar proximal tibial fractures in the same age population, postulating a hyperextension injury at the

knee with forces applied predominantly to the anterior cortex causing compressive forces with anterior cortical buckling, posterior cortical diastases, and possible anterior tilting of the proximal tibial epiphysis.[22,24]

Physeal fractures (Salter-Harris classification)
The physis provides the cartilaginous mold necessary for endochondral ossification and growth of the bone. However, the cartilaginous physis is weaker than its surrounding ossified bone and more susceptible to injury before its closure.[25] The most common location for acute physeal fractures is the distal radius.[26] Usually the physis heals

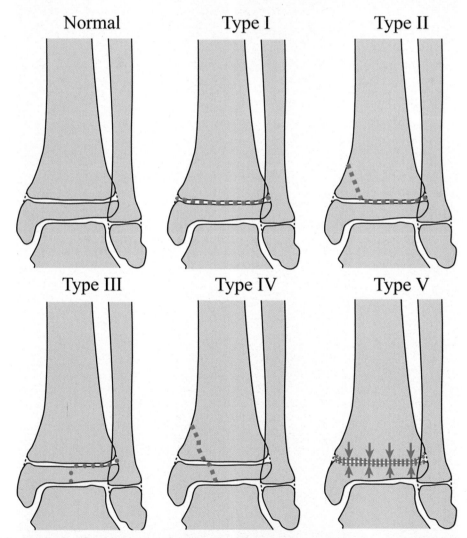

Fig. 5. Salter-Harris Classification in the distal tibia. Type I fracture demonstrates physeal distance from the metaphysis without radiographic evidence of fracture through the ossified bone. Type II fracture is the most common fracture pattern, with the fracture line extending from the physis into the metaphysis. Type III fracture is intra-articular and extends from the epiphyses into the physis. Type IV fracture is also intra-articular and involves both epiphyseal and metaphyseal components with the fracture line passing across the physis. Type V fracture is considered a crush injury of the physis and is very uncommon.

rapidly, between 3 to 6 weeks.[15] This rapid healing provides a limited window for fracture reduction because late reduction (>1 week) potentially leads to physeal damage.[27] Injury to the physis can result in growth abnormalities and premature physeal closure with progressive angular deformity, limb-length discrepancy, and joint incongruity.[13,15,28] Thus, appropriate imaging diagnosis and identification of physeal fractures is critical in limiting potential complications.

The Salter-Harris (SH) classification is the most common system for physeal fracture characterization based on the radiographic appearance of the physeal fracture (**Figs. 5–7**).[29] A more complex classification scheme has been proposed by Ogden,[30] with inclusion of 4 other mechanism of injury patterns in addition to the original 5 in the SH classification. However, it has not been widely used compared with the original SH classification.

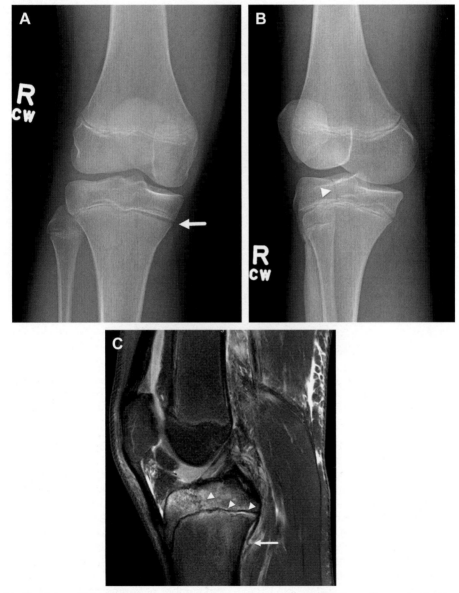

Fig. 6. Salter-Harris type III fracture of the right proximal tibia in a 15-year-old boy after soccer tackle. (*A*) Frontal and (*B*) oblique radiographs demonstrate widening of the medial physis (*arrow*) with epiphyseal lucent fracture line (*arrowhead*). (*C*) Sagittal intermediate-weighted fat-saturated MR image confirming nondisplaced fracture line (*arrowheads*) extending from the posterior physis into the epiphysis. There is disruption and superior retraction of the posterior tibial periosteum (*arrow*).

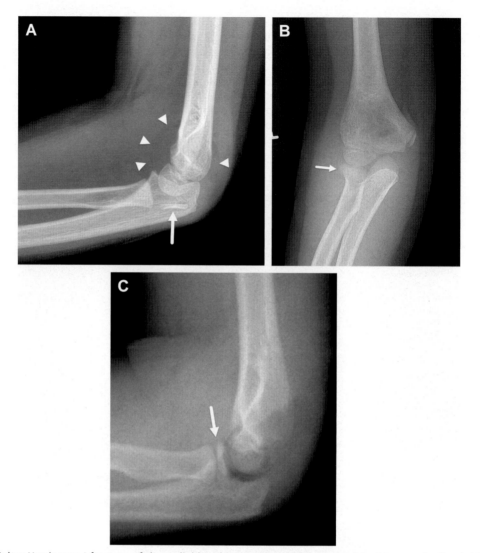

Fig. 7. Salter-Harris type I fracture of the radial head in a 10-year-old boy with blunt trauma to the right elbow after fall. (*A*) Frontal and (*B*) lateral views of the right elbow demonstrate complete physeal separation of the radial head and posterior displacement of the secondary ossification center into the joint (*arrow*) with a joint effusion (*arrowheads*). (*C*) Lateral fluoroscopic image after anatomic reduction of the fracture (*arrow*).

Transitional fractures are a particular subset of distal tibia physeal fractures that occur during the period of distal physeal closure.[31] The 2 fractures included in this specific group of fractures are the triplane fracture (SH IV fracture) and the juvenile Tillaux fracture (SH III fracture). The mechanism of injury is typically supination, external rotation, and compression stress with unpredictable multiplanar fracture patterns.[31,32] The cause of these fractures is related to the orderly asymmetric physeal closure of the distal tibia. The closure of the distal tibia begins centrally, continues medially, and terminates anterolaterally. Radiographically, the central tibial site overlying the medial edge of the talar dome where fusion begins is known as Kumps bump.[33] The type of transitional fracture is determined by the degree of physeal closure and relative weakness of the open physis. Older pediatric patients with more advanced physeal closure present with juvenile Tillaux fractures (**Fig. 8**). Juvenile Tillaux fractures are often intra-articular; thus anatomic reduction of the joint surfaces is recommended to minimize future posttraumatic arthritis. Following radiographic diagnosis, CT is indicated to determine the number of fragments, their configuration, and any displacement of the articular surface. Pediatric patients with a residual displacement of less than 2.5 mm after treatment have a uniformly good result.[32] Because these fractures present almost

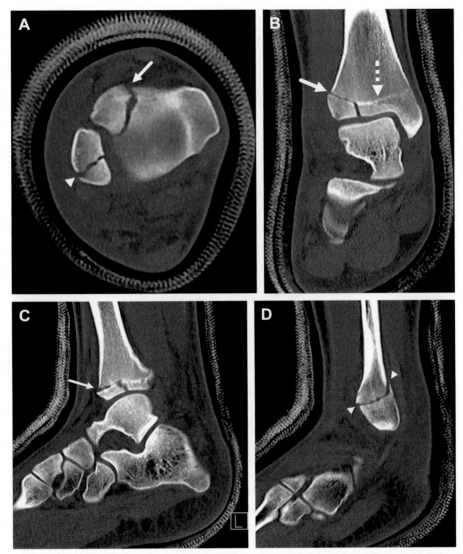

Fig. 8. Salter-Harris type III fracture of the distal tibia (Tillaux fracture) and SH type II fracture of the distal fibula in a 16-year-old female gymnast. (*A*) Axial, (*B*) coronal, and (*C*) sagittal CT images of the tibia demonstrate a SH type III fracture across the anterolateral region of the distal tibial physis with a vertical epiphyseal component (*arrows*). The medial physis demonstrate physiologic closure (*interrupted arrow*). There is approximately 3 mm of displacement of the distal tibial articular surface. (*D*) Sagittal CT image of the distal fibula demonstrates a SH type II fracture across the distal tibial physis and posterior metaphysis (*arrowheads*). The patient underwent open reduction and interval fixation of the tibial fracture.

at the end of physiologic growth, they rarely result in a growth arrest.

Complete Fractures

Fractures propagating through the entire bone can occur in children similar to adults. They are mainly described according to their orientation.

Spiral fractures

Spiral fractures are usually low-velocity injuries associated with a rotational force to the bone.

The prototypical spiral fracture is the so-called toddler's fracture of the tibia. This fracture is usually a minimally displaced short spiral oblique fracture of the distal tibial shaft in children younger than 3 years of age (**Fig. 9**).[34] The onset of limping after a minor event or without obvious injury in a young ambulating child, warrants radiographic evaluation to exclude this injury.[35] Clinically, an ankle injury is often suspected with performance of ankle radiographs with the fracture line often evident on the oblique view of the ankle.[36,37] An

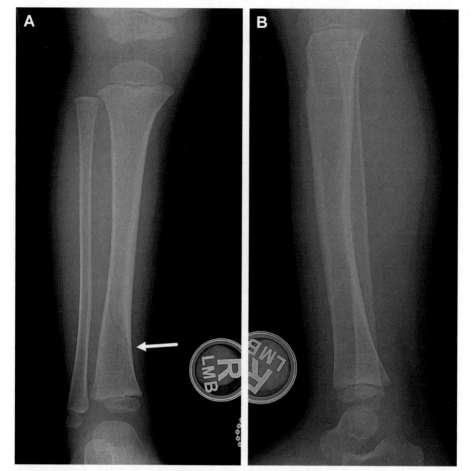

Fig. 9. Toddler fracture in a 2-year-old girl after fall. (*A*) Frontal view of the tibia demonstrates thin lucent spiral fracture line (*arrow*). (*B*) Lateral view of the tibia does not show the nondisplaced tibial fracture, which is not an usual finding in this type of fracture.

intact periosteum usually enables reduction of the fracture by reversing the rotational injury.[15] Some investigators advocate long-leg casting on young children with a history of an acute injury, inability to walk or limp, no constitutional signs, and negative radiographs with clinical concern for a toddler's fracture.[38]

Oblique fractures

Oblique fractures occur diagonally, usually at 30° to the axis, across the diaphysis of a bone. Analogous to complete fractures in the adult, these injuries usually cause more significant disruption of the soft tissues, including the periosteum.[39] These fractures are unstable and fracture reduction is attempted by immobilizing the extremity while applying traction.[15]

Transverse fractures

Transverse fractures through bone in children usually occur from 3-point bending. The periosteum on the side opposite to the force is typically torn.

Reduction is usually readily achieved by using the periosteum on the concave side of the fracture force.[39]

Apophyseal Injuries

Apophyses are secondary ossification centers that serve as insertion sites for tendons in the pediatric skeleton. The apophyses have an associated physis that models the shape of bones but does not contribute to their overall length.[11] The distraction associated with musculotendinous activity and the fragility of the physis make apophyses vulnerable to injury.[40] Trauma or unbalanced muscle contractions can cause avulsion of the apophyses with potential ligamentous injuries. Common sites for avulsion injuries include the medial epicondyle of the humerus and the ulnar styloid process of the ulna in the upper extremity, the apophyses around the pelvis, the inferior pole of the patella and tibial tuberosity in the knee, and the medial and lateral malleoli in the ankle (**Fig. 10**).[41]

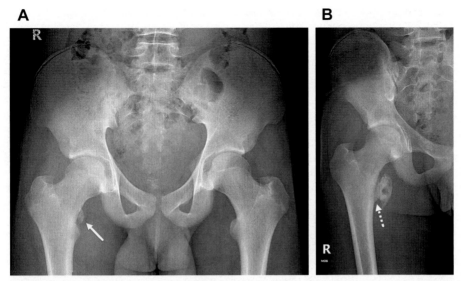

Fig. 10. Lesser trochanteric fracture in a 15-year-old girl after a fall in school gym class. (*A*) Frontal view of the pelvis and both hips during initial evaluation demonstrate superior displacement of the right lesser trochanter apophysis (*arrow*) at the distal insertion site of the iliopsoas muscle. (*B*) Frontal view of the right hip 3 months after the initial injury demonstrates solid bridging callous formation (*interrupted arrow*) in keeping with healing.

CHONDRO-OSSEOUS AND LIGAMENTOUS INJURIES IN CHILDREN

In the skeletally immature, the physis is more fragile than the ligamentous structures. Damage to the ligaments is more common with increasing age and skeletal maturity.[42] The anterior cruciate ligament (ACL) is the most common injured ligament in the knee. Avulsion of the tibial spine occurs in skeletally immature pediatric patients with similar mechanisms as those causing ACL injuries in adults (**Fig. 11**).[2] Tibial spine avulsions can be subtle in conventional radiographs or demonstrate only a joint effusion. Oblique and tunnel views are helpful for assessment of these fractures.[12,41] MR imaging allows for determination of the degree of displacement of the fracture fragment and commonly associated injuries to the collateral ligaments and menisci; crucial information for further management of these fractures.[43,44] Tibial spine avulsion fractures and ACL tears can rarely coexist.[42] However, in the experience of the

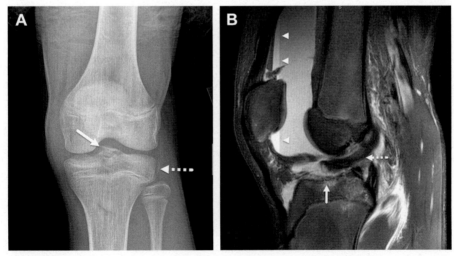

Fig. 11. Tibial spine avulsion fracture in a 14-year-old boy after a fall playing basketball. (*A*) Frontal radiograph of the knee demonstrates avulsion fracture (*arrow*) of the tibial spine (*interrupted arrow*) and Segond fracture of the lateral tibia. (*B*) Sagittal intermediate-weighted MR image confirms complete avulsion fracture (*arrow*) of the tibial spine with an intact ACL (*interrupted arrow*). Large hemarthrosis is also noted (*arrowheads*).

authors, differentiating abnormal signal intensity on MR imaging examinations secondary to ligamentous retraction of an intact ACL from a true ACL tear can be difficult and must be confirmed at the time of arthroscopic evaluation.[45]

CHRONIC SEQUELA OF MUSCULOSKELETAL TRAUMATIC INJURIES IN CHILDREN
Chronic Repetitive Injuries

Chronic repetitive injuries are caused by overuse during prolonged sports-related activities in the immature skeleton of children and adolescents.

Injuries to the physeal region from overuse can be confused with normal developmental changes in the skeletally immature.[11] The specific pattern and location of the injuries are related to the mechanical demands of individual sports. For example, chronic stress injury to the proximal humeral physis in pitchers is caused by rotational forces during overhead throwing and chronic stress injury to the distal radius in gymnasts is secondary to compressive loading during gymnastic routines.[46,47] Radiographic changes may include asymmetric widening and irregularity along the physis, and variable degrees of sclerosis and

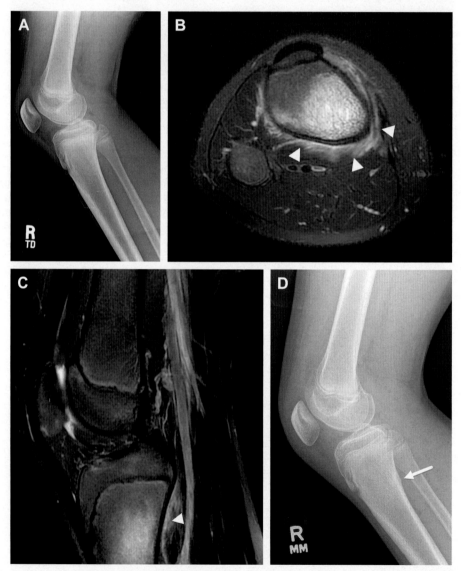

Fig. 12. Stress fracture of the proximal tibia in a 15-year-old female runner with recent increased in training regime. Patient presented with posterior knee pain. (*A*) Lateral radiograph of the knee at initial evaluation was normal. (*B*) Axial and (*C*) sagittal fat-saturated T2-weighted MR images obtained after 1 month of persistent knee pain, demonstrate bony edema within the posterior proximal tibia and pericortical soft tissue edema in a similar distribution (*arrowheads*). (*D*) Lateral radiograph of the knee obtained 2 months after (*A*) demonstrates subtle periosteal reaction with very faint cortical lucent fracture (*arrow*) in keeping with tibial stress fracture.

cystic changes in the metaphysis.[47] Similar physeal changes can be seen in the knees of young children with active participation in sports beyond the recreational level. The identification of these changes on MR imaging are important to allow for healing of the physis after cessation of the inciting activity and avoidance of potential complications such as premature physeal closure.[48]

Stress fractures are the result of long-standing workload in healthy bones. Persistent mechanical stresses cause imbalances between cortical resorption and subsequent bone deposition. Osteoblastic activity lags behind causing a failure to repair the bone and development of a stress fracture. Radiographs can be insensitive for the diagnosis of stress fractures and MR imaging is considered the best imaging modality for the presence of these injuries (**Fig. 12**).[49] Typical locations for stress fractures in young athletes include the tibia, fibula, metatarsals, and femur.[50]

Premature Physeal Closure and Growth Abnormalities

Premature physeal closure in children is most often posttraumatic.[13,51] The morbidity associated with premature physeal closure and bony bridge formation is determined by the age of the patient, bone affected, and location of the bony bridge. Younger patients with greater growth potential are at higher risk of more severe complications. For example, bony bridges on the periphery of the physis can lead to angular deformities, and bony bridges in the central portion of the physis can lead to growth arrest and limb length discrepancy (**Fig. 13**).[52] A high level of suspicion for the

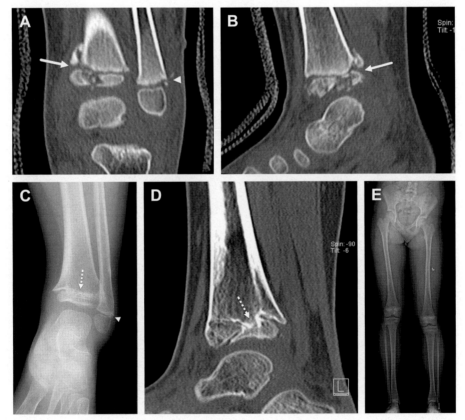

Fig. 13. Premature physeal closure of the distal tibia with angular deformity and leg length discrepancy. (*A*) Frontal and (*B*) sagittal CT images demonstrate complex comminuted Salter-Harris type IV fracture (*arrow*) of the distal tibia and small SH type II fracture (*arrowhead*) of the distal fibula at 3 years of age. (*C*) Lateral radiograph of the ankle obtained 6 months after injury shows partial premature closure of the physis (*interrupted arrow*) with varus deformity of the ankle joint related to continued growth of the open distal fibular physis (*arrowhead*). (*D*) Sagittal CT image demonstrates the bony bridge (*interrupted arrow*). The patient underwent distal fibular epiphysiodesis for correction of the angular deformity. (*E*) Orthoroentgenogram obtained 7 years after initial injury shows improvement of the left ankle varus deformity. However, there is a 3 cm leg length discrepancy (right > left) and associated right cephalad pelvic tilt; secondary to the left distal tibia premature physeal closure.

presence of premature physeal closure should be present in the follow-up of pediatric patients with known physeal fractures, particularly in the distal femur, and proximal and distal tibia. These areas have the greatest propensity for complication due to the irregular contour of the physes and greatest growth potential.[53] Conventional radiographs show bony bridges 6 to 12 months after injury. MR imaging using 3-dimensional spoiled gradient recalled echo sequences with fat

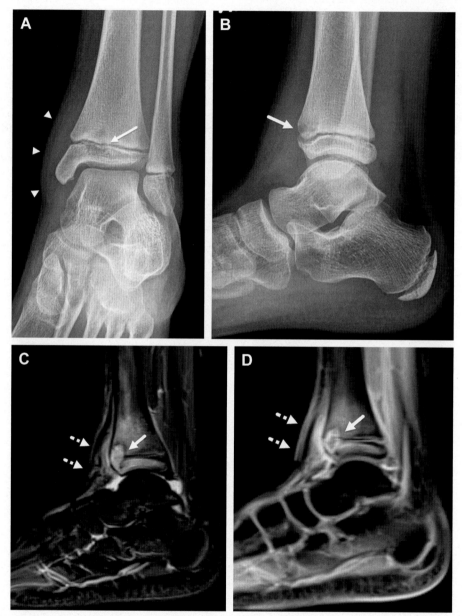

Fig. 14. An 8-year-old girl with left ankle pain and prior history of trauma 2 weeks earlier. (*A*) Frontal and (*B*) lateral radiographs of the ankle demonstrate ill-defined lucency (*arrow*) across the anterior distal tibial metaphysis and epiphysis with adjacent soft tissue swelling (*arrowheads*) concerning for osteomyelitis rather than a fracture. (*C*) Sagittal MR short-tau inversion recovery (STIR) sequence MR image demonstrates well-demarcated focal area of abnormal high signal intensity (*arrow*) corresponding to radiographic abnormality and adjacent soft tissue fluid collection (*interrupted arrows*). (*D*) Postcontrast T1 fat-saturated MR image shows a rim enhancing lesion (*arrow*) confirming osteomyelitis with anterior tibial cortical destruction and soft tissue abscess (*interrupted arrows*). Aspiration and drainage of the tibial abscess showed purulent material and growth of *Aggregatibacter aphrophilus*.

suppression demonstrates physeal discontinuity earlier and provides prognostic information regarding size and location of the bridge.[51,54,55] The general clinical recommendation for resection of a bony bridge and insertion of interposition material is the presence of less than 50% of physeal involvement in a child with 2 years or 2 cm of growth remaining.[56,57]

MIMICKERS OF MUSCULOSKELETAL TRAUMATIC INJURY IN CHILDREN
Musculoskeletal Infection

Musculoskeletal infection sometimes presents as a diagnostic challenge because it can be difficult to recognize in the early stages and can be confused with trauma or even a tumor.[58] A history of minor trauma is reported in up to one-third of children with osteomyelitis.[59] A metaphyseal hematoma due to trauma seems to predispose to bacterial colonization. Conventional radiographs are insensitive for the evaluation of osteomyelitis but are helpful to exclude traumatic injuries or tumors. MR imaging remains the primary modality for evaluation of bone infections and potential drainable abscess (**Fig. 14**).[60]

Symptomatic Anatomic Variants

There are several musculoskeletal congenital and developmental variants that can be associated with pain. Two of the most common entities associated with pain are discoid lateral meniscus in the knee joint and tarsal coalitions in the foot.

Discoid lateral meniscus can present in young patients with knee locking and lateral joint pain. Discoid lateral menisci are prone to tearing.[42,61] MR imaging criteria for the diagnosis of discoid lateral meniscus includes extension of the meniscus into the medial aspect of the joint (measuring >13 mm in transverse diameter or 2 mm greater in height in the coronal plane, and presence of 3 or more 5 mm contiguous slices showing continuity of the anterior and posterior horns in the sagittal plane; **Fig. 15**).[62]

Tarsal coalitions are common abnormalities of the hindfoot. Approximately 50% of coalitions are bilateral. Talocalcaneal and calcaneonavicular coalitions are the most common tarsal coalitions. Clinically, affected pediatric patients present with recurrent sprains and minor injuries with chronic foot pain and rigidity. The pain typically worsens with increased activity.[63] However, many tarsal coalitions can be asymptomatic without peroneal spasms or pes planovalgus deformity.[64] Radiographic features of calcaneonavicular coalition include visualization of abnormal osseous or fibrocartilaginous changes between the calcaneus and navicular in a medial oblique radiograph of the foot, and elongation of the anterior process of the calcaneus in the lateral view. Dorsal beaking of the talus and a continuous C-sign can be seen in lateral radiographs in the presence of a talocalcaneal coalition.[65] CT and MR imaging are more sensitive than radiographs and can be used effectively for treatment evaluation of subtalar coalitions (**Fig. 16**).[66]

Pathologic Fractures

Pathologic fractures can be seen with both benign and malignant bone lesions. In the pediatric population, a unicameral bone cyst is a relatively common benign lesion associated with a propensity to cause pathologic fracture. The classic radiographic features of a unicameral bone cyst include a central intramedullary location with cortical thinning adjacent to the metaphysis of the proximal humerus or femur. Following a pathologic fracture, a small cortical fallen fragment can be seen radiographically as a dependent bone fragment within the central portion of the fluid filled cavity of the cystic lesion (**Fig. 17**).[67,68]

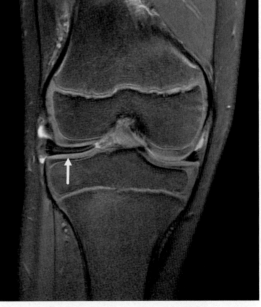

Fig. 15. A 7-year-old girl with left knee pain and locking sensation due to discoid lateral meniscus. Coronal intermediate-weighted sequence MR image at the midportion of the lateral femoral condyle shows diffuse enlargement of the lateral meniscus (*arrow*) measuring 20 mm in transverse diameter.

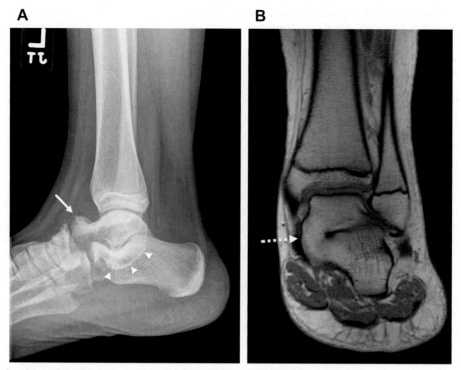

Fig. 16. Talocalcaneal coalition in a 12-year-old girl with persistent left ankle pain and cramping. (*A*) Lateral radiograph shows dorsal beaking (*arrow*) of the talus and a continuous C-sign (*arrowheads*). (*B*) Coronal T1-weighted MR image confirms complete osseous coalition (*interrupted arrow*) between the talus and calcaneus.

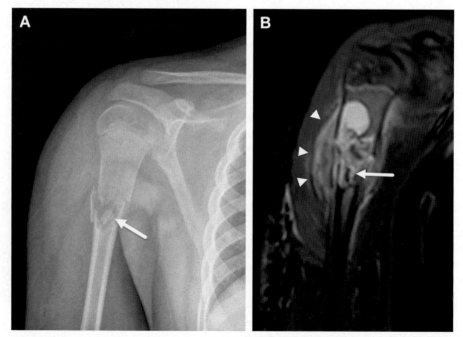

Fig. 17. A 13-year-old boy with severe right upper extremity pain after fall. (*A*) Frontal view of the right shoulder shows comminuted pathologic fracture with small cortical fragment within a cystic bone lesion (*arrow*). (*B*) Coronal STIR MR image confirms the fallen fragment (*arrow*) within a unicameral bone cyst. A pathologic fracture and subperiosteal hematoma (*arrowheads*) are also noted.

SUMMARY

Traumatic musculoskeletal injuries are a substantial source of morbidity in children and adolescents. The immature skeleton demonstrates unique injury patterns because of the presence of a growth plate and mechanical characteristics favoring plastic deformation. Clear understanding of these patterns of musculoskeletal injuries and potential for complications related to continued growth potential are essential for appropriate imaging diagnosis and optimal pediatric patient management.

REFERENCES

1. Owens PL, Zodet MW, Berdahl T, et al. Annual report on health care for children and youth in the United States: focus on injury-related emergency department utilization and expenditures. Ambul Pediatr 2008;8(4):219–40.e17.
2. Rosendahl K, Strouse PJ. Sports injury of the pediatric musculoskeletal system. Radiol Med 2016;121(5): 431–41.
3. Kissoon N, Galpin R, Gayle M, et al. Evaluation of the role of comparison radiographs in the diagnosis of traumatic elbow injuries. J Pediatr Orthop 1995; 15(4):449–53.
4. Chacon D, Kissoon N, Brown T, et al. Use of comparison radiographs in the diagnosis of traumatic injuries of the elbow. Ann Emerg Med 1992;21(8):895–9.
5. Zbojniewicz AM. US for diagnosis of musculoskeletal conditions in the young athlete: emphasis on dynamic assessment. Radiographics 2014;34(5):1145–62.
6. Hryhorczuk AL, Restrepo R, Lee EY. Pediatric musculoskeletal ultrasound: practical imaging approach. AJR Am J Roentgenol 2016;206(5):W62–72.
7. Smith-Bindman R. Is computed tomography safe? N Engl J Med 2010;363(1):1–4.
8. Brown SD, Kasser JR, Zurakowski D, et al. Analysis of 51 tibial triplane fractures using CT with multiplanar reconstruction. AJR Am J Roentgenol 2004; 183(5):1489–95.
9. Lemburg SP, Lilienthal E, Heyer CM. Growth plate fractures of the distal tibia: is CT imaging necessary? Arch Orthop Trauma Surg 2010;130(11):1411–7.
10. Frush DP, Goske MJ. Image gently: toward optimizing the practice of pediatric CT through resources and dialogue. Pediatr Radiol 2015;45(4):471–5.
11. Ho-Fung VM, Jaimes C, Jaramillo D. Magnetic resonance imaging assessment of sports-related musculoskeletal injury in children: current techniques and clinical applications. Semin Roentgenol 2012;47(2): 171–81.
12. Sanchez R, Strouse PJ. The knee: MR imaging of uniquely pediatric disorders. Magn Reson Imaging Clin N Am 2009;17(3):521–37, vii.
13. Ecklund K, Jaramillo D. Imaging of growth disturbance in children. Radiol Clin North Am 2001; 39(4):823–41.
14. McKibbin B. The biology of fracture healing in long bones. J Bone Joint Surg Br 1978;60-B(2):150–62.
15. Rodriguez-Merchan EC. Pediatric skeletal trauma: a review and historical perspective. Clin Orthop Relat Res 2005;(432):8–13.
16. Trionfo A, Cavanaugh PK, Herman MJ. Pediatric open fractures. Orthop Clin North Am 2016;47(3):565–78.
17. Mabrey JD, Fitch RD. Plastic deformation in pediatric fractures: mechanism and treatment. J Pediatr Orthop 1989;9(3):310–4.
18. Currey JD, Butler G. The mechanical properties of bone tissue in children. J Bone Joint Surg Am 1975;57(6):810–4.
19. Wilkins KE. The uniqueness of the young athlete: musculoskeletal injuries. Am J Sports Med 1980; 8(5):377–82.
20. Chamay A, Tschantz P. Mechanical influences in bone remodeling. Experimental research on Wolff's law. J Biomech 1972;5(2):173–80.
21. Crowe JE, Swischuk LE. Acute bowing fractures of the forearm in children: a frequently missed injury. AJR Am J Roentgenol 1977;128(6):981–4.
22. Swischuk LE. What is different in children? Semin Musculoskelet Radiol 2013;17(4):359–70.
23. Boyer RS, Jaffe RB, Nixon GW, et al. Trampoline fracture of the proximal tibia in children. AJR Am J Roentgenol 1986;146(1):83–5.
24. Swischuk LE, John SD, Tschoepe EJ. Upper tibial hyperextension fractures in infants: another occult toddler's fracture. Pediatr Radiol 1999;29(1):6–9.
25. Caine D, DiFiori J, Maffulli N. Physeal injuries in children's and youth sports: reasons for concern? Br J Sports Med 2006;40(9):749–60.
26. Neer CS 2nd, Horwitz BS. Fractures of the proximal humeral epiphysial plate. Clin Orthop Relat Res 1965;41:24–31.
27. Egol KA, Karunakar M, Phieffer L, et al. Early versus late reduction of a physeal fracture in an animal model. J Pediatr orthopedics 2002;22(2):208–11.
28. Jaramillo D, Shapiro F, Hoffer FA, et al. Posttraumatic growth-plate abnormalities: MR imaging of bony-bridge formation in rabbits. Radiology 1990;175(3): 767–73.
29. Salter RB, Harris R. Injuries involving the epiphyseal plate. J Bone Joint Surg 1963;45(3):587–622.
30. Ogden JA. Injury to the growth mechanisms of the immature skeleton. Skeletal Radiol 1981;6(4):237–53.
31. Crawford AH. Triplane and Tillaux fractures: is a 2 mm residual gap acceptable? J Pediatr orthopedics 2012;32(Suppl 1):S69–73.
32. Choudhry IK, Wall EJ, Eismann EA, et al. Functional outcome analysis of triplane and tillaux fractures after closed reduction and percutaneous fixation. J Pediatr orthopedics 2014;34(2):139–43.

33. Ho-Fung V, Pollock A. Triplane fracture. Pediatr Emerg Care 2011;27(1):70–2.

34. Dunbar JS, Owen HF, Nogrady MB, et al. Obscure tibial fracture of infants: the toddler's fracture. J Can Assoc Radiol 1964;15:136–44.

35. Mashru RP, Herman MJ, Pizzutillo PD. Tibial shaft fractures in children and adolescents. J Am Acad Orthop Surg 2005;13(5):345–52.

36. Jadhav SP, Swischuk LE. Commonly missed subtle skeletal injuries in children: a pictorial review. Emerg Radiol 2008;15(6):391–8.

37. Swischuk LE, Hernandez JA. Frequently missed fractures in children (value of comparative views). Emerg Radiol 2004;11(1):22–8.

38. Halsey MF, Finzel KC, Carrion WV, et al. Toddler's fracture: presumptive diagnosis and treatment. J Pediatr orthopedics 2001;21(2):152–6.

39. Frick S. Skeletal growth, development, and healing as related to pediatric trauma. In: Green N, Swiontkowski M, editors. Skeletal trauma in children: expert consult. 4th edition. Philadelphia: Saunders; 2008. p. 1–18.

40. Davis KW. Imaging pediatric sports injuries: lower extremity. Radiol Clin North Am 2010;48(6):1213–35.

41. Stevens MA, El-Khoury GY, Kathol MH, et al. Imaging features of avulsion injuries. Radiographics 1999;19(3):655–72.

42. Strouse PJ. MRI of the knee: key points in the pediatric population. Pediatr Radiol 2010;40(4):447–52.

43. Prince JS, Laor T, Bean JA. MRI of anterior cruciate ligament injuries and associated findings in the pediatric knee: changes with skeletal maturation. AJR Am J Roentgenol 2005;185(3):756–62.

44. Shea KG, Grimm NL, Laor T, et al. Bone bruises and meniscal tears on MRI in skeletally immature children with tibial eminence fractures. J Pediatr orthopedics 2011;31(2):150–2.

45. Ho-Fung VM, Jaimes C, Jaramillo D. MR imaging of ACL injuries in pediatric and adolescent patients. Clin Sports Med 2011;30(4):707–26.

46. Dwek JR, Cardoso F, Chung CB. MR imaging of overuse injuries in the skeletally immature gymnast: spectrum of soft-tissue and osseous lesions in the hand and wrist. Pediatr Radiol 2009;39(12):1310–6.

47. Davis KW. Imaging pediatric sports injuries: upper extremity. Radiol Clin North Am 2010;48(6):1199–211.

48. Laor T, Wall EJ, Vu LP. Physeal widening in the knee due to stress injury in child athletes. AJR Am J Roentgenol 2006;186(5):1260–4.

49. Anderson MW, Greenspan A. Stress fractures. Radiology 1996;199(1):1–12.

50. Niemeyer P, Weinberg A, Schmitt H, et al. Stress fractures in adolescent competitive athletes with open physis. Knee Surg Sports Traumatol Arthrosc 2006;14(8):771–7.

51. Ecklund K, Jaramillo D. Patterns of premature physeal arrest: MR imaging of 111 children. AJR Am J Roentgenol 2002;178(4):967–72.

52. Ecklund K. Magnetic resonance imaging of pediatric musculoskeletal trauma. Top Magn Reson Imaging 2002;13(4):203–17.

53. Peterson HA, Madhok R, Benson JT, et al. Physeal fractures: Part 1. Epidemiology in Olmsted County, Minnesota, 1979-1988. J Pediatr orthopedics 1994;14(4):423–30.

54. Craig JG, Cramer KE, Cody DD, et al. Premature partial closure and other deformities of the growth plate: MR imaging and three-dimensional modeling. Radiology 1999;210(3):835–43.

55. Sailhan F, Chotel F, Guibal AL, et al. Three-dimensional MR imaging in the assessment of physeal growth arrest. Eur Radiol 2004;14(9):1600–8.

56. Ogden JA. The evaluation and treatment of partial physeal arrest. J Bone Joint Surg Am 1987;69(8):1297–302.

57. Khoshhal KI, Kiefer GN. Physeal bridge resection. J Am Acad Orthop Surg 2005;13(1):47–58.

58. Ranson M. Imaging of pediatric musculoskeletal infection. Semin Musculoskelet Radiol 2009;13(3):277–99.

59. Jaramillo D, Treves ST, Kasser JR, et al. Osteomyelitis and septic arthritis in children: appropriate use of imaging to guide treatment. Am J Roentgenol 1995;165(2):399–403.

60. Jaramillo D. Infection: musculoskeletal. Pediatr Radiol 2011;41(Suppl 1):S127–34.

61. Kushare I, Klingele K, Samora W. Discoid meniscus: diagnosis and management. Orthop Clin North Am 2015;46(4):533–40.

62. Silverman JM, Mink JH, Deutsch AL. Discoid menisci of the knee: MR imaging appearance. Radiology 1989;173(2):351–4.

63. Bohne WH. Tarsal coalition. Curr Opin Pediatr 2001;13(1):29–35.

64. Cass AD, Camasta CA. A review of tarsal coalition and pes planovalgus: clinical examination, diagnostic imaging, and surgical planning. J Foot Ankle Surg 2010;49(3):274–93.

65. Mosca VS. Subtalar coalition in pediatrics. Foot Ankle Clin 2015;20(2):265–81.

66. Emery KH, Bisset GS 3rd, Johnson ND, et al. Tarsal coalition: a blinded comparison of MRI and CT. Pediatr Radiol 1998;28(8):612–6.

67. Killeen KL. The fallen fragment sign. Radiology 1998;207(1):261–2.

68. Reynolds J. The "fallen fragment sign" in the diagnosis of unicameral bone cysts. Radiology 1969;92(5):949–53. passim.

Practical Indication-Based Pediatric Nuclear Medicine Studies
Update and Review

Neha S. Kwatra, MD*, Asha Sarma, MD,
Edward Y. Lee, MD, MPH

KEYWORDS

- Radiopharmaceuticals • Pediatrics • Clinical applications • Scintigraphy

KEY POINTS

- Nuclear medicine studies provide complementary functional information to anatomic imaging modalities.
- Pediatric nuclear medicine examinations are technically challenging, requiring customization of study protocols to individual pediatric patients.
- Special emphasis on radiation dose optimization is required in pediatric practice.

INTRODUCTION

Nuclear medicine is an imaging specialty in which trace amounts of radiopharmaceuticals are used to examine different physiologic or pathologic processes in the body. Scintigraphic examinations provide useful functional information, which often complements anatomic information obtained from other radiological tests. Nuclear medicine examinations in children are often technically more difficult due to variation in body types, developmental stages, and disease conditions, as well as the need for sedation or anesthesia. Radiation dose optimization is an important concern, particularly in the pediatric population. This article reviews the current practice of diagnostic nuclear medicine in pediatrics. A discussion of radionuclide therapy and newer radiopharmaceutical agents that are predominantly investigational in the United States is beyond the scope of this article.

PEDIATRIC-SPECIFIC TECHNICAL CONSIDERATIONS
Radiopharmaceuticals

Most of the radiopharmaceuticals used in pediatric patients are labeled with technetium-99m (^{99m}Tc). Some other commonly used radionuclides include iodine-123 (^{123}I), xenon-133 (^{133}Xe), and fluorine-18 (^{18}F). In the past, there was no standardization of pediatric-administered radiopharmaceutical doses. However, in 2010, the North American consensus guidelines for administered radiopharmaceutical activities were developed for 11 radiopharmaceuticals, primarily based on patient weight.[1] These were updated in 2014 and have been harmonized with the European Association of Nuclear Medicine radiopharmaceutical pediatric dose card.[2] The commonly used radiopharmaceuticals and their dosages based on the North American consensus guidelines (if applicable) are listed in **Table 1**.

Department of Radiology, Boston Children's Hospital, Harvard Medical School, 300 Longwood Avenue, Boston, MA 02115, USA
* Corresponding author.
E-mail address: Neha.Kwatra@childrens.harvard.edu

Radiol Clin N Am 55 (2017) 803–844
http://dx.doi.org/10.1016/j.rcl.2017.02.014

Table 1
Commonly used radiopharmaceuticals in pediatric nuclear medicine

	Radiopharmaceutical	Typical Dose or Dose Range (MBq/kg, Unless Otherwise Specified), Typical Route of Administration	Indication
1.	^{99m}Tc-bicisate (ethyl cysteinate dimer [ECD])	7.4–11.1, intravenous (IV)	Brain perfusion
2.	^{99m}Tc-exametazime (hexamethylpropylene amine oxime [HMPAO])	7.4–11.1, IV	Brain perfusion
3.	^{18}F-fluorodeoxyglucose (FDG)	3.7 (brain),[a] IV 3.7–5.2 (body),[a] IV	Epilepsy imaging, myocardial viability imaging, oncology, infection or inflammation
4.	^{111}In-diethylenetriaminepentaacetic acid (DTPA)	1.85–74 MBq, intrathecal	Cerebrospinal fluid (CSF) imaging
5.	^{99m}Tc-DTPA	11.1–37 (CSF imaging) MBq, intrathecal 7.4 (brain death), IV 1.85 glomerular filtration rate (GFR), IV	CSF imaging, blood flow agent for brain death scintigraphy, GFR evaluation
6.	^{99m}Tc-sestamibi or ^{99m}Tc-tetrofosmin	9.25 (rest or stress only), IV 5.55 (rest) and 12.95 (stress) when performed on the same day, IV 11 (parathyroid scintigraphy), IV	Myocardial single-photon emission computed tomography (SPECT) perfusion, parathyroid scintigraphy
7.	^{13}N-ammonia	11.1, IV	Myocardial PET perfusion
8.	^{99m}Tc-macroaggregated albumin (MAA)	2.59 (if ^{99m}Tc-DTPA used for ventilation),[a] IV 1.11 (if ^{99m}Tc-DTPA not used for ventilation),[a] IV	Lung perfusion
9.	^{133}Xe	370–740 MBq, inhaled	Lung ventilation
10.	^{99m}Tc-sulfur colloid	11.1 MBq (salivagram), oral 7.4–37 MBq (esophageal transit), oral 9.25–37 MBq (oral liquid gastric emptying),[a] oral, naso-gastric or orogastric tube, gastrostomy tube 9.25–18.5 MBq (solid gastric emptying),[a] oral ≤37 MBq (per bladder filling cycle during cystography)[a]	Salivagram, esophageal transit, gastric emptying, cystography with augmented bladder
11.	^{99m}Tc-pertechnetate	1.85 (Meckel),[a] IV ≤37 MBq (per bladder filling cycle during cystography)[a]	Ectopic gastric mucosa, radionuclide cystogram, occasionally thyroid scintigraphy
12.	^{99m}Tc-labeled autologous red blood cells (RBC)	7.4, IV	Gastrointestinal (GI) bleeding scintigraphy
13.	^{99m}Tc-iminodiacetic acid (IDA)	1.85,[a] IV	Hepatobiliary scintigraphy
14.	^{99m}Tc-mercaptoacetyltriglycine (MAG-3)	3.7 (without flow),[a] IV 5.55 (with flow),[a] IV	Dynamic renal scintigraphy, diuretic renography, captopril renography

(*continued on next page*)

Table 1
(continued)

Radiopharmaceutical	Typical Dose or Dose Range (MBq/kg, Unless Otherwise Specified), Typical Route of Administration	Indication
15. ^{99m}Tc-dimercaptosuccinic acid (DMSA)	1.85,[a] IV	Renal cortical scintigraphy
16. ^{99m}Tc-methylene diphosphonate (MDP)	9.3,[a] IV	Skeletal scintigraphy
17. ^{18}F-sodium fluoride (NaF)	2.22,[a] IV	Skeletal scintigraphy
18. ^{123}I-sodium iodide (NaI)	0.2, oral	Thyroid uptake and scan
19. ^{123}I-metaiodobenzylguanidine (MIBG)	5.2,[a] IV	Neuroblastoma or neuroendocrine imaging
20. ^{111}In-white blood cell (WBC)	0.15–0.25, IV	Infection or inflammation
21. ^{99m}Tc-WBC	3.7–7.4, IV	Infection or inflammation
22. Filtered ^{99m}Tc-sulfur colloid	18–37 MBq, intradermal	Lymphatic imaging

[a] Dosages based on the 2014 Update of the North American Consensus Guidelines for Pediatric Administered radiopharmaceutical activities.

Imaging Protocols

Although standardized study protocols are highly recommended, pediatric imaging often necessitates a greater degree of adaptability and customization. There may be variability in radiopharmaceutical doses, scanning times, and type and number of images needed. Immobilization techniques, a quiet imaging environment, and distraction methods are commonly used in infants and young children when sedation or anesthesia is not used.[3] General anesthesia is occasionally required, especially for single-photon emission computed tomography (SPECT) and PET imaging. Typical imaging protocols for common pediatric nuclear medicine studies are summarized in **Tables 2–11**.

Instrumentation

Nuclear medicine imaging includes planar imaging, SPECT, and PET performed using their respective cameras. SPECT–computed tomography (CT) and PET/CT hybrid instruments are more commonly used than SPECT or PET alone in current practice. Simultaneous PET/MR imaging is a newer imaging modality with integrated scanners now available for clinical use.

Planar imaging (dynamic or static acquisition) is the most commonly used modality in pediatrics. Parallel-hole collimators used for planar imaging are often high-resolution and ultrahigh-resolution type. For rapid dynamic studies, low-energy converging collimators provide adequate spatial resolution and sensitivity. Magnification scintigraphy with a pinhole collimator (insert of small aperture, 2–3 mm)[4] provides the highest spatial resolution and is essential for imaging small parts in children.

SPECT imaging provides 3-dimensional (3D) information and enhanced contrast resolution. SPECT acquisition, however, can be challenging in newborns and infants. The use of customized narrow pediatric pallets allows closer positioning of the detector to the patient, leading to improved image quality.[5] New SPECT gantries and focusing, and multipinhole collimators combined with solid-state detectors used in routine cardiac imaging[6] could potentially be used in pediatric SPECT imaging.

PET imaging also provides 3D information, with a relatively smaller tradeoff between spatial resolution and sensitivity compared with SPECT and traditional gamma camera imaging.[7] Traditionally, the CT portion of a PET/CT examination was used only for photon attenuation correction of PET and anatomic localization, and an additional higher dose diagnostic CT was obtained as needed. Currently, several approaches are being used to eliminate the need for 2 CTs, including performing low-dose contrast-enhanced CT as a part of PET/CT or using the diagnostic CT for attenuation correction.[8]

Integrated PET/MR imaging combines the high soft-tissue contrast of MR imaging with the functional information of PET. Advantages of PET/MR imaging include lower radiation dose compared with PET/CT and the potential to reduce the number of sedation sessions for children requiring both PET and MR imaging studies (by using PET/MR imaging in lieu of PET/CT). However, prohibitive cost, limited insurance reimbursement, and technical limitations of attenuation correction are continued obstacles to widespread adoption of this modality.

Table 2
Central nervous system applications

Examination	Common Radiopharmaceuticals	Common Indications	Protocol Considerations	Imaging Findings
1. Ictal or interictal SPECT	99mTc-ECD 99mTc-HMPAO	• Localization of epileptogenic focus in refractory epilepsy	• Ultrahigh-resolution collimator • SPECT is obtained anytime from 30 min to 6 h postinjection	• Focal hyperperfusion in the epileptogenic region on ictal SPECT • Focal hypoperfusion or normal perfusion in the epileptogenic region on interictal SPECT
2. Interictal PET	18F-FDG	• Lateralization and general localization of epileptogenic focus in refractory epilepsy, especially in cortical dysplasia • Assessment of functional status of the remainder of the brain in cases of epilepsy in which surgical resection is being considered	• Imaging begins 30 min after intravenous injection of FDG	• Focal hypometabolism in the epileptogenic region
3. Brain PET (tumor)	18F-FDG	• Distinguish high-grade from low-grade tumors and radiation necrosis	• Imaging begins 60 min after intravenous injection of FDG	• Higher uptake in high-grade gliomas compared with low-grade tumors or radiation necrosis

4.	CSF imaging	¹¹¹In-DTPA ⁹⁹mTc-DTPA	• Assessment of delivery of chemotherapeutic agents • Assessment of ventriculoperitoneal or atrial shunt function • Localization of CSF leaks (rarely used) • Hydrocephalus (rarely used)	• Medium-energy collimator for ¹¹¹In-DTPA imaging and ultrahigh-resolution collimator for ⁹⁹mTc-DTPA imaging • Tracer is usually administered in the lumbar subarachnoid space or in the shunt valve reservoir • ⁹⁹mTc-DTPA is preferred due to its higher photon flux and lower radiation dose in younger children • In older children, ¹¹¹In-DTPA is typically used • Image over site of tracer injection to ensure adequate injection • For assessment of hydrocephalus or obstruction of CSF flow: images obtained in the anterior or posterior and lateral projections at 2, 4–6, and 24 h • For shunt function, initial dynamic and then delayed static imaging along the course of the shunt	• Normally, on the 2 and 4–6 h images, the tracer progressively migrates upward from the basal cisterns into the sylvian and interhemispheric fissures (trident appearance) • By 24 h, tracer is seen over the convexities • Filling defects or abrupt termination of CSF flow due to obstruction by tumor • With communicating hydrocephalus, radiotracer circulates in the ventricles and does not appear over the convexities
5.	Brain death scintigraphy	Brain specific agents: ⁹⁹mTc-ECD ⁹⁹mTc-HMPAO Blood flow agents: ⁹⁹mTc-DTPA ⁹⁹mTc-pertechnetate	Suspected brain death when: • Clinical examination and electroencephalography are unreliable (e.g., severe hypothermia, barbiturate coma) • The patient is under consideration for organ donation • Family members require documentation of absent blood flow	• High-resolution collimator • Radionuclide cerebral angiogram with anterior dynamic imaging for 1–2 min • Immediate static images in anterior, left lateral, right lateral projections • SPECT performed as needed	• No evidence of intracranial blood flow • Lack of tracer uptake in the brain with brain-specific agents • Blush of activity in nasal region on anterior views (hot nose sign)

Table 3
Cardiovascular applications

	Examination	Commonly Used Radiopharmaceuticals	Common Indications	Protocol Considerations	Imaging Findings
1.	Myocardial SPECT perfusion imaging	^{99m}Tc-sestamibi ^{99m}Tc-tetrofosmin	• Kawasaki disease with known coronary artery involvement • Transposition of the great arteries after arterial switch operation • Repaired tetralogy of Fallot with possibility of coronary compromise • Single ventricle with poor function • Borderline cardiac function on echocardiography • Coronary arteriopathy in heart transplant patients	• Ultrahigh-resolution collimator • Rest and stress imaging (higher dose for examination performed second if performed on the same day) • Exercise stress testing is typically preferred to pharmacologic stress with a vasodilator or dobutamine	• Reversible (ischemia) or fixed (scar or hibernating myocardium) perfusion defect in the region of the affected vascular territory • Ejection fraction may be reduced, left ventricle may be dilated • Wall motion abnormalities may be present • Abnormally increased lung activity and transient ischemic dilatation of the left ventricle (subendocardial ischemia) may be present with severe disease
2.	Cardiac PET perfusion imaging	^{13}N-ammonia ^{82}Rb ^{15}O-water	• Evaluation of myocardial perfusion (indications similar to cardiac SPECT)	• Repeat perfusion imaging (stress or rest) is typically performed at a 20–40 min interval • No dose adjustment is necessary when both studies are performed on the same day (in contradistinction to SPECT perfusion imaging) • Exercise stress may be difficult to perform because of the short half-lives of the PET perfusion agents, and requires careful planning and coordination	• Reversible (ischemia) or fixed (scar or hibernating myocardium) perfusion defect in the region of affected vascular territory

3.	FDG PET metabolic imaging (myocardial viability imaging)	^{18}F-FDG	• Evaluation of cardiac metabolism to differentiate between scarred and hibernating myocardium	• Typically, myocardial viability assessment by FDG is performed in conjunction with a resting perfusion scan • Fasting is required for at least 6 h prior • ^{18}F-FDG is administered intravenously approximately 1 h after an oral or intravenous glucose load • Imaging is performed 1 h after injection of FDG	• Hibernating myocardium presents as a perfusion-metabolism mismatch (fixed perfusion defect in an area that exhibits preserved or increased FDG uptake) • Nonviable or scarred myocardium shows no perfusion or FDG uptake
4.	FDG PET metabolic imaging (infection or inflammation)	^{18}F-FDG	• Cardiac device infection or endocarditis • Suspected cardiac sarcoidosis	• To reduce nonspecific uptake by myocardium, a ketogenic (high-fat–low-carbohydrate) diet is initiated 24 h before the study, with the patient fasting starting at midnight before the study • A high-fat breakfast is consumed the morning of the study • 10-min image with bed position over the heart	• Focally increased uptake at the site of suspected infection

Abbreviations: ^{15}O-water, Oxygen-15; ^{82}Rb, Rubidium-82.

Table 4
Pulmonary applications

Examination	Commonly Used Radiopharmaceuticals	Common Indications	Protocol Considerations	Imaging Findings
1. Lung perfusion scans	^{99m}Tc-MAA	• Differential and regional lung perfusion in patients with congenital heart disease at baseline and follow-up after intervention • Qualitative and quantitative assessment of right-to-left shunt	• Only ~10,000 particles needed for evaluation of lung perfusion in infants with CHD • Typically, MAA is administered intravenously in a supine position to minimize differential regional blood flow between the lung apex and base • Imaging is typically performed in anterior and posterior projections • Region of interest analysis is used to quantitatively assess differential or regional lung perfusion	• Differences in regional or differential lung perfusion can be assessed visually and also quantified by obtaining geometric means of perfusion on the anterior and posterior images • Systemic penetration of the tracer indicates a right-to-left shunt
2. Ventilation-perfusion (V/Q) scans	Ventilation agents ^{133}Xe ^{99m}Tc-DTPA aerosol Perfusion agent ^{99m}Tc-MAA	• Pulmonary thromboembolism (acute or chronic) • Quantification of differential pulmonary perfusion or ventilation in patients with congenital diaphragmatic hernia • Airway obstruction • Parenchymal lung disease • Chest wall deformity	• For evaluation of pulmonary embolism, perfusion images are acquired in multiple projections (anterior, posterior, lateral, and oblique projections) • With ^{133}Xe, posterior projection initial single breath, wash-in, equilibrium, and wash-out phases ventilation images are acquired • With ^{99m}Tc-DTPA aerosol, images are obtained in the same projections as perfusion images • In a combined V/Q scan, the second study is performed with a higher administered dose of radiopharmaceutical due to persistence of the tracer in the lungs from the initial study	• Prospective evaluation of pulmonary embolism diagnosis (PIOPED) II criteria are used to evaluate segmental perfusion defects mismatched with ventilation • Complete airway obstruction shows absent ventilation with variable changes in perfusion • Air trapping in partial airway obstruction shows delayed wash-in and wash-out of ^{133}Xe
3. Radionuclide salivagram	^{99m}Tc-sulfur colloid	• Recurrent infections or concern for aspiration, especially in high-risk patients such as those with congenital head and neck abnormalities and neurologic impairment	• Ultrahigh-resolution collimator • A drop of ^{99m}Tc–sulfur colloid in saline (100 μL) is placed in the oral cavity and swallowed with saliva • Typically, dynamic imaging is performed for 60 min • Tracer is readministered if there is rapid clearance from the oral cavity or esophagus • If there is high clinical suspicion for aspiration, additional delayed images may increase sensitivity	• Tracer is seen within the tracheobronchial tree with aspiration

Table 3
Gastrointestinal applications

Examination	Commonly Used Radiopharmaceuticals	Common Indications	Protocol Considerations	Imaging Findings
1. Esophageal transit scintigraphy	^{99m}Tc-sulfur colloid	• Primary (e.g., achalasia) and secondary esophageal motility disorders (postsurgical, corrosive injury) • Initial diagnosis and post-treatment follow-up, especially in cases in which esophageal manometry or contrast esophagogram are equivocal	• Ultrahigh-resolution collimator • Liquid (milk, formula, water, juice) labeled with ^{99m}Tc-sulfur colloid and/or solid or semisolid meals (scrambled eggs, pudding, yogurt) • 1–2 min dynamic supine and/or upright imaging • Delayed static imaging as needed • Qualitative and quantitative analysis • Equal regions of interest are placed in the upper, mid, and lower esophagus and the stomach and a time activity curve is generated	• Normally, rapid transit of tracer through the esophagus (<10 s) with sequential sharp peaks in the upper, mid and lower esophagus and prompt detection of gastric activity • Some characteristic dysmotility patterns include high-amplitude waves in the lower esophagus (nutcracker esophagus) and significant tracer retention in the lower esophagus in both the supine and upright positions (achalasia in absence of anatomic obstruction)
2. Gastroesophageal reflux scintigraphy (milk scan)	^{99m}Tc-sulfur colloid	• Suspected gastroesophageal reflux	• Radiolabeled milk or formula administered orally, via naso- or orogastric tube, or gastrostomy tube • Posterior dynamic imaging of the chest and upper abdomen for 60 min • Delayed static images of the chest at 2–4 h	• New appearance of tracer in the esophagus indicates reflux • Semiquantitative measurements may be obtained to grade reflux • Tracer is seen in the lung fields with secondary pulmonary aspiration
3. Gastric emptying scintigraphy	^{99m}Tc-sulfur colloid	• Delayed gastric emptying (vomiting, abdominal pain, nausea, early satiety, bloating, weight loss) • Rapid gastric emptying (dumping syndrome)	• No barium study should be performed within the prior 48 h • Medications affecting gastric motility should be discontinued • Ultrahigh-resolution collimator • Routes of administration: oral, naso- or orogastric tube, G-tube • Liquid or solid or semisolid • Dynamic imaging for 60 min • Additional delayed imaging at 2–4 h as needed • 4-h solid-phase gastric emptying protocol with imaging at 0, 1, 2, 3, and 4 h	• Gastroparesis is defined by adult criteria for a standardized solid meal as a gastric residual of >90%, 60%, 30%, and 10% at 1, 2, 3, and 4 h, respectively • Lack of standardized technique and absence of pediatric normative data limits assessment of gastric emptying

(continued on next page)

Table 5
(continued)

Examination	Commonly Used Radiopharmaceuticals	Common Indications	Protocol Considerations	Imaging Findings
4. ^{99m}Tc-pertechnetate scintigraphy (Meckel scan)	^{99m}Tc-pertechnetate	• Asymptomatic gross rectal bleeding	• Pretreatment with histamine (H_2) blockers, proton pump inhibitors, or glucagon to improve sensitivity • High-resolution or ultrahigh-resolution collimator • Dynamic anterior imaging of the abdomen or pelvis for 30–60 min • Additional static imaging as needed	• Accumulation of tracer in the abdomen (typically the right lower quadrant) that appears simultaneously with gastric activity and increases in intensity over time
5. Gastrointestinal (GI) bleeding scintigraphy	^{99m}Tc-RBC	• Detect and localize GI bleeding	• Ultrahigh-resolution collimator • Initial angiographic phase (1–3 frames/sec for 1 min) • Dynamic imaging for 60–90 min • Static imaging as needed • SPECT or SPECT/CT can increase the sensitivity and specificity of bleeding-site localization	• Key diagnostic criteria for active GI bleeding include appearance of activity outside the normal blood pool structures, change in intensity of activity, and movement of activity in a pattern consistent with bowel motility (antegrade or retrograde) • Motion is best detected on cinematic display • Small bowel bleeding is indicated by rapid distal progression of tracer through multiple, small, centrally located curvilinear segments • Large bowel bleeding has an elongated pattern with a peripheral location

Table 6
Hepatobiliary applications

Examination	Commonly Used Radiopharmaceuticals	Common Indications	Protocol Considerations	Imaging Findings
1. Hepatobiliary scintigraphy	^{99m}Tc-trimethyl bromo-iminodiacetic acid (mebrofenin) ^{99m}Tc-diisopropyl iminodiacetic acid (disofenin)	• Biliary atresia • Choledochal cyst • Cholecystitis (acute and chronic) • Biliary leak • Biliary obstruction	• Ultrahigh-resolution collimator • 60 min dynamic anterior imaging • Delayed imaging at 2, 4, 6, 8, and 24 h (as needed for biliary atresia) • Patient should be fasting, and without parenteral lipids for 4 h before study, except for biliary atresia assessment • Phenobarbital premedication in a dose of 5 mg/kg/d for 5 d, with adequacy of premedication confirmed by measurement of serum phenobarbital level ($\geq$15 mcg/mL) • Sincalide (cholecystokinin analogue) intravenous infusion of 0.02 mcg/kg with additional imaging for 30 min during infusion to assess for gallbladder contractility in suspected chronic cholecystitis or biliary dyskinesia • Delayed imaging at 4 h or after administration of intravenous morphine may be used for assessment of acute cholecystitis	• Biliary atresia: Normal hepatic uptake with no biliary excretion of tracer • Choledochal cyst: accumulation of the tracer in the expected location of choledochal cyst • Bile leak: tracer activity adjacent to the liver or in the peritoneal cavity • Acute cholecystitis: gallbladder not visualized even on delayed imaging or with morphine • Chronic cholecystitis or biliary dyskinesia: low gallbladder ejection fraction after administration of sincalide • High-grade biliary obstruction: liver scan sign of increasing activity in the liver without biliary excretion

Table 7
Genitourinary applications

Examination	Commonly Used Radiopharmaceuticals	Common Indications	Protocol Considerations	Imaging Findings
1. Dynamic renal scintigraphy	^{99m}Tc-MAG3	• Distinguish or confirm multicystic dysplastic kidney vs hydronephrosis • Renal transplant evaluation	• Ultrahigh-resolution collimator • Dynamic imaging for 20 min after intravenous injection of the tracer • Delayed static imaging as necessary	• Multicystic dysplastic kidney has no demonstrable renal function • Renal transplant evaluation • Acute tubular necrosis: normal perfusion with delayed cortical clearance of the tracer in the immediate post-transplant setting • Acute rejection: nonspecific findings including diminished cortical uptake • Graft thrombosis: lack of transplant perfusion • Obstruction: hydronephrosis or hydroureter • Urinary leak: tracer outside the urinary tract or within the surgical drain

2.	Diuretic renography	^{99m}Tc-MAG3	• Hydronephrosis or hydroureter with suspected urologic obstruction	• Ultrahigh-resolution collimator
				• Intravenous hydration
				• Bladder catheterization (particularly for younger patients)
				• Initial dynamic imaging for 20–30 min after intravenous injection of the tracer followed by postdiuretic imaging for 20–30 min (F+20 method using intravenous furosemide, 1 mg/kg)
				• Qualitative and quantitative assessment of postdiuresis drainage is performed including wash-out half time ($T^1/_2$) and residual at 30 min
				• Postvoid imaging as needed
					• Scintigraphic signs of high-grade obstruction:
					• Flat drainage curve
					• Cortical retention
					• Progressive worsening of drainage over multiple follow-up examinations
					• With the F+20 method, parameters for clearance are defined as
					  $T^1/_2$ <10 min, nonobstructive
					  $T^1/_2$ >20 min: obstructive
					  $T^1/_2$ 10–20 min, indeterminate
					• The half-time criteria should not be used in isolation because children have a dynamic drainage system that changes with growth, unlike adults
					• Evaluation of changes in $T^1/_2$ over multiple studies is more accurate than evaluation of $T^1/_2$ at a single point in time

3.	Renal cortical scintigraphy	^{99m}Tc-DMSA	• Acute pyelonephritis and renal scarring • Assessment of differential renal function • Assessment of renal number, location, and size	• Ultrahigh-resolution collimator • Images obtained 2–4 h after intravenous injection of tracer • Planar imaging for differential function • Pinhole or SPECT imaging for renal cortical detail	• In acute pyelonephritis, cortical defects have reduced or absent tracer uptake with indistinct margins that do not deform renal contour • Scan defects related to acute pyelonephritis resolve in variable amounts of time (typically 6 mo) or may progress to scarring • A cortical scar has relatively sharp edges with associated volume loss of the affected cortex

(continued on next page)

Table 7
(continued)

Examination	Commonly Used Radiopharmaceuticals	Common Indications	Protocol Considerations	Imaging Findings
4. GFR evaluation	^{99m}Tc-DTPA	• Prechemotherapy and postchemotherapy GFR evaluation in pediatric patients with malignancies • Assessment of GFR in patients undergoing bone marrow transplantation	• Adequate hydration necessary • In the plasma sample method, typically blood samples are obtained at 3 different time points after intravenous tracer injection with generation of a monoexponential curve of plasma clearance of DTPA • Following intravenous administration of ^{99m}Tc-DTPA, dynamic posterior images of the kidneys are obtained for 20 min • The images are used to visually estimate the renal function and also to quantify differential renal function • GFR in mL/min/1.73 m^2 body surface area (BSA) is calculated by standard slope-intercept technique (the gamma camera uptake method is not preferred)	• GFR calculation is normalized to adult BSA (mL/min/1.73 m^2) • Reference ranges are available in the literature

5. Direct radionuclide cystography (RNC)	^{99m}Tc-pertechnetate	• Initial study for evaluation of vesicoureteral reflux (VUR) in girls
		• Screening for familial VUR
		• Follow-up evaluation after medical or surgical management of VUR
			• Sterile urethral catheterization
			• Radiopharmaceutical mixed with saline infused into the bladder
			• Posterior dynamic imaging during filling and voiding
			• Postvoid static image as needed
				• RNC grades of VUR
				  Grade 1: activity limited to ureter
				  Grade 2: activity reaching the renal collecting system
				  Grade 3: activity reaching the renal collecting system with dilation

Table 8
Musculoskeletal applications

Examination	Commonly Used Radiopharmaceuticals	Common Indications	Protocol Considerations	Imaging Findings
1. Skeletal scintigraphy	^{99m}Tc-MDP ^{18}F-NaF	• Acute osteomyelitis • Chronic recurrent multifocal osteomyelitis (CRMO) • Trauma or fractures or stress injuries such as pars defect or spondylolysis, stress fractures, shin splints • Suspected osteoid osteoma • Detection of skeletal metastases • Nonaccidental trauma • Avascular necrosis • Typical indications of ^{18}F-NaF scan include evaluation of low back pain in athletes and problem-solving in nonaccidental trauma	• Ultrahigh-resolution collimator, with pinhole or SPECT imaging as needed • Inject tracer contralateral to site of expected pathologic finding • Routinely delayed imaging at 3–4 h following tracer injection • 3 phase scan typically performed in osteomyelitis includes dynamic angiographic phase, immediate blood pool (tissue phase), and delayed skeletal phase images at 3–4 h postinjection • Whole-body or limited body part PET/CT performed 30 min after intravenous injection of ^{18}F-NaF	• Osteomyelitis: focal hyperemia on angiographic phase, focal accumulation of tracer on tissue phase, and abnormal focal uptake on delayed skeletal phase uptake in the involved part of the bone, typically the metaphysis of a long bone • CRMO: multifocal or recurrent sites of abnormal focal skeletal uptake, typically in long bone metaphyses and the clavicle. The tibia is the most common bone involved. A significant number of children may have a single lesion • Bone stress or injury (eg, spondylolysis): Abnormal uptake at sites of bone turnover • Osteoid osteoma: Intense uptake within the nidus with less marked uptake in the surrounding reactive bone (double-density sign) • Malignancy: Abnormal uptake within the primary bone malignancy and skeletal metastatic disease. Subtle indistinctness of physeal uptake, often symmetric, may indicate metaphyseal metastases in neuroblastoma. The primary mass in neuroblastoma may also demonstrate uptake • Nonaccidental trauma: Multiple sites of abnormal uptake in the skeleton including spine, ribs, clavicles, scapulae, and sternum. Classic metaphyseal lesions and skull fractures are not well assessed • Avascular necrosis (eg, slipped capital femoral epiphysis): photopenia in the acute phase and increased uptake during the healing phase in the involved bone

Table 9
Endocrine applications

Examination	Commonly Used Radiopharmaceuticals	Common Indications	Protocol Considerations	Imaging Findings
1. Thyroid scintigraphy	^{123}I ^{99m}Tc pertechnetate	• Congenital hypothyroidism • Hyperthyroidism (to distinguish cause, aid in clinical management, and determine dose for radioiodine therapy)	• High-sensitivity (for uptake), ultrahigh-resolution, and pinhole collimators for ^{123}I • Imaging performed 4–6 h after oral administration of ^{123}I • Pinhole imaging in anterior and oblique projections images and ^{57}Co transmission images for ectopic thyroid • Radioiodine uptake performed at 4–6 and 24 h	• Graves disease (^{123}I): homogeneously increased uptake in the gland at 4 and 24 h. The gland has convex borders and a pyramidal lobe is seen • Thyroiditis (^{123}I): variable uptake depending on stage; chronic thyroiditis usually shows patchy, decreased activity and subacute thyroiditis usually shows suppressed uptake and nonvisualization of the gland • Autonomous thyroid nodules (^{123}I): high-uptake with suppression of the remainder of the gland • Cold nodules (^{123}I): differential diagnosis includes malignancy • Thyroid cancers are usually single nodules rather than diffuse or multifocal abnormalities • Congenital hypothyroidism: nonvisualized or ectopic thyroid gland

| 2. | Parathyroid scintigraphy | ^{99m}Tc-sestamibi | • Localization of parathyroid adenomas, hyperplastic parathyroids, ectopic parathyroid
• Preoperative localization can help guide the surgical approach | • Commonly, dual phase imaging is performed with a single radiopharmaceutical
• Pinhole collimator, aperture <3 mm for higher lesion conspicuity
• Additionally, ultrahigh-resolution collimator for wide field of view imaging
• Imaging begins 5 min after injection and includes static images of neck and chest, pinhole, and birds-eye image 15–30 cm from the neck
• Delayed imaging 1.5–2 h after injection should show clearance of radiotracer from thyroid tissue, with persistence in parathyroid tissue
• SPECT or SPECT/CT may be useful, in particular for localization of an ectopic gland | • Increased radiotracer uptake in parathyroid lesions that persists on delayed imaging
• Thyroid lesions may be seen on initial images but should not persist on delayed images |
| 3. | Neuroendocrine tumor imaging | ^{123}I-MIBG | • To detect and characterize neuroendocrine tumors, such as neuroblastoma and pheochromocytoma
• To identify metastatic disease related to neuroendocrine tumors | • Supersaturated potassium iodide (SSKI) drops or Lugol solution are administered 1 d prior and 3 d following ^{123}I-MIBG injection for thyroid protection
• Imaging performed 24 h after intravenous injection of tracer
• Medium energy collimator
• Planar whole-body imaging
• SPECT or SPECT/CT of the torso | • Radiotracer uptake in primary tumors and sites of metastases |

Abbreviation: ^{57}Co, Cobalt-57.

Table 10
^{18}F-fluorodeoxyglucose PET–computed tomography (oncologic and infection or inflammation applications)

Examination	Common Indications	Protocol Considerations	Imaging Findings
1. ^{18}F-FDG PET/CT	• Initial diagnosis, staging and restaging of malignancies including lymphoma, bone and soft-tissue sarcoma • Assessment of MIBG-negative neuroblastomas • Assessment for malignant degeneration of plexiform neurofibromas in neurofibromatosis-1 patients • Distinguish between high-grade and low-grade brain tumors and recurrent or residual tumor from post-therapy changes • Emerging role in initial diagnosis and follow-up of Langerhans cell histiocytosis and initial diagnosis of post-transplant lymphoproliferative disorders • Emerging adjunctive role in fever of unknown origin, device or prosthesis-associated infection, suspected large-vessel vasculitis, osteomyelitis, and inflammatory bowel disease	• Patients fast for 4–6 h before study to ensure appropriate insulin levels • Blood glucose level is checked before FDG injection • Imaging is performed around 1 h after intravenous tracer injection during which the patient is in a temperature-controlled environment to prevent brown adipose tissue uptake, which can obscure disease • Pharmacologic approaches to decrease brown adipose tissue uptake (eg, low-dose beta-blocker, benzodiazepine, or fentanyl) are less commonly used in children • Whole-body, torso, or limited body part scan performed with quiet breathing • Concurrent low-dose (for attenuation correction (AC) and localization) or diagnostic CT, or a combination, for which intravenous contrast may or may not be administered	• Increased uptake in metabolically active tissues, including sites of primary malignancy and metastases and sites of infection or inflammation • Maximum standardized uptake value (SUVmax) is the most common unit of measurement used to quantify tumor uptake • Using AC-corrected images, SUVmax of tumor is compared with blood pool or background activity • Poorly differentiated, aggressive tumors tend to have higher SUVmax • FDG uptake by malignancies in or adjacent to sites of high physiologic activity, (eg, brain, genitourinary system) may be obscured

Table 11
Lymphatic system applications

Examination	Commonly Used Radiopharmaceuticals	Common Indications	Protocol Considerations	Imaging Findings
1. Lymphoscintigraphy	Filtered ^{99m}Tc-sulfur colloid (0.22 μm filter)	• Primary or secondary lymphedema • Suspected chylous effusions or ascites or leaks • Lymphatic dysplasia • Sentinel node mapping (eg, soft-tissue sarcoma, melanoma)	• Topical lidocaine is applied before tracer injection • Intradermal web space injection in the hands or feet for suspected lymphedema (2 on each side) • Injection in the dorsum of the foot just proximal to the toes may also be performed • Ultrahigh-resolution collimator • Sequential planar images of the extremities and torso at multiple time points • Transmission images can be acquired with a ^{57}Co flood source • Peritumoral injection typically intradermal (eg, melanoma) for sentinel node mapping • SPECT or SPECT/CT may be useful in sentinel node localization, especially for head and neck tumors	• Normal lymphatic transit from feet to inguinal or pelvic region within 45–60 min and from the hands to the axillary region within 10–30 min • Lymphatic dysfunction is indicated by delayed lymphatic transit, prominent or collateral lymphatic channels, dermal backflow • Hepatic accumulation of tracer indicates intact central lymphatic drainage (typically within 4 h) • Accumulation of tracer within chylous pleural effusion or ascites

Image Processing

For both planar and SPECT imaging, filtering of raw data is performed to reduce image noise and, thus, enhance image quality. SPECT images were traditionally reconstructed using filtered back projection but, more recently, iterative reconstruction techniques similar to those used for PET emission data have been used. With iterative reconstruction, image quality is much improved and, therefore, high-quality studies can be obtained with lower radiation exposure to the patient, shorter imaging times, or a combination of both.

Image fusion registers 2 or more 3D datasets of the same or different imaging modalities in the same orientation in the same space.[4] Varying combinations of 3D image sets can also be generated. Hardware image fusion is available for PET/MR, PET/CT, and SPECT/CT equipment.

Radiation Considerations

Diagnostic nuclear medicine procedures involve relatively low levels of ionizing radiation. The clinical benefit of these procedures far outweighs potential radiation risk with appropriate use.

Nevertheless, optimizing radiation dose is the cornerstone of pediatric practice. The higher risk of radiation exposure in children is ascribed to greater radiosensitivity of their actively growing tissues and a longer remaining lifespan compared with adults.

SPECTRUM OF UNDERLYING PATHOLOGIC AND IMAGING FINDINGS

The major applications of nuclear medicine in pediatrics are briefly discussed in this section. The reader is also referred to **Tables 2–11** for a list of commonly performed nuclear medicine examinations, their indications, typical imaging protocols, and imaging findings. Important pearls and pitfalls in performance and interpretation of radionuclide examinations in pediatrics are listed in **Box 1**.

Central Nervous System Indications and Applications

Epilepsy imaging
Radionuclide epilepsy imaging is indicated in pediatric patients with refractory seizures who are being considered for surgery (**Fig. 1**). It can

---

Box 1
Pearls and pitfalls

- When imaging infants, it is important to consider that the kinetics and physiologic distribution of radiopharmaceuticals differ from those in adults and older pediatric patients due to rapid growth during first year of life.

- High-energy or medium-energy collimators should be used with ^{123}I agents because low-energy collimators are ineffective at stopping the low-abundance (2.6%) high-energy (>400 KeV) photons emitted by ^{123}I. These particles cause significant image degradation due to collimator septal penetration.

- To optimally localize a seizure focus on ictal SPECT, tracer should be injected immediately (<5 s) after seizure onset.

- For accurate interpretation of FDG PET for epilepsy, it is important to monitor with electroencephalogram (EEG) during the FDG uptake phase. Seizures that occur during FDG uptake may affect tracer distribution.

- Radionuclide epilepsy imaging is especially useful if MR imaging shows either no lesions or several lesions that may not all be epileptogenic (eg, tuberous sclerosis), or if EEG changes are equivocal.

- Except for the occasional finding of transient entry at 4 hours, any radioactivity in the ventricles on a cerebrospinal fluid (CSF) study is considered abnormal and suggests hydrocephalus.

- For brain tumor imaging with ^{18}F-FDG PET/CT, delayed imaging at 3 to 4 hours improves the tumor-to-brain uptake ratio.

- Minimal dural sinus activity may be seen in cases of brain death.

- Real myocardial perfusion defects should be visible on at least 2 views. A defect seen at the base of the heart is frequently artifactual unless it extends to the apex.

- Misregistration between the PET and CT portions of a myocardial perfusion PET/CT may produce artifactual perfusion defects.

- Injection of fewer ^{99m}Tc-macroaggregated albumin (MAA) particles is recommended for patients with pulmonary hypertension and those with suspected right-to left shunt. When a smaller number of particles are administered, a higher specific activity preparation of ^{99m}Tc-MAA is typically prepared to obtain adequate counts.

- Care must be taken to avoid drawing blood into ^{99m}Tc-MAA injection syringe because it could lead to clot formation that can impair the diagnostic utility of lung perfusion imaging.

- In a patient with bidirectional Glenn shunt, venous return from the upper extremities flows to the lungs, whereas venous return from the inferior vena cava is returned to the systemic circulation. The pattern of perfusion seen on a perfusion lung scan depends on the site of tracer administration.

- External contamination by labeled saliva should not be mistaken for aspiration on a salivagram.

- In assessment for endocarditis or cardiac device infection, normal myocardial uptake needs to be suppressed using a high-fat–low-carbohydrate diet.

- On a gastric emptying study, not accounting for emptying during feeding may result in overestimated gastric residuals causing improper classification of emptying as delayed.

- A lateral image may be useful to differentiate Meckel diverticulum from genitourinary activity.

- ^{99m}Tc-pertechnetate that is secreted by the gastric mucosa will gradually accumulate in the small bowel. This activity can be distinguished from a Meckel diverticulum by its delayed appearance as a poorly defined area of mildly increased activity.

- False-positive radiopharmaceutical activity suggestive of Meckel diverticula can result from bowel inflammation, intussusception or small-bowel obstruction, peptic ulcer and vascular lesions with increased blood pool, focal pooling in the urinary tract, or uterine blush. A false-negative result may occur with prior barium fluoroscopy examination, prior administration of perchlorate, brisk gastrointestinal bleeding or if the focus of ectopic mucosa is small.

- Gastrointestinal bleeding scintigraphy is best performed with in vitro ^{99m}Tc-labeled autologous red blood cells.

- Normal hepatic uptake of tracer is used to distinguish biliary atresia from severe neonatal hepatitis. Biliary excretion of tracer is not demonstrated in either case.

- To differentiate gallbladder activity from duodenal activity on hepatobiliary scintigraphy, a right lateral or left anterior oblique view may be performed (gallbladder anterior).

- Optimal hydration and bladder catheterization are necessary prerequisites to diuretic renography in infants and young children.

- Poor renal function precludes adequate assessment of postdiuretic drainage or urinary obstruction.

- With augmented bladder, ^{99m}Tc-sulfur colloid is used for radionuclide cystography instead of ^{99m}Tc-pertechenetate to avoid absorption of the tracer into the circulation through gastric or intestinal mucosa used for augmentation.

- In infants and young children, the need for sedation can be avoided by using multispot instead of whole-body imaging.

- Skeletal scintigraphy (^{18}F-sodium fluoride [NaF] PET) is complementary to the radiographic skeletal survey in nonaccidental trauma. It is more sensitive in detecting fractures in the chest, including those of the spine, ribs, clavicles, scapulae, and sternum; however, it has limited sensitivity for classic metaphyseal lesions.

- Atypical thyroid adenomas are the most common cause for a false-positive result on parathyroid scintigraphy.

- False-positive metaiodobenzylguanidine (MIBG) studies for neuroblastoma can result from misinterpretation of physiologic foci of uptake or MIBG uptake by mature ganglioneuromas or other neuroendocrine tumors. Most false-negative MIBG studies are seen in patients with minimal residual disease after therapy.

- To reduce the effect of post-therapy inflammation or edema, ^{18}F-FDG PET for assessment of brain tumors should be performed 3 months after the end of therapy.

- Diffuse marrow uptake of ^{18}F-FDG typically represents treatment or non–treatment-related marrow stimulation, such as the response to anemia or a systemic inflammatory process.

- On PET/CT imaging, the standardized uptake value of lesions smaller than scanner resolution is underestimated.

- ^{18}F-FDG PET imaging is sensitive for detecting infection and inflammation but does not reliably distinguish between the two.

- In some cases of chylous effusions, it may be helpful to perform injection in the right arm as a separate study and compare the pattern of drainage after injection in the left arm or the feet.

- In patients with lymphedema, instead of typical intradermal injections in the web spaces, injections placed in the dorsum of the feet may cause less discomfort.

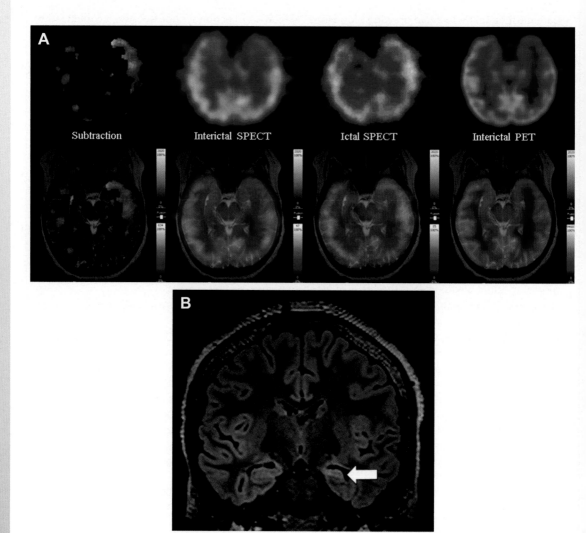

Fig. 1. A 17-year-old girl with complex partial seizures due to mesial temporal sclerosis. (*A*) Axial SPECT and PET images without (*top row*) and with (*bottom row*) MR fusion demonstrate focally decreased perfusion (SPECT) and metabolism (PET) in the left temporal lobe in the interictal phase and increased perfusion in the ictal phase. (*B*) Coronal FLAIR MR imaging demonstrates small size and hyperintensity of the left hippocampus (*arrow*).

be performed with interictal ^{18}F-fluorodeoxyglucose (FDG) PET and/or interictal and ictal SPECT. FDG PET has a high-sensitivity of 85% to 90% for detecting the epileptogenic focus in temporal lobe epilepsy, with lower sensitivity for extratemporal epilepsy (~55% in frontal lobe epilepsy). Ictal SPECT can accurately localize the epileptogenic focus in 70% to 90% of unilateral temporal lobe epilepsy, whereas the sensitivity for interictal SPECT is very low (<50%).[9] Subtraction ictal SPECT coregistered to MR imaging (SISCOM), in which the interictal SPECT images are digitally subtracted from the ictal images with the results coregistered with MR images can increase the focus detection rate up to 93% compared with 74% without it.[10]

Cerebrospinal fluid imaging

With the advent of CT and MR imaging, there has been a significant reduction in the use of radionuclide cerebrospinal fluid (CSF) imaging, particularly for evaluation of CSF leaks. The major clinical applications include assessment of delivery of intrathecal chemotherapy (**Fig. 2**) and ventricular shunt function and patency.[11]

Brain death scintigraphy

Radionuclide techniques only provide corroborative (not diagnostic) evidence of brain death in the appropriate clinical setting. Blood flow agents or brain-specific lipophilic perfusion agents can be used. Typically, only planar imaging is used but SPECT imaging can be used to improve sensitivity.

A   **B**

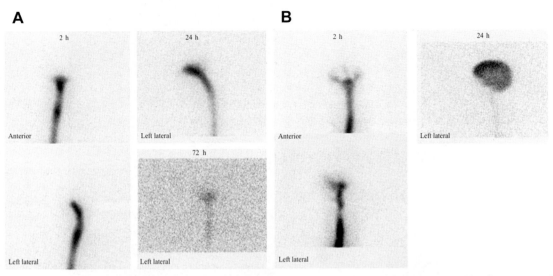

Fig. 2. An 11-year-old boy with acute lymphoblastic leukemia and a history of severe meningitis who presented for assessment of patency of the CSF spaces before possible intrathecal chemotherapy. (*A*) Planar images from an [111]In- diethylenetriaminepentaacetic acid (DTPA) CSF study demonstrate radiotracer within the spinal intrathecal space, without transit of radiotracer into the basilar cisterns or over the cerebral convexities over the course of 72 hours. (*B*) A normal study in a different patient is provided for comparison.

Cardiovascular Indication and Applications

Myocardial perfusion single-photon emission computed tomography imaging

Myocardial perfusion imaging (MPI) is not used very frequently in pediatrics but can be used to evaluate for ischemia in patients with congenital heart disease and coronary artery abnormalities. Understanding the prior surgical and percutaneous procedures that the patient may have undergone helps to distinguish normal from true pathologic variants because prosthetic material and atypical locations of outflow tracts can mimic myocardial infarcts.[12]

Myocardial perfusion PET imaging

In general, the clinical indications for PET MPI in children (**Fig. 3**) are similar to those for SPECT MPI. PET can offer significantly lower radiation dose compared with SPECT. Stress-only PET MPI can be performed with less than 1.5 mSv total-body effective dose in most patients.[13]

Cardiac device infection and endocarditis

^{18}F-FDG PET/CT is useful in the setting of suspected cardiac device infection when conventional imaging is negative or equivocal (**Fig. 4**).[14] Although ^{18}F-FDG PET/CT imaging is highly sensitive in evaluating infection, its specificity is low due to nonspecific inflammatory uptake in the early postoperative period (4–8 weeks) and interference from normal myocardial uptake.

Pulmonary Indications and Applications

Lung perfusion scintigraphy

The major clinical indications for lung perfusion scintigraphy in the pediatric population are qualitative and quantitative assessment of differential and regional pulmonary blood flow, and assessment of right-to-left shunts in congenital heart disease, which can be performed preintervention and postintervention (**Fig. 5**).[15,16]

Ventilation-perfusion scintigraphy

Ventilation-perfusion scintigraphy (V/Q) is performed in children with suspected pulmonary thromboembolism, usually in the setting of contraindications to CT angiography, such as contrast allergy or renal disease, or when there are radiation concerns.[17]

In repaired congenital diaphragmatic hernia, V/Q scintigraphy is useful to assess ventilation and perfusion abnormalities (**Fig. 6**). Typically, ventilation improves over time but perfusion remains decreased, probably related to underlying vascular hypoplasia. A V/Q scintigraphy performed in infancy is useful for identifying patients who may have greater ongoing needs and those who require interventions to preserve pulmonary function.[18–20]

Less commonly, V/Q scintigraphy is performed in pediatric patients with airway disorders (e.g., asthma, mucous plugs) and pulmonary parenchymal diseases, such as cystic fibrosis and pulmonary fibrosis.[21]

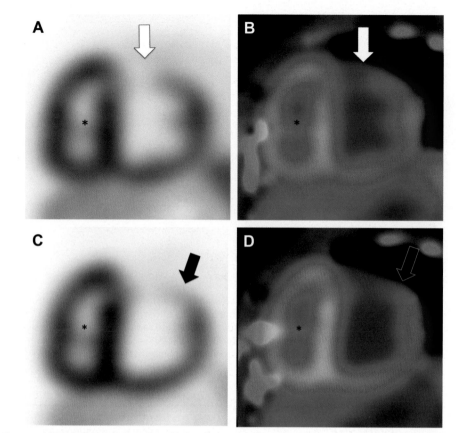

Fig. 3. A 5-year-old boy with left anterior descending artery injury during attempted operative repair of transposition of the great arteries and ventricular septal defect. (*A*) ^{13}N-ammonia cardiac rest PET and (*B*) PET/CT demonstrate a myocardial perfusion defect in the anterior wall of the left ventricle (*white arrow*) and intense uptake in the hypertrophic right ventricle (*asterisk*). After pharmacologic stress with an intravenous infusion of adenosine, (*C*) stress PET and (*D*) PET-CT demonstrate a small reversible myocardial perfusion defect in the mid-anterolateral wall adjacent to the fixed anterior wall defect (*black arrow*), indicating peri-infarct ischemia.

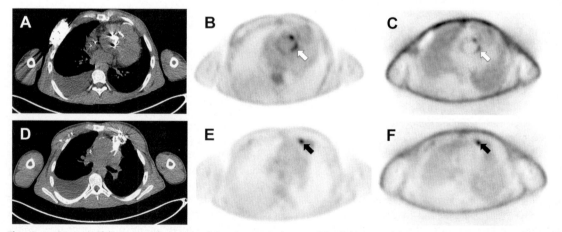

Fig. 4. A 24-year-old man with repaired truncus arteriosus with right ventricle to pulmonary artery (RV–PA) conduit, prosthetic aortic valve, and intracardiac defibrillator, with suspected endocarditis. (*A*) Axial CT and (*B*) attenuation-corrected and (*C*) nonattenuation-corrected ^{18}F-FDG PET images at the level of the aortic valve prosthesis (*white arrows*) reveal abnormal focal FDG uptake, suggesting infection. (*D–F*) Abnormal uptake is also seen at the level of the RV-PA conduit (*black arrows*). No abnormal uptake was identified at the pacemaker leads (figure not shown). The presence of uptake on the nonattenuation-corrected image confirms that the abnormality is not an artifact of attenuation correction related to the presence of metal.

A　**B**

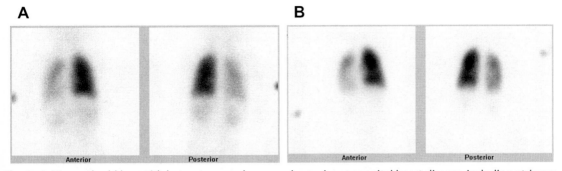

Fig. 5. A 16-month-old boy with heterotaxy syndrome and complex congenital heart disease, including atrioventricular canal defect, with stenosis at the origin of the right pulmonary artery. (*A*) Anterior and posterior images from a [99mTc]- macroaggregated albumin (MAA) perfusion scan demonstrate markedly reduced radiotracer uptake in the right compared with the left lung. Systemic penetration of the tracer is consistent with a right-to-left shunt. (*B*) At a later date, after repair of the atrioventricular canal defect and dilation of the right pulmonary artery, perfusion of the right lung is improved, with decreased right-to-left shunting.

Combined assessment of pulmonary perfusion and ventilation also may be useful in pediatric patients with chest wall deformities, such as pectus excavatum or severe spinal scoliosis.[22–24]

Salivagram

Recurrent pneumonias may be related to repeated aspiration of oral secretions, commonly in neurologically impaired pediatric patients. Radionuclide salivagram is a simple, very low-dose, physiologic scintigraphic test use to detect salivary aspiration that provides complementary information to fluoroscopic barium swallow (**Fig. 7**).

Gastrointestinal Applications

Esophageal motility

Esophageal transit scintigraphy is a simple noninvasive scintigraphic technique for assessment of esophageal motility. Both the provided qualitative and quantitative information on esophageal transit of a labeled bolus may be particularly useful (**Fig. 8**) in cases in which esophageal manometry or contrast esophagogram are equivocal.

Gastroesophageal reflux scintigraphy (milk scan) and gastric emptying scintigraphy

Gastroesophageal reflux (GER) scintigraphy, also known as milk scan, is a highly sensitive scintigraphic test for GER and pulmonary aspiration secondary to reflux. This examination is typically coupled with gastric emptying scintigraphy (**Fig. 9**).

Gastric emptying scintigraphy is a commonly used test in pediatric practice. Variability in techniques and lack of normative data, however, limit its utility. Most normal values have been provided by studies of subjects with suspected GER referred for gastric emptying scintigraphy.[25,26] Meals can be liquid (typically in infants and young children when coupled with GER scintigraphy) or solid or semisolid.

Technetium-99m–pertechnetate scintigraphy (Meckel scan)

Meckel diverticulum is the most common cause of lower gastrointestinal (GI) bleeding in previously healthy infants.[4] Almost all bleeding Meckel diverticula contain ectopic gastric mucosa, which can be evaluated with [99mTc]-pertechnetate scintigraphy (**Fig. 10**). The bleeding is related to mucosal ulceration in the diverticulum or adjacent ileum caused by hydrochloric acid secreted from the ectopic gastric mucosa. Meckel scintigraphy should only be used when the patient is not actively bleeding.[27]

Gastrointestinal bleeding scintigraphy

GI bleeding scintigraphy is indicated for evaluation of overt mid-GI or lower-GI bleeding. [99mTc]-labeled autologous red blood cells ([99mTc]-RBCs) are the radiopharmaceutical of choice. [99mTc]-RBCs can detect GI bleeding at a rate as low as 0.1 mL per minute.[28] The purpose of this examination is to determine whether the patient has active GI hemorrhage, to localize the site of hemorrhage, and to estimate the rate of blood loss.[28]

Hepatobiliary Applications

In infants, hepatobiliary scintigraphy is primarily used to distinguish hepatocellular disease from biliary atresia (**Fig. 11**) and diagnose choledochal cysts. Hepatobiliary scintigraphy with phenobarbital pretreatment is 100% sensitive, 93% specific, and 94.6% accurate in differentiating biliary atresia from other causes of neonatal cholestasis when both biliary excretion and quality of hepatic

A

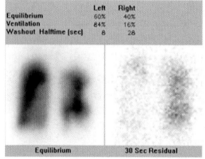

0 seconds	4	8	12	16	20	24
28	32	36	40	44	48	52
56	60	64	68	72	76	80
84	88	92	96	100	104	108
112	116	120	124	128	132	136

Page: 2 of 3

B

	Left	Right
Equilibrium	60%	40%
Ventilation	84%	16%
Washout Halftime (sec)	8	28

Equilibrium   30 Sec Residual

C

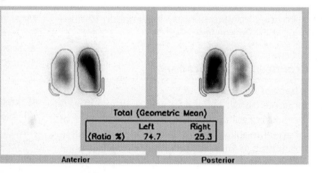

Total (Geometric Mean)		
(Ratio %)	Left	Right
	74.7	25.3

Anterior   Posterior

D

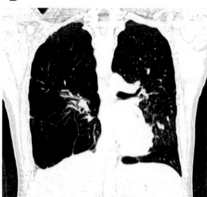

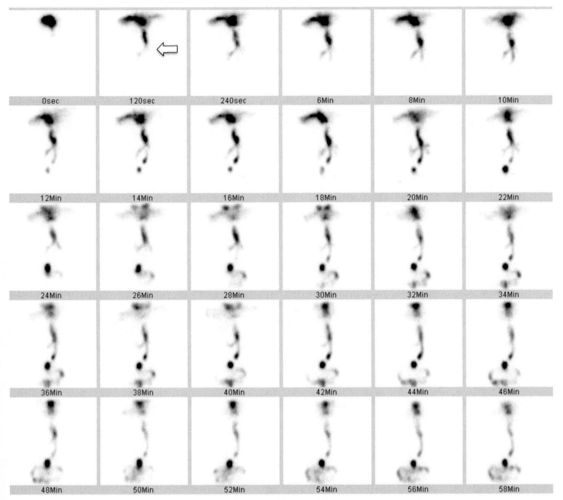

Fig. 7. A 5-year-old boy with cerebral palsy and recurrent aspiration pneumonia. Dynamic images from a saliva-gram show aspirated radiotracer within the trachea and bronchi starting at 120 seconds (arrow), persisting to 48 minutes.

uptake are considered in interpretation of the scans.[29] In older children and adolescents, hepa-tobiliary scintigraphy is used for diagnosis of acute cholecystitis[17] or chronic cholecystitis or biliary dyskinesia.[30,31] Hepatobiliary scintigraphy may also be used for evaluation of biliary leaks in the postoperative or post-traumatic setting.[32–34]

Genitourinary Applications

Dynamic renal scintigraphy and diuresis renography

Dynamic renal scintigraphy is used to assess renal perfusion, tubular function, and collecting system drainage in renal transplantation, either routinely within 24 to 72 hours of transplantation (**Fig. 12**)

Fig. 6. A 14-year-old girl with a history of repaired right-sided congenital diaphragmatic hernia. (A, B) Posterior ^{133}Xe ventilation images demonstrate marked air trapping in the right lung. At approximate ventilation equilib-rium, differential localization of radiotracer is 60% for the left and 40% for the right lung. The perfusion images (C) demonstrate that the pulmonary blood flow abnormality to the affected right side is more severe than the ventilation abnormality, with differential perfusion being 75% to the left and 25% to the right lung. A coronal CT image of the lungs (D) demonstrates correlating hyperlucency and architectural distortion throughout the hy-poplastic right lung, most prominent in the right lower lobe, due to compensatory hyperinflation.

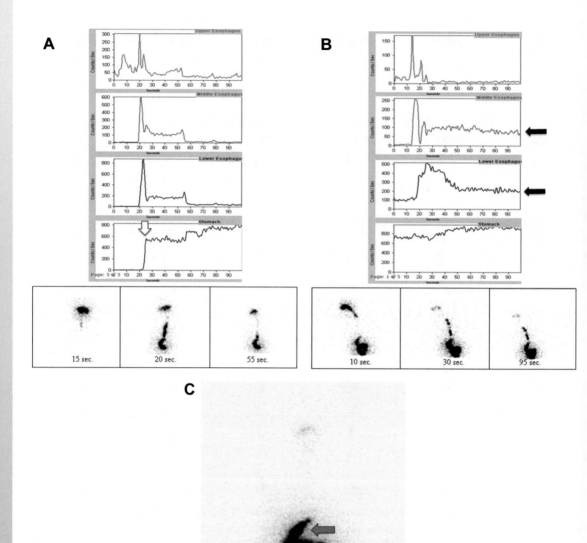

Fig. 8. A 5-year-old boy with a history of Nissen fundoplication and odynophagia. (*A*) Time activity curves and dynamic images from a ⁹⁹ᵐTc-sulfur colloid esophageal transit study demonstrate prompt, near-complete passage of radiotracer mixed with dextrose water through the esophagus into the stomach (*white arrow*). (*B*) Solid phase imaging obtained after swallowing of radiotracer mixed with egg demonstrates delayed transit through the mid to lower esophagus (*black arrows*). (*C*) Static solid phase image obtained at approximately 2 minutes demonstrates a small amount of tracer retention at the gastroesophageal junction in the region of the wrap (*gray arrow*). The patient subsequently underwent a dilation procedure with symptomatic improvement.

or on follow-up with suspected transplant dysfunction or rejection.[17]

Dynamic renal scintigraphy is also combined with diuretic renography in pediatric patients with suspected ureteropelvic junction obstruction to assess postdiuretic drainage and the need for surgical intervention (**Fig. 13**). In North America, the diuretic furosemide is most commonly administered intravenously after completion of the initial 20 to 30 minutes of dynamic imaging. This scan is referred to as the F+20 diuretic renogram.[35]

Dynamic renal scintigraphy may be combined with captopril renography in patients with suspected renovascular hypertension to assess for functionally significant renal artery stenosis, although this examination is not commonly performed.[36]

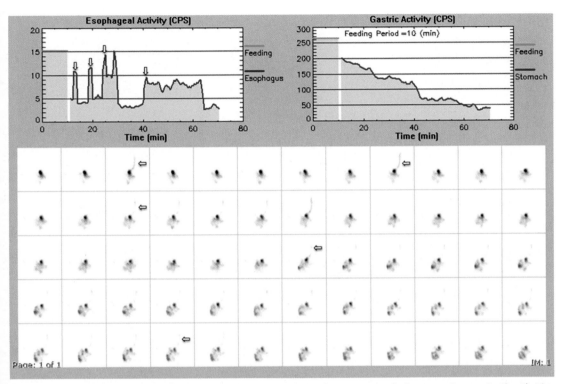

Fig. 9. A 5-year-old boy with cerebral palsy and recurrent aspiration pneumonia (same patient as in **Fig. 7**). Time activity curves and dynamic images from a gastric emptying study (performed with radiotracer mixed with formula administered via gastrostomy) demonstrate several episodes of GER (*arrows*). At 1 hour, 13% of the radiotracer remains in the stomach. No aspiration is observed.

Renal cortical scintigraphy

[99m]Tc-dimercaptosuccinic acid (DMSA) renal cortical scintigraphy is considered the gold standard for detection of acute pyelonephritis and renal scarring (**Fig. 14**).[37] The sensitivity and specificity of DMSA cortical imaging using SPECT in an experimental piglet model for detection and localization of pyelonephritic lesions were found to be 94.1% and 95.4%, respectively.[38] DMSA scintigraphy may be used when solitary kidney is suspected by ultrasound to assess for small amounts of ectopic functional renal tissue that may not have been detected sonographically.[39]

Glomerular filtration rate evaluation

Nuclear medicine assessment of glomerular filtration rate (GFR) is typically performed in pediatric patients undergoing chemotherapy or bone marrow transplantation. GFR is best estimated by measuring plasma clearance of tracers that are cleared exclusively or predominantly by glomerular filtration. ^{99m}Tc-diethylenetriaminepentaacetic acid (DTPA) is used most commonly in the United States. Of the several available methods for calculating GFR plasma clearance, the slope-intercept technique provides the best compromise between accuracy and simplicity.[40] The plasma sample method is considered more accurate than the gamma camera uptake method.[41]

Radionuclide cystography

Radionuclide cystography (RNC) is a simple technique for the assessment of vesicoureteral reflux (VUR) (**Fig. 15**). It is typically used in follow-up rather than for initial diagnosis of VUR because it is very sensitive but has limited anatomic resolution to assess for genitourinary anomalies.[42]

Musculoskeletal Applications

When compared with ^{99m}Tc-methylene diphosphonate (^{99m}Tc-MDP) bone scan, ^{18}F-sodium fluoride (^{18}F-NaF) PET/CT provides higher quality imaging.[43] While interpreting skeletal scintigraphy, it is important to be aware of the variations in pediatric skeletal development. In infants, there is absence of tracer uptake in structures that have not yet ossified. The physeal growth centers, on the other hand, have intense radiotracer uptake.[4] For example, 2-phase or 3-phase bone scan can be performed in

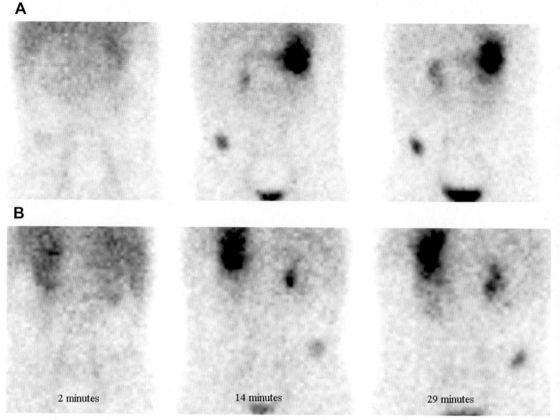

Fig. 10. A 7-year-old boy with hematochezia. (*A*) Anterior and (*B*) posterior planar images from a ^{99m}Tc-sodium pertechnetate scan demonstrate progressive focal right lower quadrant radiotracer accumulation in a Meckel diverticulum containing gastric mucosa, which parallels uptake by normal gastric mucosa in the left upper quadrant.

osteomyelitis. Marrow abnormalities are poorly detected on the skeletal phase and are more evident with blood pool imaging.[44] Skeletal scintigraphy may be preferred over MR imaging when a site of osteomyelitis is not clinically localized; for example, in a patient with bacteremia and refusal to bear weight.[45] Its sensitivity and specificity in diagnosing osteomyelitis are approximately 94% and 95%, respectively.[46] Bone scan is also used to assess a wide variety of other skeletal pathologic conditions, including benign and malignant bone tumors or skeletal metastases (**Fig. 16**), chronic recurrent multifocal osteomyelitis, trauma or sports injuries, and nonaccidental trauma.[47] The most common indication of ^{18}F-NaF PET/CT in children is evaluation of back pain related to sports injuries, scoliosis, or trauma (**Fig. 17**). It is also used in the postsurgical setting.[48]

Endocrine Applications

Thyroid scintigraphy

Thyroid scintigraphy is typically performed with ^{123}I-sodium iodide (NaI), with normal uptake being 6% to 18% at 4 to 6 hours and 10% to 35% at 24 hours.[49] It is useful for detecting causes of congenital hypothyroidism, such as agenesis and ectopia.[50] Thyroid scintigraphy is also useful for differentiating Graves disease from toxic or autonomous nodule or multinodular goiter, a distinction that is important in determining a therapeutic dose of radioiodine (**Fig. 18**). When read in conjunction with thyroid function tests, it is helpful in differentiating Graves disease from other causes of thyrotoxicosis (eg, subacute thyroiditis and factitious hyperthyroidism).[51] Though uptake is typically increased in patients with Graves disease, it may occasionally be normal in mild cases.[52]

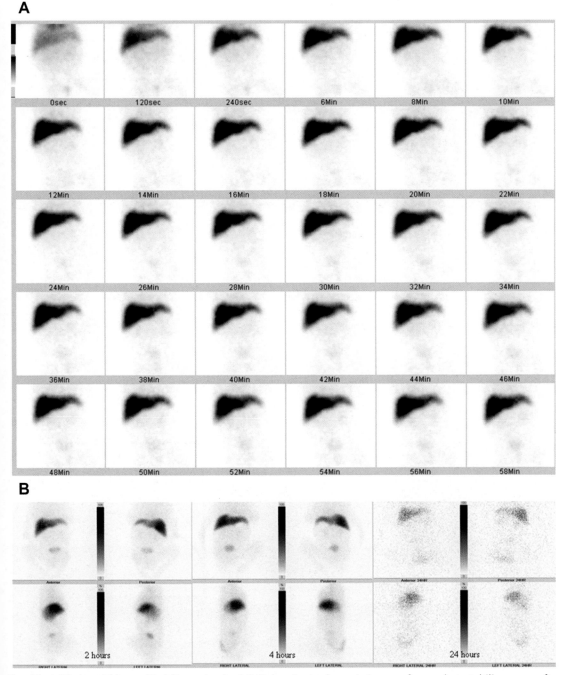

Fig. 11. A 20-day-old boy with biliary atresia. (*A*) Sixty-minute dynamic images from a hepatobiliary scan after pretreatment with phenobarbital demonstrate prompt hepatic uptake and blood pool clearance of radiotracer with no biliary or bowel excretion. (*B*) No bowel activity is seen on 2-, 4-, and 24-hour delayed static images, with persistence of radiotracer in the liver. Urinary clearance of radiotracer is indicated by activity in the renal collecting system, bladder, and diaper.

A

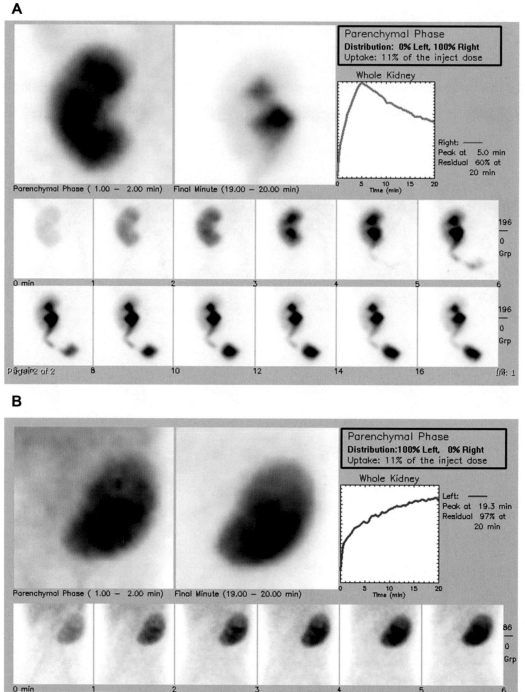

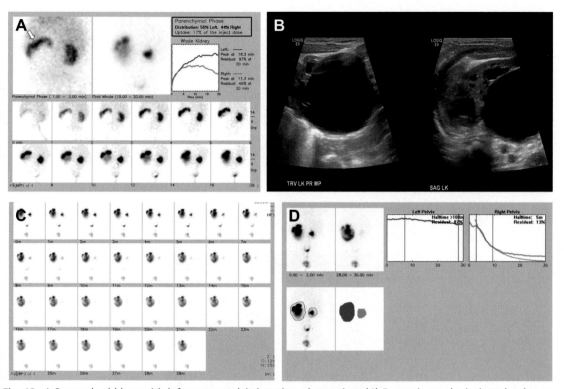

Fig. 13. A 3-month-old boy with left ureteropelvic junction obstruction. (*A*) Dynamic renal scintigraphy demonstrates marked enlargement of the left kidney with rotation of the parenchyma around the severely dilated collecting system (*arrow*). There is gradual accumulation of tracer in the collecting system with no significant drainage over 20 minutes. (*B*) Analogous findings are seen on transverse and sagittal grayscale ultrasound of the left kidney. (*C, D*) After administration of furosemide, essentially no additional clearance is observed. In contrast, the right kidney shows delayed spontaneous drainage with pooling of tracer in a prominent extrarenal pelvis but normal drainage with diuresis. A 6-month follow-up study (not pictured) did not demonstrate any significant change in postdiuretic drainage parameters, and open left pyeloplasty was performed.

Parathyroid scintigraphy

Parathyroid scintigraphy is used in the setting of hypercalcemia and suspected hyperparathyroidism. The sensitivity of ^{99m}Tc-sestamibi is between 80% and 90% for a single adenoma but lower (40%–60%) in cases of multiple adenomas or hyperplasia.[53]

Neuroendocrine tumor imaging (^{123}I-metaiodobenzylguanidine scintigraphy)

^{123}I-metaiodobenzylguanidine (MIBG) scintigraphy has a sensitivity of 88% to 93% and a specificity of 83% to 92% for neuroblastoma.[54] Approximately 10% of neuroblastomas do not show MIBG uptake. In these patients, ^{18}F-FDG PET scan is an additional tool for whole-body staging.[55] ^{123}I-MIBG scintigraphy is also used in the setting of opsoclonus-myoclonus[56] (**Fig. 19**) and biochemical evidence of sympathochromaffin tumors, such as pheochromocytoma and an adrenal mass on cross-sectional imaging.[53]

Somatostatin receptor scintigraphy using ^{111}In-pentetreotide could also be performed to image neuroendocrine tumors, such as

Fig. 12. Two pediatric patients, both 1 day status postrenal transplant. (*A*) Dynamic renography in a 10-year-old boy with a right lower quadrant transplant demonstrates rapid cortical perfusion with persistent cortical retention of tracer after 20 minutes of imaging. (*B*) The same study in a 2-year-old girl with a left lower quadrant transplant shows rapid cortical perfusion with more markedly decreased cortical clearance over 20 minutes. No tracer is seen outside the collecting system to indicate urinary leak, and no segmental perfusion abnormalities are demonstrated to indicate ischemia in either study. Prolonged cortical retention is a nonspecific indicator of renal dysfunction and may indicate a degree of acute tubular necrosis in the immediate post-transplant setting.

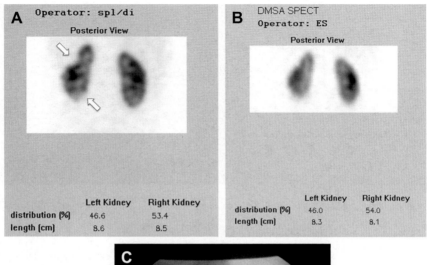

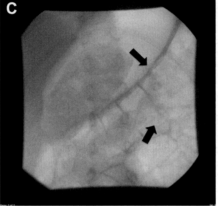

Fig. 14. A 4-year-old girl with pyelonephritis and vesicoureteral reflux. (*A*) An initial DMSA scan demonstrates a large focal defect in the upper pole and a small focal defect in the lower pole of the right kidney (*white arrows*). (*B*) Follow-up at 7 months demonstrates a small focal scar in the upper pole and a probable scar in the lower pole at sites of prior pyelonephritis. (*C*) A fluoroscopic image from a voiding cystourethrogram demonstrates vesicoureteral reflux into a nondilated collecting system (*black arrows*).

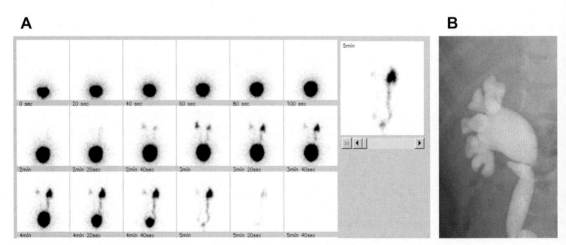

Fig. 15. A 3-year-girl with right hydronephrosis incidentally identified on ultrasound. (*A*) Posterior dynamic images of a radionuclide cystogram (RNC) demonstrate reflux into both renal collecting systems (RNC grade 3 on the right and RNC grade 2 on the left). (*B*) A prior voiding cystourethrogram had demonstrated grade IV right-sided reflux and no left-sided reflux (not pictured).

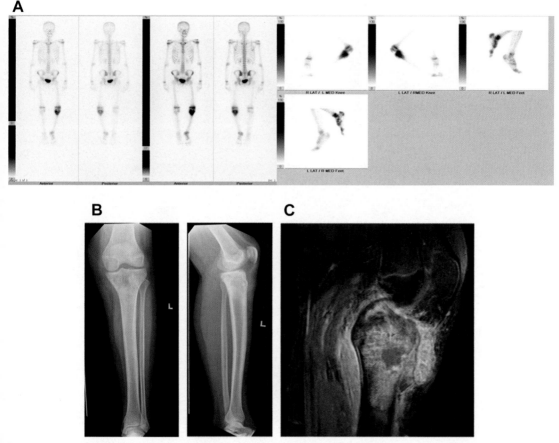

Fig. 16. A 14-year-old girl with proximal tibial osteosarcoma. (*A*) A ^{99m}Tc-MDP bone scan demonstrates increased uptake in the left proximal tibia. No skeletal metastases are identified. Increased uptake in the ipsilateral distal femoral physis and left foot is due to stress changes from altered weight-bearing. (*B*) PA and lateral radiographs and (*C*) sagittal postcontrast T1-weighted MR imaging demonstrate the aggressive proximal tibial lesion with adjacent soft-tissue extension.

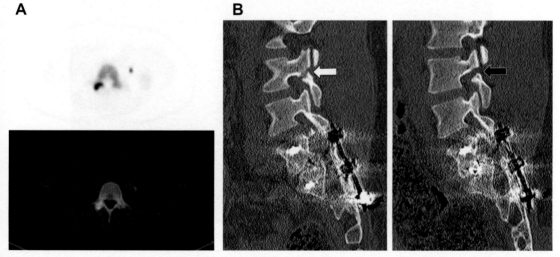

Fig. 17. A 16-year-old boy with a history of spondylolisthesis status post lumbosacral fusion presenting with back pain. (*A*) Axial ^{18}F-NaF PET and PET/CT images demonstrate increased radiotracer uptake denoting high bone turnover in the right but not the left L3 pars interarticularis. (*B*) Sagittal CT images of the lumbar spine demonstrate bilateral diastatic pars defects. The right-sided defect (*white arrow*) appears irregular, whereas the left-sided defect (*black arrow*) appears smoothly corticated, suggesting chronicity.

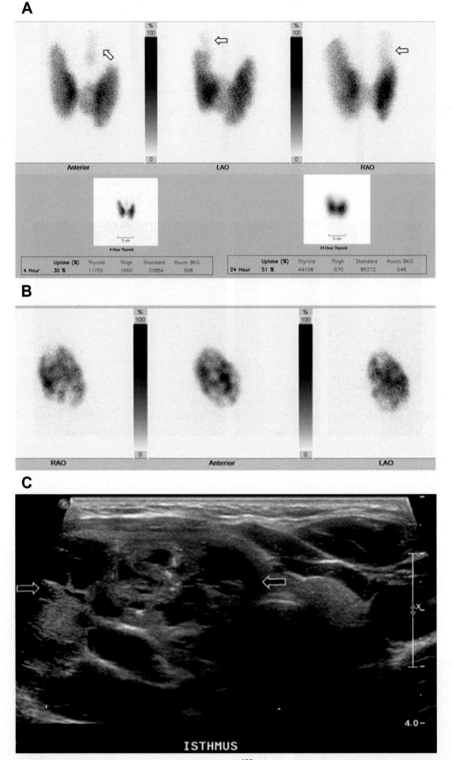

Fig. 18. Two pediatric patients with thyrotoxicosis. (*A*) An ^{123}I thyroid scan in a 15-year-old boy with thyrotoxicosis due to Graves disease demonstrates a homogeneously enlarged thyroid gland with convex borders and a prominent pyramidal lobe (*white arrows*). Radioiodine uptake was 30% at 4 hours and 51% at 24 hours. (*B*) In a 19-year-old woman with thyrotoxicosis due to an autonomous nodule, ^{123}I scan demonstrates heterogeneous uptake within a thyroid nodule. No activity is seen in the remainder of the gland, which is suppressed. (*C*) In the latter patient, ultrasound of the thyroid demonstrates a large, heterogeneous nodule in the right lobe and isthmus (*black arrows*).

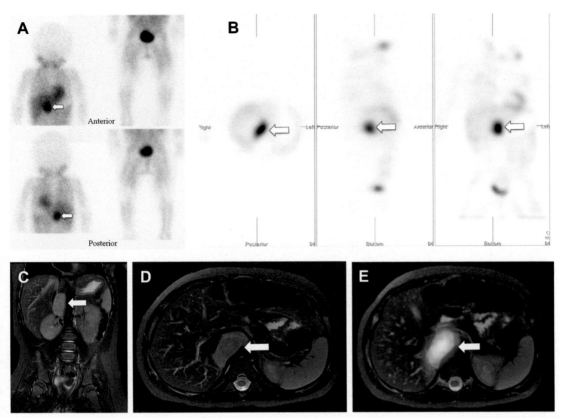

Fig. 19. A 13-month-old girl with neuroblastoma who presented with opsoclonus-myoclonus. (*A*) Planar and (*B*) SPECT images from an MIBG scan reveal focal uptake by a neuroblastoma in the right suprarenal region (*arrows*). No additional sites of disease are identified. (*C, D*) Coronal and axial T2-weighted MR imaging and (*E*) axial PET/MR fusion confirm the presence of a hyperintense oval right suprarenal mass with increased MIBG uptake.

insulinoma or carcinoid, but is not further discussed because it is not commonly performed in pediatrics.

Oncologic Applications

^{18}F-fluorodeoxyglucose PET–computed tomography

^{18}F-FDG PET/CT is the most commonly used nuclear medicine study for diagnosis, initial staging, response assessment, and tumor surveillance of various pediatric malignancies. The sensitivity and specificity of ^{18}F-FDG PET/CT for tumor staging in common pediatric cancers are 90% to 97% and 99% to 100%, respectively.[57] The most common malignancies in which ^{18}F-FDG PET/CT is routinely used in pediatrics are lymphoma (**Fig. 20**) and bone and soft-tissue sarcomas. It can also be used for assessment of MIBG-negative neuroblastoma[55] and malignant degeneration within peripheral nerve sheath tumors in pediatric patients with neurofibromatosis.[58] ^{18}F-FDG PET may be helpful in grading brain tumors such

as gliomas, determining the optimal site for biopsy, and distinguishing residual or recurrent tumor from post-treatment changes.[59] A major limitation in the evaluation of brain tumors is physiologic uptake in the normal brain.

Similar to ^{18}F-FDG PET/CT, simultaneous ^{18}F-FDG PET/MR imaging (**Fig. 21**) has great potential to improve evaluation of common pediatric malignancies.[60]

Inflammation and Infection

Traditionally, white blood cells (WBCs) labeled with either ^{99m}Tc or ^{111}In, have been used for imaging of suspected soft-tissue and bone infections, fever of unknown origin (FUO), and inflammatory bowel disease (IBD).[61] In practice, ultrasound, CT, and/or MR imaging are used as first-line for suspected soft-tissue, intra-abdominal, and lung infections, whereas bone scan and/or MR imaging are used for osteomyelitis. There is an emerging role for ^{18}F-FDG PET in

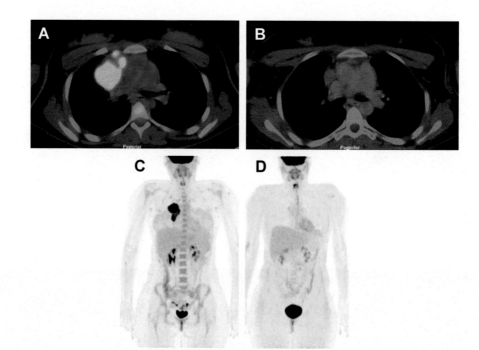

Fig. 20. A 16-year-old girl with Hodgkin lymphoma. (*A*) Fused ¹⁸F-FDG PET/CT and (*C*) SUV$_{max}$ maximum intensity projection PET images from the initial staging scan reveal right-sided mediastinal adenopathy. (*B*, *D*) Interim PET/CT after 2 cycles of chemotherapy demonstrates treatment response, with significant reduction in size of the adenopathy and only low-level residual FDG uptake, similar to or slightly less than liver uptake. Diffuse marrow uptake on the initial PET is likely reactive and is not uncommonly seen in patients with Hodgkin disease presenting with B symptoms.

FUO, osteomyelitis (**Fig. 22**), vasculitis, device or prosthesis-associated infections, and IBD.[61,62]

Lymphatic Imaging

Lymphoscintigraphy is the first-line test for assessment of lymphatic function. In children, it is typically used in diagnosing primary lymphedema (**Fig. 23**). It should be strongly considered in all pediatric patients with signs of lymphatic dysplasia, including those with minimal or early signs of lymphatic impairment, for quickly obtaining a diagnosis and initiating treatment.[63,64] A less common indication is sentinel lymph node localization.

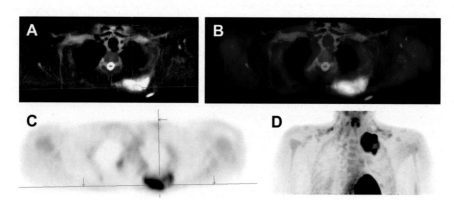

Fig. 21. A 19-year-old male patient with soft-tissue sarcoma of left posterior back. (*A*) Axial T2 HASTE MR, (*B*) ¹⁸F-FDG PET/MR, and (*C*, *D*) axial and MIP ¹⁸F-FDG images demonstrate an intensely FDG-avid mass in the left posterior chest wall. HASTE, half-Fourier single-shot turbo spin-echo; MIP, maximum intensity projection. (*Courtesy of* Ruth Lim, MD, Massachusetts General Hospital.)

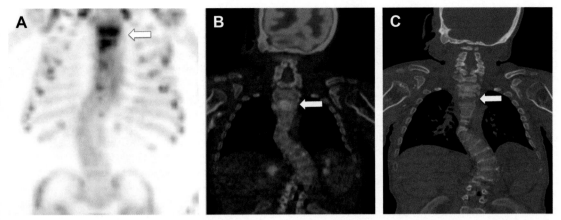

Fig. 22. A 29-year-old man with spondyloepiphyseal skeletal dysplasia and previous thoracic spinal fusion who presented with cervicothoracic spinal osteomyelitis. (A) A coronal image from a ^{99m}Tc-MDP bone scan demonstrates increased radiotracer uptake in the C7, T1, and T2 vertebral bodies (arrow). The differential diagnosis included osteomyelitis and reactive mechanical changes due to spinal fusion at a lower level. (B) A coronal ^{18}F-FDG PET/CT image obtained approximately 1 week after the bone scan demonstrates increased radiotracer uptake (arrow) in the affected vertebrae and adjacent soft tissues, consistent with osteomyelitis. (C) Coronal CT shows lysis and sclerosis of the affected vertebral bodies (arrow).

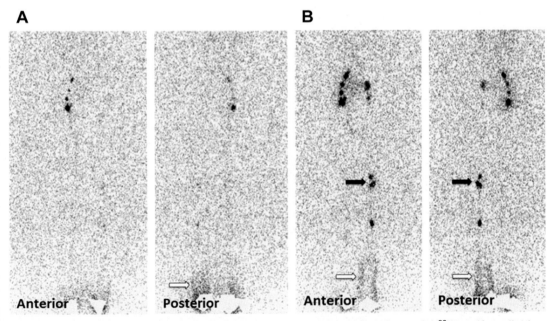

Fig. 23. A 16-year-old girl with lymphedema related to Phelan-McDermid syndrome. (A) ^{99m}Tc-sulfur colloid scan 45-minute planar images demonstrate delayed proximal lymphatic transit and dermal backflow (white arrows) in the left lower extremity. (B) Planar images obtained at 4 hours demonstrate a paucity of left inguinal lymph nodes compared with the normal right side and tracer uptake within left popliteal lymph nodes (black arrows), which supports the diagnosis of lymphedema. Dermal back flow (white arrows) is more evident. Shielding of the injection sites (between the first and second digits of both feet) was performed to reduce artifact.

SUMMARY

Nuclear medicine is indispensable in diagnosing a variety of diseases in children. With the advent of more modern equipment and newer radiopharmaceuticals, conventional gamma camera imaging may have lost some ground in current pediatric nuclear medicine practice but largely remains relevant. Simultaneous PET/MR imaging will be an extremely useful tool in pediatrics once its limitations are overcome. Nuclear medicine examinations in children typically result in very low radiation doses, especially with recent efforts at radiopharmaceutical dose standardization, continued advances in imaging equipment, and more sophisticated postprocessing techniques. It remains critical, however, to be mindful of the potential risks of radiation exposure in the vulnerable pediatric population.

REFERENCES

1. Gelfand MJ, Parisi MT, Treves ST. Pediatric radiopharmaceutical administered doses: 2010 North American consensus guidelines. J Nucl Med 2011; 52(2):318–22.

2. Lassmann M, Treves ST, EANM/SNMMI Paediatric Dosage Harmonization Working Group. Paediatric radiopharmaceutical administration: harmonization of the 2007 EANM paediatric dosage card (version 1.5.2008) and the 2010 North American consensus guidelines. Eur J Nucl Med Mol Imaging 2014; 41(5):1036–41.

3. Treves ST, Grant FD. General aspects of pediatric nuclear medicine. In: Treves ST, Fahey FH, Grant FD, editors. Pediatric nuclear medicine and molecular imaging. 4th edition. New York: Springer; 2014. p. 1–20.

4. Treves ST, Baker A, Fahey FH, et al. Nuclear Medicine in the First Year of Life. J Nucl Med 2011; 52(6):905–25.

5. Cooper JA, McCandless BK. Improved renal cortical SPECT of neonates and young infants using narrow imaging pallets. J Nucl Med Technol 1999;27(2): 127–31.

6. Slomka PJ, Pan T, Berman DS, et al. Advances in SPECT and PET Hardware. Prog Cardiovasc Dis 2015;57(6):566–78.

7. Fahey FH, Lim R, El-Fakhri G. Physical aspects of pediatric nuclear medicine imaging. In: Treves ST, editor. Pediatric nuclear medicine and molecular imaging. 4th edition. New York: Springer; 2014. p. 621–43.

8. Daldrup-Link HE, Gambhir SS. Pediatric molecular imaging. In: Treves ST, Fahey FH, Grant FD, editors. Pediatric nuclear medicine and molecular imaging. 4th edition. New York: Springer; 2014. p. 571–95.

9. Kumar A, Chugani HT. The role of radionuclide imaging in epilepsy, Part 1: sporadic temporal and extratemporal lobe epilepsy. J Nucl Med 2013; 54(10):1775–81.

10. O'Brien TJ, So EL, Mullan BP, et al. Subtraction SPECT co-registered to MRI improves postictal SPECT localization of seizure foci. Neurology 1999; 52(1):137–46.

11. Treves ST, Chugani HT, Bourgeois BFD, et al. Central nervous system: the brain and cerebrospinal fluid. In: Treves ST, Fahey FH, Grant FD, editors. Pediatric nuclear medicine and molecular imaging. 4th edition. New York: Springer; 2014. p. 47–97.

12. Partington SL, Valente AM, Landzberg M, et al. Clinical applications of radionuclide imaging in the evaluation and management of patients with congenital heart disease. J Nucl Cardiol 2015;23: 45–63.

13. Dorbala S, Di Carli MF, Delbeke D, et al. SNMMI/ ASNC/SCCT guideline for cardiac SPECT/CT and PET/CT 1.0. J Nucl Med 2013;54(8):1485–507.

14. Musso M, Petrosillo N. Nuclear medicine in diagnosis of prosthetic valve endocarditis: an update. Biomed Res Int 2015;2015:127325.

15. Tamir A, Melloul M, Berant M, et al. Lung perfusion scans in patients with congenital heart defects. J Am Coll Cardiol 1992;19(2):383–8.

16. Dae MW. Pediatric nuclear cardiology. Semin Nucl Med 2007;37(5):382–90.

17. Shammas A, Vali R, Charron M. Pediatric nuclear medicine in acute care. Semin Nucl Med 2013; 43(2):139–56.

18. Jeandot R, Lambert B, Brendel AJ, et al. Lung ventilation and perfusion scintigraphy in the follow up of repaired congenital diaphragmatic hernia. Eur J Nucl Med 1989;15(9):591–6.

19. Hayward MJ, Kharasch V, Sheils C, et al. Predicting inadequate long-term lung development in children with congenital diaphragmatic hernia: an analysis of longitudinal changes in ventilation and perfusion. J Pediatr Surg 2007;42(1):112–6.

20. Pal K, Gupta DK. Serial perfusion study depicts pulmonary vascular growth in the survivors of non-extracorporeal membrane oxygenation-treated congenital diaphragmatic hernia. Neonatology 2010;98(3):254–9.

21. Johnson K. Ventilation and perfusion scanning in children. Paediatr Respir Rev 2000;1(4):347–53.

22. Shimoyama S, Kobayashi T, Inoue Y, et al. Left displacement of the mediastinum determines the imbalance in the pulmonary vascular bed and lung volume in children with pectus excavatum. Pediatr Surg Int 2008;24(5):549–53.

23. Blickman JG, Rosen PR, Welch KJ, et al. Pectus excavatum in children: pulmonary scintigraphy before and after corrective surgery. Radiology 1985;156(3):781–2.

24. Kinuya K, Ueno T, Kobayashi T, et al. Tc-99m MAA SPECT in pectus excavatum: assessment of

perfusion volume changes after correction by the Nuss procedure. Clin Nucl Med 2005;30(12): 779–82.

25. Argon M, Duygun U, Daglioz G, et al. Relationship between gastric emptying and gastroesophageal reflux in infants and children. Clin Nucl Med 2006; 31(5):262–5.

26. Aktaş A, Ciftçi I, Caner B. The relation between the degree of gastro-oesophageal reflux and the rate of gastric emptying. Nucl Med Commun 1999; 20(10):907–10.

27. Spottswood SE, Pfluger T, Bartold SP, et al. SNMMI and EANM practice guideline for meckel diverticulum scintigraphy 2.0. J Nucl Med Technol 2014; 42(3):163–9.

28. Dam HQ, Brandon DC, Grantham VV, et al. The SNMMI Procedure Standard/EANM Practice Guideline for Gastrointestinal Bleeding Scintigraphy 2.0. J Nucl Med Technol 2014;42(4):308–17.

29. Kwatra N, Shalaby-Rana E, Narayanan S, et al. Phenobarbital-enhanced hepatobiliary scintigraphy in the diagnosis of biliary atresia: two decades of experience at a tertiary center. Pediatr Radiol 2013;43(10):1365–75.

30. Mahida JB, Sulkowski JP, Cooper JN, et al. Prediction of symptom improvement in children with biliary dyskinesia. J Surg Res 2015;198(2):393–9.

31. Ziessman HA. Functional hepatobiliary disease: chronic acalculous gallbladder and chronic acalculous biliary disease. Semin Nucl Med 2006;36(2): 119–32.

32. Kulaylat AN, Stokes AL, Engbrecht BW, et al. Traumatic bile leaks from blunt liver injury in children: a multidisciplinary and minimally invasive approach to management. J Pediatr Surg 2014;49(3):424–7.

33. Mortazavi N, Chaumet-Riffaud P, Chauffet-Riffaud P, et al. Biliary leak in a child after liver transplant and value of delayed images. Clin Nucl Med 2008;33(1): 44–5.

34. Ziessman HA. Hepatobiliary Scintigraphy in 2014. J Nucl Med 2014;55(6):967–75.

35. Shulkin BL, Mandell GA, Copper JA et al. Procedure guideline for diuretic renography in children 3.0. In: SNMMI procedure standards 2008. Available at: http://snmmi.files.cms-plus.com/docs/162.pdf. Accessed October 8, 2016.

36. Lagomarsino E, Orellana P, Muñoz J, et al. Captopril scintigraphy in the study of arterial hypertension in pediatrics. Pediatr Nephrol 2004;19(1):66–70.

37. Rossleigh MA. Scintigraphic imaging in renal infections. Q J Nucl Med Mol Imaging 2009;53(1): 72–7.

38. Majd M, Nussbaum Blask AR, Markle BM, et al. Acute pyelonephritis: comparison of diagnosis with 99mTc-DMSA, SPECT, spiral CT, MR imaging, and power Doppler US in an experimental pig model. Radiology 2001;218(1):101–8.

39. Rossleigh MA. Renal cortical scintigraphy and diuresis renography in infants and children. J Nucl Med 2001;42(1):91–5.

40. Fleming JS, Zivanovic MA, Blake GM, et al. British Nuclear Medicine Society. Guidelines for the measurement of glomerular filtration rate using plasma sampling. Nucl Med Commun 2004;25(8):759–69.

41. Itoh K. 99mTc-MAG3: review of pharmacokinetics, clinical application to renal diseases and quantification of renal function. Ann Nucl Med 2001;15(3):179–90.

42. Piepsz A, Ham HR. Pediatric applications of renal nuclear medicine. Semin Nucl Med 2006;36(1):16–35.

43. Grant FD, Fahey FH, Packard AB, et al. Skeletal PET with 18F-fluoride: applying new technology to an old tracer. J Nucl Med 2008;49(1):68–78.

44. Kwatra N, Shalaby-Rana E, Majd M. Two-phase whole-body skeletal scintigraphy in children–revisiting the usefulness of the early blood pool phase. Pediatr Radiol 2013;43(10):1376–84.

45. DiPoce J, Jbara ME, Brenner AI. Pediatric osteomyelitis: a scintigraphic case-based review. Radiographics 2012;32(3):865–78.

46. Schauwecker DS. The scintigraphic diagnosis of osteomyelitis. AJR Am J Roentgenol 1992;158(1): 9–18.

47. Shammas A. Nuclear medicine imaging of the pediatric musculoskeletal system. Semin Musculoskelet Radiol 2009;13(3):159–80.

48. Grant FD. ^{18}F-fluoride PET and PET/CT in children and young adults. PET Clin 2014;9(3):287–97.

49. Balon HR, Silberstein EB, Meier DA. Society of Nuclear Medicine Procedure Guideline for Thyroid Uptake Measurement. In: SNMMI procedure standards. 2006. Available at: http://snmmi.files.cms-plus.com/docs/Thyroid%20Uptake%20Measure%20v3%200.pdf. Accessed October 2, 2016.

50. Williams JL, Paul DL, Bisset G. Thyroid disease in children: part 1: State-of-the-art imaging in pediatric hypothyroidism. Pediatr Radiol 2013;43(10): 1244–53.

51. Williams JL, Paul D, Bisset G. Thyroid disease in children: part 2: State-of-the-art imaging in pediatric hyperthyroidism. Pediatr Radiol 2013;43(10): 1254–64.

52. Grant FD, Treves ST. Thyroid. In: Treves ST, Fahey FH, Grant FD, editors. Pediatric Nuclear Medicine and Molecular Imaging. 4th edition. New York: Springer; 2014. p. 99–129.

53. Grant FD. Imaging parathyroid and neuroendocrine tumors. In: Treves ST, editor. Pediatric nuclear medicine and molecular imaging. 4th edition. New York: Springer; 2014. p. 447–78.

54. Vik TA, Pfluger T, Kadota R, et al. (123)I-mIBG scintigraphy in patients with known or suspected neuroblastoma: results from a prospective multicenter trial. Pediatr Blood Cancer 2009;52(7): 784–90.

55. Sharp SE, Gelfand MJ, Shulkin BL. Pediatrics: diagnosis of neuroblastoma. Semin Nucl Med 2011; 41(5):345–53.

56. Parisi MT, Hattner RS, Matthay KK, et al. Optimized diagnostic strategy for neuroblastoma in opsoclonus-myoclonus. J Nucl Med 1993;34(11):1922–6.

57. Uslu L, Donig J, Link M, et al. Value of 18F-FDG PET and PET/CT for evaluation of pediatric malignancies. J Nucl Med 2015;56(2):274–86.

58. Tsai LL, Drubach L, Fahey F, et al. [18F]-Fluorodeoxyglucose positron emission tomography in children with neurofibromatosis type 1 and plexiform neurofibromas: correlation with malignant transformation. J Neurooncol 2012;108(3):469–75.

59. Biermann M, Schwarzlmüller T, Fasmer KE, et al. Is there a role for PET-CT and SPECT-CT in pediatric oncology? Acta Radiol 2013;54(9):1037–45.

60. Gatidis S, la Fougère C, Schaefer JF. Pediatric oncologic imaging: a key application of combined PET/MRI. RöFo 2016;188(4):359–64.

61. Palestro CJ. Infection and inflammation. In: Treves ST, Fahey FH, Grant FD, editors. Pediatric nuclear medicine and molecular imaging. 4th edition. New York: Springer; 2014. p. 541–69.

62. Vaidyanathan S, Patel CN, Scarsbrook AF, et al. FDG PET/CT in infection and inflammation–current and emerging clinical applications. Clin Radiol 2015; 70(7):787–800.

63. Bellini C, Villa G, Sambuceti G, et al. Lymphoscintigraphy patterns in newborns and children with congenital lymphatic dysplasia. Lymphology 2014; 47(1):28–39.

64. Bellini C, Boccardo F, Campisi C, et al. Lymphatic dysplasias in newborns and children: the role of lymphoscintigraphy. J Pediatr 2008;152(4):587–9, 589–3.

Practical Imaging Evaluation of Foreign Bodies in Children: An Update

Bernard F. Laya, MD, DO[a],*, Ricardo Restrepo, MD[b],
Edward Y. Lee, MD, MPH[c,d]

KEYWORDS

- Foreign bodies in children • Foreign body aspiration • Foreign body ingestion
- Foreign body insertion • Foreign body complications

KEY POINTS

- Foreign bodies in children can be inhaled, ingested, or inserted in natural body cavities or tissues.
- Most ingested foreign bodies pass the pylorus without sequelae.
- Foreign bodies can cause severe and even life-threatening complications.
- Radiologic imaging helps in detection, characterization, localization, and assessment of complications of foreign bodies in children.
- Not all foreign bodies are visible on radiographs.

INTRODUCTION

The typical mechanisms of entry for a foreign body (FB) include aspiration, ingestion, insertion, penetrating trauma, or even iatrogenic. When the event is witnessed, diagnosis and management are usually expedited and less problematic in the pediatric population. However, unrecognized FB may present long after the initiating incident, and the symptoms may even mimic other conditions.[1] The Susy Safe database, a large database describing all pediatric FB-related injuries in children, showed that 74% of objects were inorganic and were mostly represented by pearls and balls, followed by coins.[2] FB injuries may be asymptomatic and, if symptoms are present, they may be nonspecific. FB injuries can be misinterpreted as a gastrointestinal or respiratory infection or other conditions, contributing to delayed diagnosis and increased risk of complications.[3] Therefore, history with documentation of the possible object is of outmost importance when witnessed.

Accidental aspiration of FBs into the respiratory system is commonly encountered in children younger than 3 years old and is an important cause of morbidity and mortality in children. A diagnosis of FB aspiration is often missed or delayed because the causative event is usually unobserved and the symptoms are often nonspecific in children.[4] FB can also be ingested and many pass naturally through the gastrointestinal tract without complications. However, severe potential complications, including obstruction, mucosal injury, or perforation can occur. These complications depend on the characteristics of the FB, its

Disclosure Statement: The authors have nothing to disclose.
[a] Institute of Radiology, St. Luke's Medical Center-Global City, 32nd Street Corner, Rizal Drive, Bonifacio Global City, Taguig City, Metro Manila 1634, Philippines; [b] Nicklaus Children's Hospital, 3100 Southwest 62nd Avenue, Miami, FL 33155, USA; [c] Division of Thoracic Imaging, Department of Radiology, Boston Children's Hospital, Harvard Medical School, 300 Longwood Avenue, Boston, MA 02115, USA; [d] Pulmonary Division, Department of Medicine, Boston Children's Hospital, Harvard Medical School, 300 Longwood Avenue, Boston, MA 02115, USA
* Corresponding author.
E-mail address: Bernielaya@gmail.com

Radiol Clin N Am 55 (2017) 845–867
http://dx.doi.org/10.1016/j.rcl.2017.02.012

anatomic location, the child's age, and delay in diagnosis.[3] Insertion of FBs in various natural body cavities also occurs in children. Aural FB placement can be a response to irritation or could be a child's way of exploring the ear cavity. Although accidental and traumatic insertion of FB in the vaginal and urethrovesical cavity can occur, intentional insertion is the more common cause, believed to be due to body exploration or for sexual gratification. In either case, sexual abuse or psychiatric disorder has to be excluded.

Various medical imaging modalities have been used in the evaluation of FBs. Radiographs can be helpful in localizing radiopaque FBs such as coins, buttons, pins, and batteries. However, radiographic visibility of a foreign object depends on its inherent composition and its location in the human body. FBs might be radiographically visible in 1 body part but not visible if located in another, much thicker, body part. The same FB might be visible in a superficial extremity soft-tissue but invisible in the abdomen. This also means that not all radiopaque objects are detected by radiography.[5] Fluoroscopy with oral administration of contrast can be a useful tool, particularly in outlining nonradiopaque FB ingestions. Ultrasound (US) is also used to evaluate FBs in the gastrointestinal tract, as well as vagina and the urinary bladder. Computed tomography (CT) has become more valuable by virtue of its wide availability; high resolution; and the multiplanar, 3-dimensional (3D), and other image reconstruction capabilities. CT can establish the diagnosis of FB, indicate its exact location, and detect associated complications. Because of its great soft tissue differentiation capability, MR imaging has been used for FB evaluation in the genitourinary tract.

It is often that radiologists are the first to raise the possibility or report presence of FB, particularly in the pediatric population. Thus, it is important for a radiologist to confirm its presence, as well as to describe associated secondary findings or complications related to long-standing FBs.

AIRWAY FOREIGN BODIES
Overview and Etiologic Factors

Inhalation of FBs in children is a frequent complaint in the pediatric emergency department. Most FB inhalations occur in children less than 3 years old, with a peak incidence between 10 to 24 months of age.[6,7] Serious complications can occur, such as severe airway obstruction and death, especially in younger children and infants because of the small caliber of their airways. FB aspiration is ranked sixth most common cause of accidental deaths in children.[8]

Younger children are predisposed to FB inhalation for 3 main reasons. First, they have a tendency to explore by placing objects into their mouths; second, they are unable to adequately chew certain foods due to lack of molars that can grind food into smaller, smoother particles; and third, they have immature or poorly coordinated swallowing mechanisms.[9–11] Additionally, there may be less adult supervision as children increase ambulation and thus the likelihood of aspiration is higher.[11] Most aspirated FBs are organic or food objects, including peanuts and sunflower seeds, which together account for almost 80% of aspirated FBs. Organic FBs cause more tissue reaction and tend to produce more complications.[12] Nonorganic or nonfood objects, such as whistles, soil, and plastic objects, including musical mouth pieces, pen tops, and LEGO toy pieces, have also been retrieved and are more likely culprits in older children.[6,11–13] Inert FBs are more likely to remain in 1 place for a longer period of time and are less likely to cause complications.[12]

Location and Symptoms

Upper airway
Aspirated FB can lodge anywhere along the upper airway that lies above the thoracic inlet. Nasal FBs tend to be located on the floor of the nasal passage, just below the inferior turbinate, or in the upper nasal fossa anterior to the middle turbinate (**Fig. 1**). Affected pediatric patients often present with unilateral, foul-smelling nasal discharge.[14] Approximately 3% of aspirated FBs lodge in the larynx, and are usually bulky, irregularly shaped, or sharp (even penetrating) objects (**Figs. 2 and 3**).[13,15] They produce symptoms that are abrupt and severe, with an acute event noted in 90% of cases.[1] Signs and symptoms of FB lodged in the supraglottic region are cough, dyspnea, salivation, and voice changes. When in the larynx, there is stridor, cough, voice changes, and severe breathing difficulty. When in the extrathoracic trachea, inspiratory stridor and expiratory rhonchi are observed.[16,17]

Lower airway
Most aspirated FBs (75%) in the lower airway are lodged below the thoracic inlet, most frequently in the bronchi,[1,15] especially in the right main bronchus, which is larger than the left main bronchus and directly aligned with the trachea in upright patients (**Fig. 4**).[9,10] Recent studies state that the difference in occurrence of FB lodged in the right and the left bronchus is less pronounced because the airway in children is immature and that the

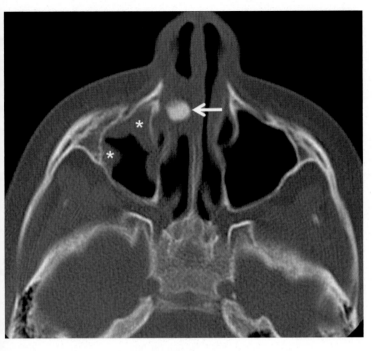

Fig. 1. Nasal foreign body in a 6-year-old girl who presented with fever, nasal congestion, and discharge. Axial bone window CT image of the paranasal sinuses shows a small rectangular FB (*arrow*), later found to be a pencil eraser in the anterior aspect of the right nasal passage. Note the inflammatory soft tissue changes surrounding the FB and the mucoperiosteal thickening (*asterisks*) of the ipsilateral maxillary sinus.

differences between the right and left bronchial trees are not significant.[11]

Symptoms of FB aspiration are related to its size, shape, nature, and duration since aspiration. Organic FB causes more airway inflammation, whereas an inorganic FB may go undetected for a long time.[8] Sharp objects may cause direct injury to the airway or even perforation. The clinical presentation has a wide spectrum from no symptoms in small objects to respiratory failure when large

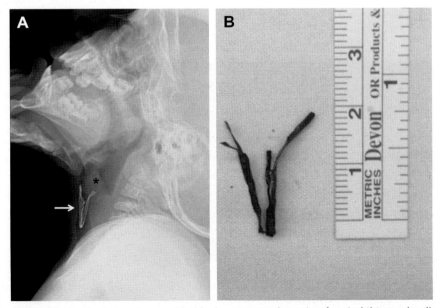

Fig. 2. Upper airway foreign body in a 4-year-old girl who presented gasping for air. (*A*) Lateral radiograph of the airway shows a curvilinear metallic FB (*arrow*) lodged in the subglottic airway along with edema of the aryepiglottic folds (*asterisk*). (*B*) Photograph of the endoscopically retrieved specimen reveals a twisted metallic wire.

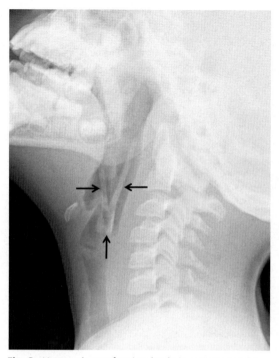

Fig. 3. Upper airway foreign body in a 9-year-old boy who presented with dysphagia and FB sensation after eating chicken. Lateral neck radiograph shows a V-shape radiopaque structure (*arrows*) lodged in the hypopharynx, compatible with a chicken bone.

to suspect FB aspiration.[16–19] Wheezing in the absence of known pulmonary disease such as asthma, especially if unilateral, should be considered to be due to FB aspiration until proven otherwise.[20] Initial symptoms may subside and the child become asymptomatic for days or weeks and at times, the child's symptoms may not be easily understood and the diagnosis delayed for weeks or even months.[11]

Mimics, Complications, and Treatment

Prompt diagnosis and management of FB aspiration are crucial but, unfortunately, the time lapse between aspiration and seeking medical consultation ranges from 30 minutes to 6 months,[11,12] or even years.[17] Correct diagnosis of FB aspiration in the first 24 hours following the incident is made in only 50%[21] to 59% of cases.[6,22] One of the main reasons for delayed diagnosis is because many FB aspirations in children are unobserved and unwitnessed.[11,23] In addition, the symptoms of FB aspiration are nonspecific and can be manifested by other conditions.

Mucous plug from inspissated bronchial secretions can cause partial or complete airway obstruction that mimics FB aspiration.[18,24] External airway compression from enlarged lymph nodes, mediastinal neoplasms, vascular rings, or cardiomegaly can also have similar symptoms. Other differential considerations include intraluminal tracheobronchial pathologies, neoplasm, granulation tissue (as in tuberculosis), asthma, pulmonary abscess, or croup.[25] Delayed or even missed diagnosis can result in respiratory complications ranging from chronic cough and wheezing,

objects lodge into the carina.[16,17] Choking followed by an acute episode of coughing is the most common presentation.[15] Wheezing, dyspnea, cyanosis, reduced air entry, and chronic or recurrent pulmonary infections are subtle clues

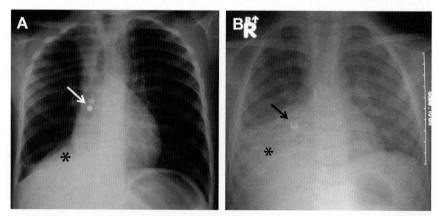

Fig. 4. Lower airway foreign body in 2 pediatric patients. (*A*) Frontal radiograph, in an 8-year-old boy who presented with developmental delay and respiratory distress demonstrates a metallic earring (*arrow*) within the right lower lobe bronchus, along with atelectasis (*asterisk*). (*B*) Frontal radiograph in a 5-year-old boy who presented with fever and persistent right middle and lower lobe pneumonia reveals a radiopaque FB (*arrow*) in the bronchus intermedius, which was proven to be a pencil eraser holder on surgery. Also noted is a combination of postobstructive pneumonitis and atelectasis (*asterisk*) in the right middle and lower lobes.

bronchiectasis, recurrent pneumonias, hemoptysis, and failure to thrive, to more severe conditions, including lung abscess,[11,12,17,22,26] drowned lung due to obstructive emphysema,[27] and bronchoesophageal fistula.[17] Bronchoscopy is often performed for definitive diagnosis and treatment, even when there is little suspicion or doubtful history. It has a diagnostic accuracy of 94.5%[26] and successful FB retrieval rate of 97% to 99.7%.[26,28]

Imaging Evaluation

Chest radiography

When FB inhalation is suspected, radiographs are usually obtained because they are widely available and relatively inexpensive. Frontal and lateral chest radiographs are often performed, and both frontal and lateral neck radiographs are included, depending on the symptoms. Radiographic diagnosis is challenging for 3 main reasons: (1) only 10% of all airway FBs are radiopaque,[18,29,30] (2) up to 80% of children with laryngotracheal foreign bodies[29,31] and 30% to 50% of children with endoscopically proven bronchial FBs have normal radiographs,[6,19,22,29–31] and (3) because most FBs are radiolucent so diagnosis can only be suggested by secondary changes.

In the upper airway, indirect signs of airway obstruction include overdistention of the hypopharynx[13] and prevertebral soft tissue swelling.[1,13,29] In the lower airway, secondary signs include unilateral emphysema or localized air trapping of the affected side (**Fig. 5**), bilateral emphysema, focal airspace disease such as pneumonia and/or atelectasis,[6,9,10,19,31] pleural effusion, subcutaneous emphysema, pneumothorax, and mediastinal shift.[9,10,31] These secondary findings are nonspecific and may also occur in patients without FB aspiration.[22,32] Although chest radiography may help, it seems neither sufficiently sensitive nor specific for the diagnosis of FB aspiration given its low sensitivity of 60% to 85%, and specificity of 32% to 68% in the detection of FB aspiration.[20,22,33,34]

Unilateral air-trapping detection in FB aspiration can be enhanced with expiratory or bilateral decubitus radiographs.[6,19,35] An expiratory radiograph allows visualization of air trapped by a ball-and-valve–like mechanism due to partial obstruction of the bronchial lumen, resulting in a hyperinflated lucent lobe or lung distal to the affected airway.[3,16,19,31,36] Expiratory radiographs increase the number of true positives but its accuracy is low and its benefit remains unclear.[31] It is also technically challenging to obtain, especially in a young child, prompting multiple repeats.[9,10,31] Unilateral radiolucencies could also be misleading because it could be due to imperfect positioning in an irritated child.[19] Bilateral decubitus views have been used to simulate expiratory radiography (**Fig. 6**) but showed no clear additional diagnostic benefit in recent studies.[9,10,31] However, this latter technique may be more helpful in the young and less helpful in cooperative children.

Fluoroscopy

Fluoroscopy has been traditionally used as an adjunct to radiographs in pediatric patients suspected to have FB aspiration.[1,19,29] Evaluation is accomplished in supine position on the fluoroscopic table. Although a dynamic study, the use of last-image hold, available in most modern fluoroscopy machines, enables static images with minimal radiation exposure. Diaphragmatic motion

Fig. 5. Nonradiopaque foreign body in a 22-month-old boy who presented with an acute onset of wheezing. (*A*) Frontal radiograph demonstrates hyperaeration of the left lung (*asterisk*) raising the possibility of nonradiopaque foreign body in the left bronchus. (*B*) Coronal reconstruction from a low-dose computed tomography scan of the chest confirms the left lung hyperaeration (*asterisk*). Bronchoschopy revealed a popcorn kernel in the left bronchus. (*Courtesy of* Dr. Elizabeth H. Ey, Dayton, Ohio).

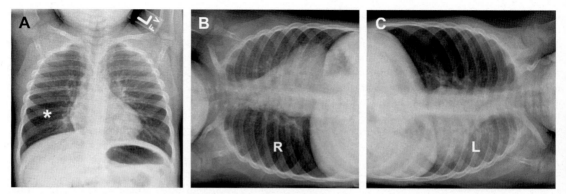

Fig. 6. Nonradiopaque foreign body in a 2-year-old boy who presented with an acute onset of wheezing and respiratory distress. (*A*) Frontal radiograph obtained in full inspiration shows mild focal hyperlucency (*asterisk*) to the right lower lobe. (*B*) Right lateral decubitus radiograph shows no collapse of the abnormal right lung (R), confirming the presence of a FB in a right bronchus. (*C*) Left lateral decubitus radiograph demonstrates the expected collapse of the normal dependent left lung (L).

and mediastinal side-to-side shifting during inspiration and expiration is observed.[18] Abnormal mediastinal shift with decreased excursion of the diaphragm could represent air trapping on the side of FB obstruction.[19,28] Digital subtraction fluoroscopy has been shown to be a sensitive method for the demonstration of tracheal and bronchial narrowing secondary to the presence of a radiolucent aspirated FB.[37] However, fluoroscopy findings are abnormal in only 47% of children with FB aspiration.[38] This technique could be difficult in irritated and uncooperative children and is also highly operator-dependent, needing expertise to develop. It has been safely used as a guide in bronchoscopic retrieval.[39]

Computed tomography

Multidetector CT (MDCT) has been established as an excellent imaging modality for lung and airway evaluation in children. MDCT can delineate airway defects formed by FBs, even when objects are small or radiolucent.[20] Indications for MDCT include clinical suspicion of FB aspiration, in pediatric patients with negative chest radiograph, in atypical presentation, and if there is discrepancy between clinical and radiological findings (**Fig. 7**).[40] MDCT is able to delineate the exact shape, location, volume, and form of an airway FB.[11,41] The foreign object demonstrates variable attenuation depending on its composition.[9,10,42] Intravenous contrast administration enhances discrimination between an intraluminal FB and other endobronchial, bronchial wall, or extrinsic findings. MDCT is also able to accurately demonstrate important secondary signs, including air trapping and lung collapse or atelectasis (**Fig. 8**),[9–11,18,41,42] as well as complications such as pneumomediastinum and pneumothorax,[31]

bronchiectasis, or recurrent infections. MDCT is superior in demonstrating lung parenchymal abnormalities, as well as other airway pathologic conditions, including tracheobronchial congenital anomalies, extrinsic compressions, and intraluminal lesions and vascular anomalies that may mimic a FB aspiration.[9,18,34,43]

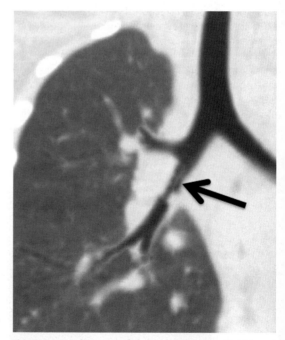

Fig. 7. Nonradiopaque foreign body in the right bronchus intermedius detected on CT in a 3-year-old boy who presented with respiratory distress. Frontal chest radiograph of this child reveals no significant findings (not shown). Coronal lung window CT image demonstrates a thin linear structure (*arrow*) in the bronchus intermedius, which was endoscopically retrieved and found to be a piece of hard plastic.

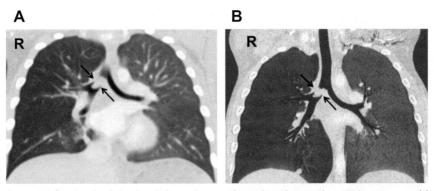

Fig. 8. Nonradiopaque foreign body in the right main-stem bronchus detected on CT in a 4-year-old girl who presented with respiratory distress. (*A*) Coronal lung window CT image shows an FB (*arrows*) in the right main bronchus and hyperlucent right lung, compared with the left, due to air trapping. (*B*) Coronal minimal intensity projection CT image better shows the FB (*arrows*), which was later found to be a carbon tip of a pencil. Hyperinflated and lucent right lung is also seen.

MDCT can be obtained as a single phase at end-inspiration or in 2 phases during end-inspiration and end-expiration.[9] Because of the inherent contrast between the air-filled tracheobronchial tree and adjacent structures, low radiation techniques are possible and are adequate for imaging. Tube current can be reduced to as low as 25 to 30 mA, and kV can be reduced to as low as 80 to 90, depending on child age and weight. For infants and toddlers, 2-mm collimation with 1-mm reconstructions can be used but for older children and adolescents, 3-mm collimation at 3-mm reconstructions can be used with the smallest possible field of view.[22,41] Multiplanar reformatted and curved coronal reconstruction can also be created for better view of the large airways. A 3D volume-rendered imaging of the large airway from the external perspective (virtual bronchography) and the internal perspective (virtual bronchoscopy) can be generated using the axial CT data set.[9,11] Additional advantage of the MDCT includes shorter examination time, which has substantially decreased the frequency of sedation required to image children.[18] MDCT is a highly accurate tool with sensitivity of 99.83% and specificity of 99.89% in evaluating the presence of airway FB.[11]

It must be noted, however, that mucous plug within the airway may be difficult to differentiate from a FB in CT.[18,44] In addition, CT cannot show the mucosal morphology and vascularity.[11] CT also carries some risk from radiation, although the dose has been decreased using a low-tube-current technique and rapid table speed.[22]

MR imaging

MR imaging has multiplanar capability and excellent tissue differentiation, which is helpful in accurate location of airway FBs.[45,46] A few studies have described the utility of MR imaging in peanut inhalation. Peanuts have a high fat-rich content, which has high signal on T1-weighted MR images in comparison with surrounding low-signal air in the lung, allowing high contrast differentiation. MR imaging also allows differentiation between peanuts and associated indirect findings such as granulation or atelectasis.[45] However, MR imaging studies are rarely used for suspected FB aspiration because of sedation, which is almost mandatory in younger children, the same age group most prone to FB inhalation.

Practical imaging algorithm

If clinical suspicion of an airway FB is present and the affected pediatric patient is stable enough to have imaging tests, plain radiographs of the chest in frontal (anteroposterior or posteroanterior) and lateral views are recommended. Depending on clinical symptoms, a frontal and lateral view of the neck may be included to evaluate the upper airway. If there is visualization of a radiopaque FB, or if there are secondary changes (air trapping, atelectasis, or consolidation), the patient can proceed to bronchoscopy for further evaluation and retrieval. If the radiographs are normal or unremarkable in symptomatic pediatric patients, CT can be subsequently obtained. If CT is not available, inspiratory-expiratory ($\geq$5 years of age) or bilateral decubitus radiographs (<5 years of age) and fluoroscopy may be obtained. For suspected peanut inhalation, MR imaging can be considered.

GASTROINTESTINAL FOREIGN BODIES
Overview and Etiologic Factors

Pediatric FB ingestion is a worldwide problem. According to the Susy Safe project, a large database describing pediatric FB injury in children, about 18% of these involved FB ingestion.[2] Of all reported FB ingestions, 80% involve children from 6 months to 3 years of age, which is the oral developmental period when children explore their surroundings, often leading to the accidental swallowing of the object being explored.[47] Repeated episodes of FB ingestion are also observed in children with a history of pica, developmental delay, psychiatric disorder, or mental retardation.[47–49] There are variable reports regarding the incidence of witnessed FB ingestion, which ranges from 23%[49] to 74%.[50] Although the types of ingested objects by children are unlimited, coins are the most commonly ingested FBs in children (**Fig. 9**).[48,51] Other frequently encountered objects include crayons, marbles, small toys, keys, stones, safety pins, batteries, magnets, and bones of meat, fish, or chicken (**Figs. 10 and 11**).[47,48,52] There is also a geographic and cultural influence on the type of FB ingested. Most children presented within 48 hours of ingestion.[49] Most (80%–90%) ingested foreign objects that reach the stomach pass uneventfully without intervention[1,48] but the remainder may become blocked in the esophagus or other region of the alimentary tract, which can lead to significant complications (see **Fig. 11**).[48]

Location and Symptoms

Although uncommon, an ingested FB can become impacted in the oropharynx. Children younger than 6 months are rarely able to get a foreign object into the oropharynx but they can do so with the assistance of a sibling.[48] The esophagus is a common site for FB impaction and there are 3 common locations of esophageal obstruction, namely (1) the C6 vertebral level at the upper esophageal sphincter or cricopharyngeus muscle, which is the most common site of obstruction (**Fig. 12**)[49,52,53]; (2) the T4 level where the distal aortic arch descends posterior to the midesophagus (**Fig. 13**); and (3) at the lower esophageal sphincter. Areas with acquired or congenital esophageal strictures are also frequent sites of FB lodgment (**Fig. 14A**).[48] Other potential blockage sites in the gastrointestinal tract are at the pylorus, duodenal sweep, ileocecal valve, rectosigmoid colon, and anus.[52,53] If the object has irregular or sharp edges, the FB may lodge anywhere in the gastrointestinal tract, especially at areas of anatomic narrowing or physiologic angulation. Objects longer than 5 cm or more than 2 cm in diameter are less likely to pass through the pylorus. Longer objects that pass from the stomach are also at risk for entrapment in areas such as the duodenal sweep, the ligament of Treitz area, and at the ileocecal valve.[48]

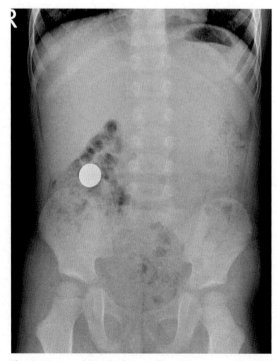

Fig. 9. 5-year old girl who swallowed a penny. Frontal supine abdominal radiograph reveals a round metallic object in the right hemiabdomen, compatible with a coin in the ascending colon.

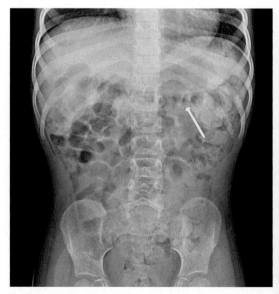

Fig. 10. Radio-opaque foreign body in a 3-year-old girl who presented with irritability and abdominal pain. Abdominal radiograph shows a sharp tubular radiopaque object (nail) in the left upper quadrant.

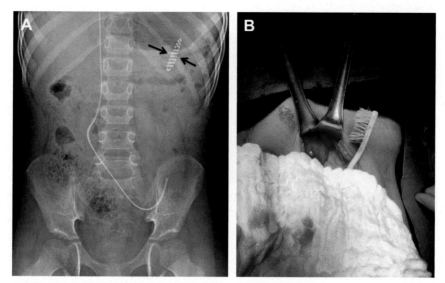

Fig. 11. Unusual foreign body in an 8-year-old developmentally delayed boy who presented with abdominal pain. (*A*) Abdominal radiograph shows a cluster of radiopaque dots (*arrows*) in the left upper quadrant corresponding to the bristles of a toothbrush. (*B*) Intraoperative image reveals that the toothbrush was free in the peritoneal cavity, raising the possibility of neglect.

Children with esophageal FBs may present with drooling, inability to swallow solids, refusal to eat, choking or gagging, vomiting, chest pain, or respiratory distress.[48,49,53] Up to 5% can present with airway obstruction symptoms when the bolus is impacted near the upper esophageal sphincter with secondary compression of the trachea.[54,55] Physical examination is normal in most children (76%) with ingested FBs. In patients with abnormal examinations, tenderness to palpation is the most frequent finding (25%).[49] Careful examination should assess for signs of perforation, such as subcutaneous emphysema or peritoneal signs.[53]

Rectal foreign bodies may also be encountered but are uncommon among children (**Fig. 15**). Unless witnessed, children may not confess to placement of object in the rectum. In any case, sexual abuse should be excluded. They may complain of pelvic, abdominal, or rectal pain, pruritus, or bleeding.[56,57] In the case of suspected or known sexual assault, the appropriate legal authority or child protective services should be notified immediately.[56]

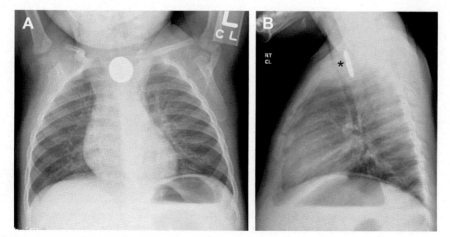

Fig. 12. Coin in upper esophagus of an 18-month-old boy who presented with drooling, refusal to accept food, and fever. Frontal (*A*) and lateral (*B*) radiographs of the chest show a metallic coin lodged in the proximal third of the esophagus. The lateral radiograph (*B*) shows a substantial thickening of the tracheoesophageal stripe (*asterisk*), indicating inflammation and long-standing foreign body (coin) lodgment in the area.

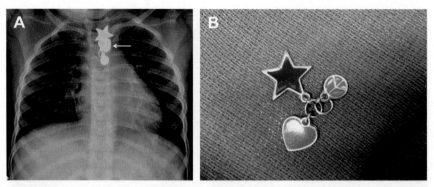

Fig. 13. Radio-opaque foreign body in the midesophagus of a 3- year-old girl who presented with gagging. Frontal (*A*) chest radiographs shows a cluster of radio-opaque FBs (*arrow*) in the region of the middle esophagus, proven to be a necklace pendant (*B*).

Type of Foreign Body, Complications, and Treatment

Of the FBs brought to the attention of physicians, 80% to 90% pass through the gastrointestinal tract spontaneously,[53,54] 10% to 20% require endoscopic removal, and about 1% require surgery.[53] It is estimated that up to 1500 deaths occur annually in the United States owing to ingestion of FBs, most of these cases are children.[58] Potential complications include obstruction, ulceration,

perforation (particularly at areas of acute angulations or physiologic narrowing; see **Fig. 11**),[50,55] bleeding, abscess formation, peritonitis, or even fistula formation.[17,50,58] Chronic esophageal FB may result in tracheal compression with several mechanisms, including direct compression, formation of granulomatous inflammatory mass, or esophageal dilatation.[1]

Ingestion of disk (button) batteries by children became more frequent in recent years due to the increasing accessibility of electronic toys and

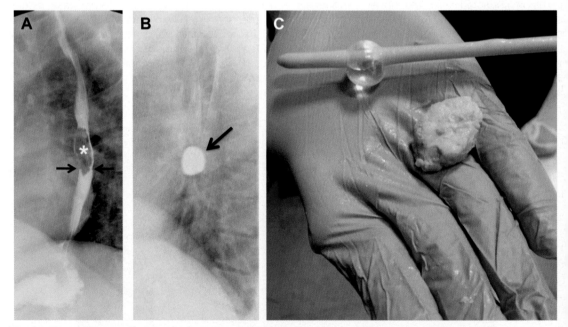

Fig. 14. Nonradiopaque foreign body in the esophagus of a 12-year-old boy who presented with a history of chronic esophageal stricture. (*A*) Fluoroscopic spot image of the esophagus from an esophagram study shows a slightly irregular oval filling defect (*asterisk*), compatible with an ingested FB in the midesophagus proximal to a focal esophageal stricture (*arrows*). (*B*) Fluoroscopic-guided FB retrieval image shows an inflated, contrast-filled Foley catheter balloon (*arrow*) pass the FB. (*C*) Post-Foley catheter retrieval image showed the FB to be a chicken nugget.

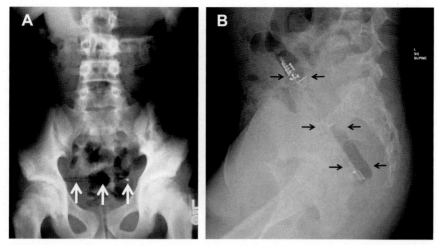

Fig. 15. Rectal foreign bodies in 2 pediatric patients. (*A*) Frontal abdominal radiograph in a 16-year-old boy demonstrates an elongated lucent structure with a small radiopaque tip (*arrows*), compatible with a pen inserted in the rectum. (*B*) A lateral radiograph of the pelvis in a 17-year-old body reveals a rectangular object (*arrows*) with internal linear wire-like opacities, later proven to be a television remote control inserted in the rectum.

devices to children (**Fig. 16**). When ingested, there is potential leakage of toxic substance, which may lead to mucosal burns, pressure necrosis, perforation, and systemic toxicity from heavy metal poisoning.[13,52,57,59] There has also been an alarming increase in magnet ingestion in children[60] because of the availability of small, spherical magnet sets in toys, jewelry, and novelty items.[61] A single piece of magnet is expected to behave like other foreign objects, often observed to pass spontaneously but ingestion of multiple magnet pieces is known to cause potential complications when located in different bowel loops by attracting each other and cause pressure necrosis of the bowel wall and subsequent perforation (**Fig. 17**).[3,62,63]

Pica is the abnormal craving or eating of items that are not food. Usually, pica is only recognized when it results in complications that lead to seek medical attention (**Fig. 18**).[64] Pediatric patients may consume soil, clay, sand, stones, bricks, and other nonfood items. Lead exposure is a problem for children who ingest lead-based paint chips from old houses.[64] Pica is associated with increased risk for anemia and micronutrient deficiency, although the mechanism for the latter remains unknown.[65] It can also damage the teeth as they chew on hard objects.[64]

Bezoars are foreign bodies that have accumulated in the alimentary tract over a period of time. Although affected children may present with a wide diversity of ingested materials, the

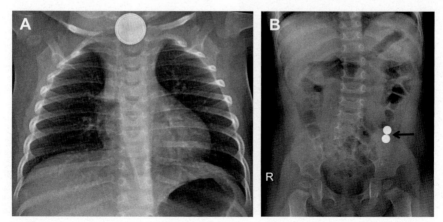

Fig. 16. Ingested battery in 2 pediatric patients. (*A*) Frontal chest radiograph in a 1-year-old boy shows a round radio-opaque foreign body with a peripheral lucent line, compatible with a button battery in the upper esophagus. (*B*) Abdominal radiograph in a 7-year-old boy demonstrates 2 button batteries (*arrow*) in the left lower abdomen.

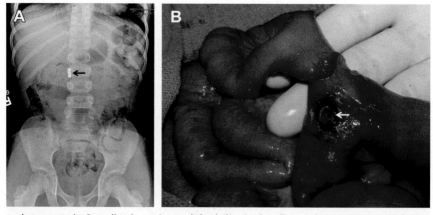

Fig. 17. Ingested magnets in 2 pediatric patients. (*A*) Abdominal radiograph in a 7-year-old boy reveals 3 small round radio-opaque foreign bodies stuck to each other (*arrow*) in the region of the gastric antrum. (*B*) Operative image of a 3-year-old girl demonstrates small bowel perforation (*arrow*) due to pressure necrosis after swallowing several magnets.

most common types are poorly digested vegetable or plant matter (phytobezoar), hair (trichobezoar) (**Fig. 19**), milk concretions (lactobezoar) (**Fig. 20**), and persimmons (disopyrobezoar). These indigestible materials can accumulate in the stomach because of their size and can cause delayed gastric emptying time or gastric outlet obstruction.[57,66] Affected pediatric patients present with a chronic history of unexplained abdominal pain, vomiting, dyspepsia, weight loss,

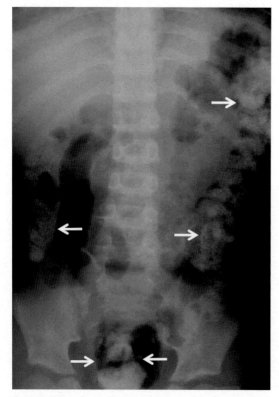

Fig. 18. Pica in a 3-year-old boy who eats sand. Abdominal radiograph shows slightly radiopaque material (*arrows*) casting the colon and rectum corresponding to the ingested sand.

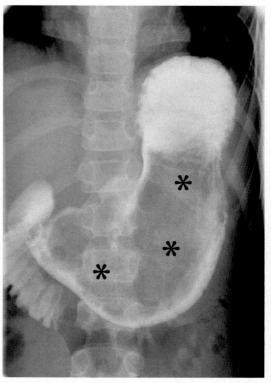

Fig. 19. Trichobezoar in a 16-year-old girl. Fluoroscopic spot image of an upper gastrointestinal study reveals a large, mobile filling defect (*asterisks*) within the stomach, later confirmed to be a trichobezoar.

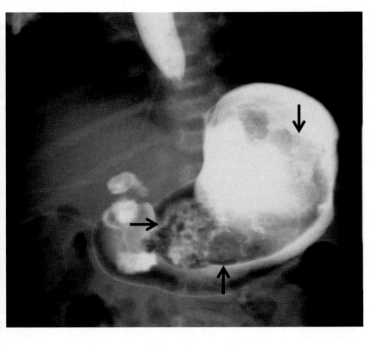

Fig. 20. Lactobezoar in a 3-month-old girl who presented with failure to thrive on formula. Fluoroscopic image of the stomach shows a large filling defect (*arrows*) within the stomach corresponding to accumulated concretion of formula powder.

halitosis, or palpable abdominal mass.[67] Bezoars may occur as a result of eating other foreign objects, especially in mentally retarded children[67]; therefore, psychiatric evaluation is needed for pediatric patients with recurrent bezoars.[57] History of trichotillomania (hair pulling) with trichophagia (hair eating) should be sought in a patient with trichobezoar.[68] Lactobezoars in children can be initially managed by withholding oral feeds, parenteral fluids for several days, and gentle gastric lavage.[67] In phytobezoars, enzymatic digestion can be initiated. Endoscopic removal might be attempted in selected bezoars but most necessitate surgical intervention, preferably laparotomy or gastrostomy, with excellent outcome.[53,57,68]

Because most ingested FBs pass through the gastrointestinal tract without a problem, intervention is only recommended when significant symptoms develop or if the object fails to progress through the gastrointestinal tract in 3 to 4 weeks.[47] Therapeutic techniques for FB ingestion include (1) Foley catheter removal, (2) bougienage, (3) endoscopic retrieval, and (4) surgery. Foley catheter retrieval is generally successful with a high success rate for smooth objects (see **Fig. 14**B, C) but there remains a potential for airway compromise, risk of esophageal injury, and discomfort. Sedatives are avoided to minimize the risk of aspiration during the procedure. Radiographic signs of chronic FB lodgment, such as tracheoesophageal interphase thickening or posterior tracheal

compression, are contraindications to Foley catheter removal.[69]

Bougienage is the method of pushing smooth objects into the stomach with the expectation that approximately 90% to 95% of them eventually evacuate. Criteria include single coin ingestion, less than 24 hours, no history of esophageal abnormalities, no history of prior ingestion, and no respiratory distress. If strict criteria are followed, there is high success rate with little morbidity.[57] Endoscopic retrieval is currently the most complete and thorough technique for removal of foreign bodies in the esophagus with success rate greater than 95%.[53] The affected pediatric patient is under general anesthesia, and careful evaluation of the FB and esophagus can be done. For foreign bodies that had been lodged for more than 2 to 3 days or for unknown duration, sharp objects, or if there is obstruction or distress, endoscopic retrieval should be the primary option.[57] If endoscopic retrieval is unsuccessful, surgical removal is considered if FB remains in the same location for 3 days.[47] In the rectum, small items can be easily retrieved but large foreign bodies may require anesthesia for removal. Rarely, a laparotomy is required to retrieve a rectal FB that has migrated into the colon or peritoneal cavity.[57]

Disk batteries lodged in the esophagus require urgent endoscopic intervention because of burns and injury as early as 4 hours. Batteries in the stomach or the rest of alimentary tract maybe observed because most spontaneously evacuate without sequelae. Surgical intervention is warranted if there are signs of gastrointestinal injury, multiple batteries, or a large battery that fail to traverse the pylorus.[57] Early surgical intervention is also recommended in cases of suspected ingestion of multiple magnets or multiple metallic FBs.[62]

Imaging Evaluation

Radiographs

The first imaging tool for the evaluation of suspected FB ingestion is radiography. Radiographs play an important role because most (83%) ingested FBs are radiopaque.[49] However, some metallic objects, including tin foil and the aluminum commonly used in soda cans are nonradiopaque. Radiographs should be obtained regardless of whether symptoms are present to confirm that the FB has passed into the stomach.[1] Frontal and lateral neck, frontal and lateral chest, and abdominal radiographs are obtained. Two views are important because some FBs may not be identified only in 1 projection.[48,54] In addition, some radiopaque objects overlying the vertebral column may only be visible on the lateral view. When the FB is projecting in the pelvis, a lateral radiograph of abdomen or pelvis may be useful to confirm a possible rectal location. The visibility of low-opacity FBs can be improved using a low peak kilovoltage technique that helps increase the contrast between tissues and radiopaque objects.[48]

On frontal chest radiographs, coins in the esophagus are most frequently seen enface (see **Fig. 12A**), whereas coins in the trachea are seen in tangent because of a posterior gap in the tracheal cartilage rings.[70] However, occasionally, a sagittal orientation of the coin can be seen when in the esophagus.[71] Other radiographic features in the upper alimentary tract include prevertebral soft-tissue swelling, loss of cervical lordosis, and the presence of an air-fluid level.[48,54] Thickening of the tracheoesophageal interphase or posterior tracheal compression are considered signs of chronic FB impaction (see **Fig. 12B**).[69] An abdominal radiograph is useful to exclude the presence of pneumoperitoneum after ingestion of sharp or pointed objects.[48] Pediatric patients who have swallowed blunt, radiopaque objects and are asymptomatic are usually followed with serial radiographs, and parents are instructed to watch for the passage of the FB in stool. If a patient presents with unwitnessed metallic FB ingestion, clinical suspicion of magnet ingestion should be raised. In such cases, gaps between these metallic objects or absence of movement on a follow-up radiograph should raise the suspicion of entrapment and ischemic damage to interposed bowel wall. Bowel obstruction, perforation, and free air are radiographic signs of complicated magnet ingestion.[62]

Fluoroscopy

Objects composed of plastic and most fish bones are radiolucent and their diagnosis may be challenging.[48] In such cases, administration of oral contrast can be given to outline the radiolucent object (see **Fig. 14A**). Diluted (thin) barium is used because residual barium in the esophagus obscures visualization if a subsequent endoscopy is to be performed. An upper gastrointestinal tract barium study can be used to outline bezoars in the stomach and small bowel (see **Figs. 19** and **20**).[53,57,66,68] To avoid barium spillage into the mediastinum or pleural space, barium should be avoided if there is clinical evidence of high-grade obstruction or when there is suspicion of esophageal perforation.[54,55] In such cases, low-osmolar, water-soluble contrast can be used, such as CystoConray. If patient refuses to drink CystoConray due to the bitter flavor, undiluted nonionic contrast, such as Omnipaque or Optiray, which are tasteless, maybe a more suitable alternative. Gastrografin, which also has a bitter taste, is not recommended because it is hypertonic and can lead to pulmonary edema if aspirated.[53] Fluoroscopy can also be done after retrieval of the battery from the esophagus to evaluate mucosal injury, strictures, erosions, and fistulas.[13,59] Similarly, evaluation of rectal mucosa by contrast enema study can be done after removal of large or sharp objects in the rectosigmoid region.[57]

Ultrasound

US examination of a water-filled stomach can be useful in diagnostic workup of gastric foreign bodies in children, especially radiolucent ones.[47] It is safe, can be performed quickly with least discomfort to the child, and can obviate serial radiographs, thereby reducing radiation exposure.[47] US is also a reliable method for detecting bezoars as hyperechoic intraluminal mass with marked acoustic shadow (**Fig. 21**).[66] Ingestion of water before or during the US examination is done to get the appropriate acoustic window. The patient is positioned in the oblique right decubitus position to allow water and FB to move toward the distal body of the stomach and antrum. A 2.5 to 6 MHz convex transducer is initially used to survey the stomach and the rest of the abdomen, followed by a 5 to 10 MHz linear transducer for more detailed evaluation.[47]

Computed tomography

MDCT is superior to plain radiography and identifies the foreign bodies in 70% to 100% of

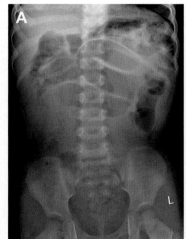
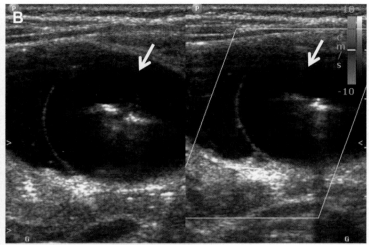
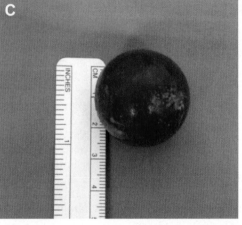

Fig. 21. Intestinal foreign body detected in US in a 3-year-old boy. (*A*) Abdominal radiograph demonstrates an obstructed bowel gas pattern with several dilated bowel loops located in the upper abdomen. (*B*) US of the upper abdomen reveals a round heterogeneously hypoechoic, nonvascular structure (*arrows*) within a dilated intestinal segment. (*C*) Postoperative image reveals an ingested small crystal ball lodged and obstructing the jejunum. (*Courtesy of* Dr Hamzaini Abdul Hamid, Kuala Lumpur, Malaysia.)

affected patients.[53] If the location of the ingested object in the body is indeterminate according to radiographs, MDCT examination provides more precise information.[48] CT is more accurate than other imaging tools in detecting bezoars and exhibits a quite characteristic well-defined heterogeneous intraluminal mass with mottled air pattern (**Fig. 22**).[66,68] MDCT can detect slightly calcified objects and fish bones that are missed by conventional radiographs (**Fig. 23**). It is also sensitive in detecting small objects trapped in the appendix that could lead to appendiceal inflammation, such as the case in screw appendicitis (**Fig. 24**).[72] It is also helpful in detecting complications such as perforation, fistula, or abscess. In the abdomen, the region of perforation may appear as a thickened focal segment, associated with localized pneumoperitoneum, regional fatty infiltration, and

associated intestinal obstruction. Intravenous contrast may be helpful for better soft-tissue detail. To maximize radiation dose reduction, the use of low-radiation dose parameters should be observed in children.

Practical imaging algorithm

The initial imaging tool for suspected FB ingestion is radiography because most ingested objects are radiopaque. The views obtained should include frontal and lateral neck, frontal and lateral chest, and a frontal abdominal radiographs. Asymptomatic pediatric patients who have blunt, radiopaque objects are usually followed with serial radiographs in the area of concern, and parents are instructed to watch for the rectal passage. If suspicion is present yet no radiopaque FB is seen on radiographs, MDCT is the most accurate imaging

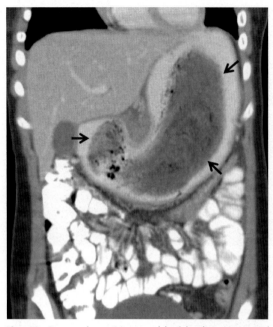

Fig. 22. Bezoar in a 14-year-old girl who presented with anorexia nervosa and alopecia. Coronal CT image of the abdomen confirms the presence of a large hypodense filling defect mixed with air (*arrows*) casting the distended stomach, compatible with a trichobezoar.

test for confirmation of FB and for assessment of complications. US can be used if the FB is in the stomach, although this has lower sensitivity compared with CT. In the absence of cross-sectional imaging, fluoroscopic evaluation with oral contrast can be obtained to assess nonradiopaque FB as well as to assess presence of mucosal irregularities, ulceration, and perforation or fistula formation. Low-osmolar, water-soluble contrast is preferred in cases of suspected

perforation. Fluoroscopic study (upper gastrointestinal or lower intestinal route) with water-soluble contrast may also be done after endoscopic retrieval of the FB.

FOREIGN BODIES IN OTHER BODY CAVITIES
Aural Foreign Bodies

Etiologic factors and clinical considerations
FB insertion in to the aural cavity, from the external auditory canal to the middle ear is not uncommon. Several factors may lead children to insert FBs intentionally into their ears, including curiosity; the wish to explore the orifices of the body; irritation caused by otalgia; attraction to small, round objects; or simply for fun.[73,74] Otitis media, which causes earache, also prompts children to use any readily available object to scratch or insert into their ears to relieve the irritation.[75] FBs are more frequently on the right side due to the preference of right-handed individuals to insert objects in their right ear.[74] Retrieved FBs are usually objects available at home, including beads, buttons, plastic toys, pebbles, eraser, paper, seeds, and popcorn kernels. Insects are more common in patients older than 10 years.[4,76]

Children with aural FBs are mostly asymptomatic and, often, the finding is incidental. However, other patients may present with ear pain, symptoms of otitis media, bleeding, tinnitus, hearing loss, or a sense of ear fullness.[4,76] Most aural FBs are clinically silent, which poses a diagnostic problem and may not be readily recognized. Long-standing aural FBs can cause extensive damage, especially those objects with sharp edges, which can perforate the tympanic membrane or cause canal laceration.[74,77,78] FBs can even be pushed medially and become impacted in the middle ear cleft.[79,80]

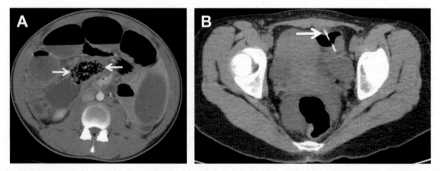

Fig. 23. Foreign bodies not detected on radiographs but seen on CT in 2 pediatric patients. (*A*) Axial CT image in a 16-year-old boy with developmental delay who presented with abdominal pain, reveals an obstructed bowel gas pattern and an irregular structure mixed with air (*arrows*) in a jejunal loop, later proven to be an ingested glove. (*B*) Axial CT image, in a 15-year-old girl, reveals a sharp elongated structure puncturing the ileum (*arrow*), proven to be an ingested fishbone.

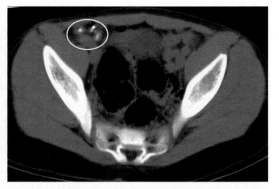

Fig. 24. Screw appendicitis in a 9-year-old boy who presented with chronic abdominal pain. Axial CT image shows a radiopaque foreign body with metallic artifact (*circle*) in the right lower quadrant within the appendix. The appendix has thickened wall but without periappendiceal fat stranding. During appendectomy, a screw was found inside the chronically inflamed appendix.

Imaging evaluation

Radiologic imaging is not routinely obtained in aural insertion of FBs because many are detected through direct visual inspection. Imaging is obtained to confirm a clinical suspicion despite a questionable physical evaluation, characterize the FB, evaluate complications, and assess anatomic integrity in preparation for retrieval. Radiographs can be helpful in metallic FB but are limited in nonradiopaque objects, commonly discovered in children's ears.

There have been numerous case reports in which the use of CT imaging, which seems to be the imaging study of choice, was helpful in detection of FBs.[79,80] A noncontrast-enhanced CT may be sufficient to accurately define the FB position, important in deciding the best therapeutic strategy (**Figs. 25** and **26**). High-resolution images with multiplanar reconstruction are important to evaluate the aural cavity. The axial raw CT image data can be reconstructed with a section thickness as small as 0.3 mm to obtain high-quality coronal and sagittal reformatted CT images. A 512 by 512 matrix is used, and the images are reviewed in both high-resolution bone and soft tissue displays. Advance reconstruction algorithms are now available to diminish artifacts associated with metallic objects. Moreover, high-resolution images can be obtained using lower dose radiation reduction methods.[81]

MR imaging is used for the evaluation of various anomalies of the ear; however, MR imaging is not used as the initial imaging tool, especially if a metallic FB is suspected for which MR imaging is

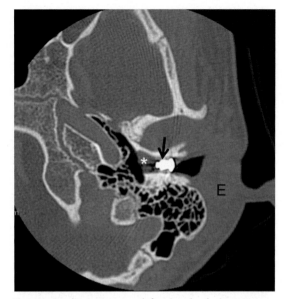

Fig. 25. Radiopaque aural foreign body in a 3-year-old boy who presented with worsening earache and purulent discharge. Axial bone window CT image of the left mastoid shows a tubular metallic structure (*black arrow*) in the external auditory canal along with associated soft tissue opacity (*asterisk*) found to represent pus. Preauricular soft tissue edema (E) indicating inflammation is also present. A piece of an earring was removed.

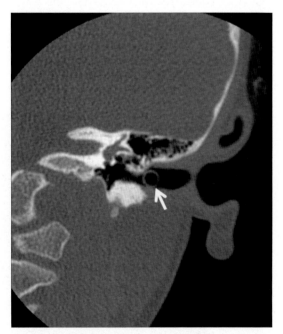

Fig. 26. Nonradiopaque aural foreign body in a 4-year-old girl who presented with ear discomfort. Coronal bone window CT image of the left mastoid shows a cylindrical structure (*arrow*) in the left external auditory canal. A tiny plastic cylinder was removed.

contraindicated because of possible complications, including intracranial migration.[76]

Vaginal Foreign Bodies

Etiologic factors and clinical considerations

FBs in the vagina can cause intense local irritation and inflammation, producing the classic symptoms of vaginal bleeding and foul smelling vaginal discharge.[82–86] The most common vaginal FB in a prepubertal girl is toilet tissue (**Fig. 27**).[86,87] However, various objects, including grains, peanuts, small plastic objects, and buttons, have been reported.[83] The prevalence of vaginal FBs in girls younger than 13 years of age with gynecologic disorders was found to be 4.0%.[88] Children rarely recount how the FB was inserted, who inserted it, or what motivated the insertion but previous reports state that most are inserted by the child during natural body exploration or during masturbatory play.[86] Association between vaginal FB and sexual abuse has been previously been established and thus it is important that this is given consideration during the examination.[82,86] FBs in the vagina cause intense inflammation but long-standing FB can result in damage to the vaginal mucosa, further inflammation, urinary and dermatologic inflammation, adhesions, perforation, or severe urinary or enteric fistulas.[83–85] There are other causes for vaginal bleeding that should be considered in prepubertal girls and it is important to arrive at a proper diagnosis promptly to avoid complications. Vaginoscopy under general anesthesia has been used as an important diagnostic and therapeutic tool at the onset of presentation[84,87] but for young girls

noninvasive techniques play a role in the initial examination.

Imaging evaluation

Pelvic plain radiography may contribute to early diagnosis, which can provide information regarding the type, size, and identity if the vaginal FB is metallic (see **Fig. 27**).[89] However, vaginal FBs in children are predominantly nonradiopaque and can be easily missed in radiographs.[84] Pelvic ultrasonography is usually the first imaging modality in the evaluation of the pediatric pelvis. It is helpful in determining the pubertal stage of the internal genitalia and exclude ovarian or uterine masses. A retained FB in the vagina can show an abnormal echogenic structure with posterior acoustic shadowing and may also show the characteristic indentation along the posterior bladder wall (**Fig. 28**).[83–85] However, the FB must be large enough to lead to the characteristic sonographic findings. Sonography has obvious advantages due to its noninvasive nature, high specificity, lack of radiation, and low cost; therefore, it can be the first choice for imaging detection of vaginal foreign bodies.[83] MR imaging allows visualization of nonmetallic objects missed by other conventional radiological examinations.[90] It precisely reveals the number of vaginal FBs, which is essential for proper treatment. Given its excellent soft tissue differentiation, MR imaging can reveal the surrounding anatomy, including vaginal mucosal injury, granulation tissue, fistulas, and other complications of long-standing vaginal lodgment of the FB.[90]

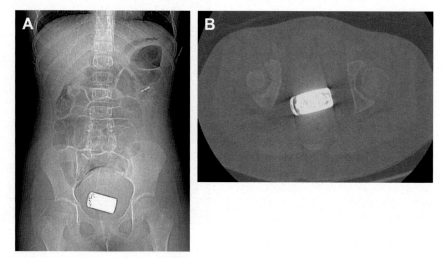

Fig. 27. Vaginal foreign body in a 10-year-old girl who presented with worsening abdominal pain, fever, vomiting, and vaginal discharge. Abdominal radiograph (*A*) and axial CT image (*B*) show a large FB, compatible with a battery within the vagina. (*Courtesy of* Dr Sanjay P. Prabhu, Boston, MA.)

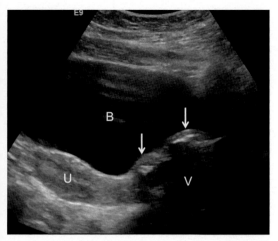

Fig. 28. Vaginal foreign body in a 10-year old girl with purulent vaginal discharge. Sagittal US image of the pelvis shows a distended vagina (V) containing a mixed echogenicity object (*arrows*) with posterior acoustic shadow proved to be a clump of toilet paper. B, bladder; U, uterus.

Urethrovesical Foreign Bodies

Etiologic factors and clinical considerations

FBs in the lower urinary tract are rare in children. They may result from self-insertion or migration from adjacent sites that may be iatrogenic or traumatic. There are several reasons for introduction of objects into the urinary tract, including psychiatric disorder; accident; sexual stimulation; curiosity, especially among children; or therapeutic.[91] The types of FBs include plastic caps, hooked wire, paper clips, metal objects, glass rods, shells, light bulbs, and many other objects.[91–93] Affected pediatric patients usually present with dysuria, difficulty in voiding, hematuria, pain, swelling of genitalia, extravasations of urine, abscess formation, or purulent discharge without other explanations.[91,93,94] Urethrovesical FBs can be a diagnostic dilemma because most pediatric patients are too ashamed to admit the insertion or application of any object and usually present when a complication is already present.[93,94] Definitive treatment is removal of FB through minimally invasive cystoscopy but occasionally surgery is required if the object is too large or in complicated cases.[92,94,95] Complications to long-standing urethrovesical FBs are urinary tract infection, bladder perforation, calcification, bleeding, sepsis, and outflow obstruction.[91,96]

Imaging evaluation

When a FB is suspected, imaging is indicated to differentiate between urethral or vesicular location of the FB and to assess the composition, size, and shape of the FB.[93] A plain abdominal radiograph usually suffices to confirm the presence and the location of radiopaque urethrovesical FB (**Fig. 29**A).[91] A cystogram could help identify radiolucent objects.[93] However, US as a noninvasive imaging tool has been used and can visualize both radiopaque and nonradiopaque objects (**Fig. 29**B).[91,92,97] Much like a FB in another location, it demonstrates hyperechogenicity with posterior acoustic shadowing on US. In some cases, CT may be required to assess complications,

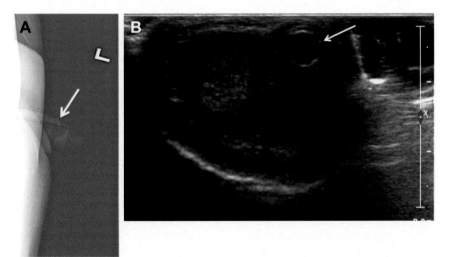

Fig. 29. Urethral foreign body in a 14-year-old boy with psychiatric illness. (*A*) Lateral radiograph of the penis reveals a rectangular density within the penis with a tapering tip (*arrow*). (*B*) US of penis shows an elongated object (*arrow*) within the urethra with acoustic shadowing. It has a transverse diameter of 1.4 cm, about 6 to 7 cm long, compatible with a pen or pencil. (*Courtesy of* Dr Sanjay P. Prabhu, Boston, MA.)

including perforation and rectal impalement injuries associated with features of peritonitis, other organ injury, or fistula formation.[92] Occasionally, cystourethrography is needed.

SUMMARY

FB aspiration, ingestion, or insertion in natural body cavities or tissues is not uncommon in children. FB-related complications can be severe or even life-threatening, and prompt recognition and management is crucial. Radiologic imaging plays an important role in the detection, characterization, and localization of these FBs but it also aids in the assessment of complications, as a guide in therapeutic management, and for follow-up assessment after treatment.

REFERENCES

1. Donnelly LF, Frush DP, Bisset GS. The multiple presentations of foreign bodies in children. AJR Am J Roentgenol 1998;170:471–9.
2. Susy Safe Working Group. The Susy Safe project overview after the first four years of activity. Int J Pediatr Otorhinolaryngol 2012;76(Suppl 1):S3–11.
3. Passali D, Gregori D, Lorenzoni G, et al. Foreign body injuries in children: a review. Acta Otorhinolaryngol Ital 2015;35(4):265–71.
4. Heim SW, Maughan KL. Foreign bodies in the ear, nose, and throat. Am Fam Physician 2007;76(8):1185–9.
5. Halverson M, Servaes S. Foreign bodies: radiopaque compared to what? Pediatr Radiol 2013;43(9):1103–7.
6. Applegate KE, Dardinger JT, Lieber ML, et al. Spiral CT scanning technique in the detection of aspiration of LEGO foreign bodies. Pediatr Radiol 2001;31(12):836–40.
7. Zhijun C, Fugao Z, Niankai Z, et al. Therapeutic experience from 1428 patients with pediatric tracheobronchial foreign body. J Pediatr Surg 2008;43(4):718–21.
8. Sahin A, Meteroglu F, Eren S, et al. Inhalation of foreign bodies in children: experience of 22 years. J Trauma Acute Care Surg 2013;74(2):658–63.
9. Lee EY, Greenberg SB, Boiselle PM. Multidetector computed tomography of pediatric large airway diseases: state-of-the-art. Radiol Clin North Am 2011;49(5):869–93.
10. Lee EY, Restrepo R, Dillman JR, et al. Imaging evaluation of pediatric trachea and bronchi: systemic review and updates. Semin Roentgenol 2012;47(2):182–96.
11. Yang C, Hua R, Xu K, et al. The role of 3D computed tomography (CT) imaging in the diagnosis of foreign body aspiration in children. Eur Rev Med Pharmacol Sci 2015;19(2):265–73.
12. Karakoc F, Karadag B, Akbenlioglu C, et al. Foreign body aspiration: what is the outcome? Pediatr Pulmonol 2002;34(1):30–6.
13. Darras KE, Roston AT, Yewchuk LK. Imaging acute airway obstruction in infants and children. Radiographics 2015;35(7):2064–79.
14. Laya BF, Lee EY. Upper airway disease. In: Coley BD, editor. Caffeys. 12th edition. Philadelphia: Elsevier Saunders; 2013. p. 527–38.
15. Eren S, Balci AE, Dikici B, et al. Foreign body aspiration in children: experience of 1160 cases. Ann Trop Paediatr 2003;23(1):31–7.
16. Lima JA, Fisher GB. Foreign body aspiration in children. Paediatr Respir Rev 2002;3(4):303–7.
17. Grassi R, Faggian A, Somma F, et al. Application of imaging guidelines in patients with foreign body ingestion or inhalation: literature review. Semin Ultrasound CT MR 2015;36(1):48–56.
18. Hegde SV, Hui PK, Lee EY. Tacheobronchial foreign bodies in children: imaging assessment. Semin Ultrasound CT MR 2015;36(1):8–20.
19. Upreti L, Gupta N. Imaging for diagnosis of foreign body aspiration in children? Indian Pediatr 2015;52(8):659–60.
20. Huang HJ, Fang HY, Chen HC, et al. Three-dimensional computed tomography for detection of tracheobronchial foreign body aspiration in children. Pediatr Surg Int 2008;24(2):157–60.
21. Muth D, Schefermeyer RW. All that wheezes. Pediatr Emerg Care 1990;6(2):110–2.
22. Koşucu P, Ahmetoğlu A, Koramaz I, et al. Low-dose MDCT and virtual bronchoscopy in pediatric patients with foreign body aspiration. AJR Am J Roentgenol 2004;183(6):1771–7.
23. Tang LF, Xu YC, Wang YS, et al. Airway foreign body removal by flexible bronchoscopy: experience with 1027 children during 2000-2008. World J Pediatr 2009;5(3):191–5.
24. Xue FS, Luo MP, Liao X, et al. Delayed endendotracheal tube obstruction by mucus plug in a child. Chin Med J 2009;122(7):870–2.
25. Tokar B, Ozkan R, Ilhan H. Tracheobronchial foreign bodies in children; importance of accurate history and plain chest radiography in delayed presentation. Clin Radiol 2004;59(7):609–15.
26. Gang W, Zhengxia P, Hongbo L, et al. Diagnosis and treatment of tracheobronchial foreign bodies in 1024 children. J Pediatr Surg 2012;47(11):2004–10.
27. Arun Babu T, Ananthakrishnan S. Unusual presentation of sand aspiration in a 14-month-old child. Indian J Pediatr 2013;80(9):786–8.
28. Hitter A, Hullo E, Durand C, et al. Diagnostic value of various investigations in children with suspected foreign body aspiration: review. Eur Ann Otorhinolaryngol Head Neck Dis 2011;128(5):248–52.

29. Mu L, Sun D, He P. Radiological diagnosis of aspirated foreign bodies in children: review of 343 cases. J Laryngol Otol 1990;l04(10):778–82.
30. Swischuk LE. Emergency radiology of the acutely ill or injured child. 3rd edition. Baltimore (MD): Williams and Wilkins; 1994. p. 113–22.
31. Brown JC, Chapman T, Klein EJ, et al. The utility of adding expiratory or decubitus chest radiographs to the radiographic evaluation of suspected pediatric airway foreign bodies. Ann Emerg Med 2013; 61(1):19–26.
32. Dunn GR, Wardrop P, Lo S, et al. Management of suspected foreign body aspiration in children. Clin Otolaryngol Allied Sci 2004;29(3):286.
33. Svedstrom E, Puhakka H, Kero P. How accurate is chest radiography in the diagnosis of tracheobronchial foreign bodies in children? Pediatr Radiol 1989;19(8):520–2.
34. Haliloglu M, Ciftci AO, Oto A, et al. CT virtual bronchoscopy in the evaluation of children with suspected foreign body aspiration. Eur J Radiol 2003; 48(2):188–92.
35. Kim IG, Brummit WM, Humphry A, et al. Foreign body in the airway: a review of 202 cases. Laryngoscope 1973;83(3):347–54.
36. Girardi G, Contador AM, Castro-Rodriguez JA. Two new radiological findings to improve the diagnosis of bronchial foreign-body aspiration in children. Pediatr Pulmonol 2004;38(3):261–4.
37. Ikeda M, Himi K, Yamauchi Y, et al. Use of digital subtraction fluoroscopy to diagnose radiolucent aspirated foreign bodies in infants and children. Int J Pediatr Otorhinolaryngol 2001;61(3): 233–42.
38. Even L, Heno N, Talmon Y, et al. Diagnostic evaluation of foreign body aspiration in children: a prospective study. J Pediatr Surg 2005;40(7):1122–7.
39. Yuksel M, Ozyurtkan MO, Lacin T, et al. The role of fluoroscopy in the removal of tracheobronchial pin aspiration. Int J Clin Pract 2006;60(11):1451–3.
40. Pinto A, Scaglione M, Pinto F, et al. Tracheobronchial aspiration of foreign bodies: Current indications for emergency plain chest radiography. Radiol Med 2006;111(4):497–506.
41. Bai W, Zhou X, Gao X, et al. Value of chest CT in the diagnosis and management of tracheobronchial foreign bodies. Pediatr Int 2011;53(4):515–8.
42. Shin SM, Kim WS, Cheon JE, et al. CT in Children with suspected residual foreign body in airway after bronchoscopy. AJR Am J Roentgenol 2009;192(6): 1744–51.
43. Jung SY, Pae SY, Chung SM, et al. Three-dimensional CT with virtual bronchoscopy: a useful modality for bronchial foreign bodies in pediatric patients. Eur Arch Otorhinolaryngol 2012;269(1):223–8.
44. Hong WS, Im SA, Kim HL, et al. CT evaluation of airway foreign bodies in children: emphasis on the delayed diagnosis and differentiation from airway mucus plugs. Jpn J Radiol 2013;31(1):31–8.
45. Imaizumi H, Kaneko M, Nara S, et al. Definitive diagnosis and location of peanuts in the airways using magnetic resonance imaging techniques. Ann Emerg Med 1994;23(6):1379–82.
46. Morijiri M, Seto H, Kageyama M, et al. Assessment of peanut aspiration by MRI and lung perfusion scintigram. J Comput Assist Tomogr 1994;18(5): 836–8.
47. Jeckovic M, Anupindi SA, Barbir SB, et al. Is ultrasound useful in detection and follow up of gastric foreign bodies in children? Clin Imaging 2013;37: 1043–7.
48. Pinto A, Lanza C, Pinto F, et al. Role of plain radiography in the assessment of ingested foreign bodies in pediatric patients. Semin Ultrasound CT MR 2015; 36:21–7.
49. Sink JR, Kitsko DJ, Mehta DK, et al. Diagnosis of pediatric foreign body ingestion: clinical presentation, physical examination, and radiologic findings. Ann Otol Rhinol Laryngol 2016;125(4):342–50.
50. Altokhais TI, Al-Saleem A, Gado A, et al. Esophageal foreign bodies in children: emphasis on complicated cases. Asian J Surg 2016. http://dx.doi.org/10.1016/j.asjsur.2015.12.008.
51. Conners GP, Chamberlain JM, Weiner PR. Pediatric coin ingestion: a home-based survey. Am J Emerg Med 1995;13(6):638–40.
52. Dereci S, Koca T, Serdaroglu F, et al. Foreign body ingestions in children. Turk Pediatri Ars 2015;50: 234–40.
53. Sugawa C, Ono H, Taleb M, et al. Endoscopic management of foreign bodies in the upper gastrointestinal tract: a review. World J Gastrointest Endosc 2014;6(10):475–81.
54. Pinto A, Muzj C, Gagliardi N, et al. Role of imaging in the assessment of impacted foreign bodies in the hypopharynx and cervical esophagus. Semin Ultrasound CT MR 2012;33(5):463–70.
55. Smith MT, Wong RK. Foreign bodies. Gastrointest Endosc Clin N Am 2007;17:361–82.
56. Cheng W, Tam PK. Foreign-body ingestion in children: experience with 1,265 cases. J Pediatr Surg 1999;34(10):1472–6.
57. Chen MK, Beierle EA. Gastrointestinal foreign bodies. Pediatr Ann 2001;30(12):736–42.
58. Sung SH, Jeon SW, Kim HK, et al. Factor predictive of risk for complications in patients with esophageal foreign bodies. Dig Liver Dis 2011;43(8):632–5.
59. Marom T, Goldfarb A, Russo E, et al. Battery ingestion in children. Int J Pediatr Otorhinolaryngol 2010; 74(8):849–54.
60. Abbas MI, Oliva-Hemker M, Choi J, et al. Magnet ingestions in children presenting to US emergency departments, 2002-2011. J Pediatr Gastroenterol Nutr 2013;57(1):18–22.

61. Brown JC, Otjen JP, Drugas GT. Too attractive: the growing problem of magnet ingestions in children. Pediatr Emerg Care 2013;29(11):1170–4.

62. Kirscher M, Milla S, Callahan MJ. Ingestion of magnetic foreign bodies causing multiple bowel perforations. Pediatr Radiol 2007;37:933–6.

63. Mandhan P, Alsalihi M, Mammoo S, et al. Troubling toys: rare-earth magnet ingestion in children causing bowel perforations. Case Rep Pediatr 2014;2014:908730.

64. Advani A, Kochhar G, Chachra S, et al. Eating everything except food (PICA): a rare case report and review. J Int Soc Prev Community Dent 2014; 4(1):1–4.

65. Miao D, Young SL, Golden CD. A meta-analysis of pica and micronutrient status. Am J Hum Biol 2015;27(1):84–93.

66. Ripolles T, Garcia-Aguayo J, Martinez MJ, et al. Gastrointestinal bezoars: sonographic and CT characteristics. AJR Am J Roentgenol 2001;177: 65–9.

67. Castle SL, Zmora O, Papillon S, et al. Management of complicated gastric bezoars in children and adolescents. Isr Med Assoc J 2015;17(9):541–4.

68. Sanneerappa PBJ, Hayes HM, Daly E, et al. Trichobezoar: a diagnosis which is hard to swallow and harder to digest. BMJ Case Rep 2014. http://dx. doi.org/10.1136/bcr-2013-201569.

69. Towbin R, Lederman HM, Dunbar JS, et al. Esophageal edema as a predictor of unsuccessful balloon extraction of esophageal foreign body. Pediatr Radiol 1989;19:359–62.

70. John SD, Swischuk LE. Stridor and upper airway obstruction in infants and children. Radiographics 1992;12:625–43.

71. Schlesinger AE, Crowe JE. Sagittal orientation of ingested coins in the esophagus in children. AJR Am J Roentgenol 2011;196(3):670–2.

72. Sarkar RR, Bisht J, Sinha Roy SK. Ingested metallic foreign body in the appendix. J Indian Assoc Pediatr Surg 2011;16(1):29–30.

73. Balbani AP, Sanchez TG, Butugan O, et al. Ear and nose foreign body removal in children. Int J Pediatr Otorhinolaryngol 1998;46:37–42.

74. Chinski A, Foltran F, Gregori D, et al. Foreign bodies in the ears in children: the experience of buenos-aires pediatric ORL clinic. Turk J Pediatr 2011;53: 425–9.

75. Sarkar S, Sadhukhan M, Roychoudhury A, et al. Otitis media with effusion in children and its correlation with foreign body in the external auditory canal. Indian J Otolaryngol Head Neck Surg 2010;62(4): 346–9.

76. Ray R, Dutta M, Mukherjee M, et al. Foreign body in ear, nose, and throat: experience in a tertiary hospital. Indian J Otolaryngol Head Neck Surg 2014; 66(1):13–6.

77. Al-juboori AN. Aural foreign bodies: descriptive study of 224 patients in Al-Fallujah general hospital, Iraq. Int J Otolaryngol 2013;2013:401289.

78. Oreh AC, Folorunsho D, Ibekwe TS. Actualities of management of aural, nasal, and throat foreign bodies. Ann Med Health Sci Res 2015;5(2): 108–14.

79. Dutta M, Ghatak S, Biswas G. Chronic discharging ear in a child: are we missing something? Med J Malaysia 2013;68(4):368–71.

80. Eleftheriadou A, Chalastras T, Kyrmizakis D, et al. Metallic foreign body in middle ear: an unusual cause of hearing loss. Head Face Med 2007;3:23.

81. Reginelli A, Santagata M, Urrano F, et al. Foreign bodies in the maxillofacial region: assessment with multidetector computed tomography. Semin Ultrasound CT MR 2015;36(1):2–7.

82. Stricker T, Navratil F, Sennhauser FH. Vaginal foreign bodies. J Paediatr Child Health 2004;40:205–7.

83. Wang ZX, Tang Y, Xiao H. Abdominal sonography for diagnosis of vaginal grains in Chinese children. J Ultrasound Med 2013;32:361–3.

84. Nayak S, Witchel AF, Sanfilillo JS. Vaginal foreign body: a delayed diagnosis. J Pediatr Adolesc Gynecol 2014;27(6):e127–9.

85. Caspi B, Zalel Y, Katz Z, et al. The role of sonography in the detection of vaginal foreign bodies in young girls: the bladder indentation sign. Pediatr Radiol 1995;25(Suppl 1):S60–1.

86. Closson FT, Lichenstein R. Vaginal foreign bodies and child sexual abuse: an important consideration. West J Emerg Med 2013;14(5):437–9.

87. Yildiz S, Ekin M, Cengiz H, et al. Vaginal foreign body: successful management with vaginoscopy. J Turk Ger Gynecol Assoc 2013;14:46–7.

88. Paradise JE, Willis ED. Probability of vaginal foreign body in girls with genital complaints. Am J Dis Child 1985;139:472–6.

89. Kyrgios I, Emmanouilidou E, Theodoridis T, et al. An unexpected cause of vaginal bleeding: the role of pelvic radiography. BMJ Case Rep 2014. http://dx. doi.org/10.1136/bcr-2013-202958.

90. Kihara M, Sato N, Kimura H, et al. Magnetic resonance imaging in the evaluation of vaginal foreign bodies in a young girl. Arch Gynecol Obstet 2001; 265:221–2.

91. Ceran C, Uguralp S. Self-inflicted urethrovesical foreign bodies in children. Case Rep Urol 2012; 2012:134358.

92. Mahapatra RS, Priyadarshi V, Madduri VK, et al. Transrectal impalement of an incense stick in a child presenting as foreign body in the urinary bladder. BMJ Case Rep 2014. http://dx.doi.org/10.1136/bcr-2014-204689.

93. Robey TE, Kaimakliotis HZ, Hittelman AB, et al. An unusual destination for magnetic foreign bodies. Pediatr Emer Care 2014;30:643–5.

94. Rafique M. Case report: an unusual intravesical foreign body: cause of recurrent urinary tract infections. Int J Nephrol 2002;34(2):205–6.

95. De Bernardis G, Haecker FM. Curious foreign body in the bladder of an adolescent. J Pediatr Surg 2012; 47(12):e39–41.

96. Benz MR, Stehr M, Kammer B, et al. Foreign body in the bladder mimicking nephritis. Pediatr Nephrol 2007;22:467–70.

97. Barzilai M, Cohen I, Stein A. Sonographic detection of a foreign body in the urethra and urinary bladder. Urol Int 2000;64(3):178–80.

Spectrum of Syndromic Disorders Associated with Pediatric Tumors
Evolving Role of Practical Imaging Assessment

Shreya Sood, MD[a],*, Anastasia L. Hryhorczuk, MD[a],
Julia Rissmiller, MD[a], Edward Y. Lee, MD, MPH[b]

KEYWORDS

• Syndromic disorders • Pediatric tumors • Imaging • Assessment

KEY POINTS

• Multi-organ system abnormalities in pediatric patients should alert to syndromic associations and trigger genetic counseling.
• Despite chromosomal localization and gene identification, phenotypic manifestations of these syndromes are highly variable.
• Early and accurate diagnosis of the syndrome allows better appropriation of care and prompt life-saving surveillance. A multidisciplinary team approach is essential.
• Radiologic imaging plays a pivotal role in surveillance, diagnosis, and treatment in these syndromic tumors as lesions may be disparate and spatially broad in span.
• Future advancements in whole-body MR imaging and potentially PET/MR imaging may mitigate ionizing radiation in the imaging evaluation of syndromic tumors in pediatric patients.

INTRODUCTION

Although most pediatric tumors develop sporadically, advancements in genetic testing and improved understanding of familial association with certain type of neoplasms have expanded the range of cancer predisposition syndromes that contribute to specific tumors in the pediatric population. Although these syndromic tumors still represent a minority of incidences of total pediatric tumors, recognition of these syndromes is growing rapidly. Most syndromic disorders associated with pediatric tumors demonstrate a clear genetic mode of transmission, such as autosomal dominant or x-linked transmission. Others show distinctive familial tendencies without identification of a causal gene. In general, many of these syndromes occur because of errors in gene functioning that impact tumor suppressor genes, oncogenes, or DNA stability repair genes.

Recognition of these syndromes is crucial to optimize clinical care and family counseling. Generally, this requires a multidisciplinary team including genetic counselors, pediatric oncologists, radiologists, and surgeons who are able to tailor biochemical and imaging surveillance strategies to the specific needs of pediatric patients. In

[a] Department of Pediatric Radiology, Floating Hospital for Children at Tufts Medical Center, 800 Washington Street, Boston, MA 02111, USA; [b] Department of Radiology, Boston Children's Hospital, Harvard Medical School, 300 Longwood Avenue, Boston, MA 02115, USA
* Corresponding author.
E-mail address: SSood@tuftsmedicalcenter.org

Radiol Clin N Am 55 (2017) 869–893
http://dx.doi.org/10.1016/j.rcl.2017.02.013
0033-8389/17/Published by Elsevier Inc.

certain situations, prophylactic surgery may be considered to prevent expected cancers. The aim of these strategies should be to aid in early detection and treatment of childhood cancers. Appropriate, early screening is even more critical in pediatric patients given their long-expected life span in which to manifest these tumors.

Although the list of genetic tumor predisposition syndromes is ever increasing with better understanding of genetics and transmission, for the scope of this review, the authors focus on the relatively commonly encountered syndromes with attention to key genetic traits, clinical features, imaging findings, and treatment as well as current management options.

IMAGING TECHNIQUES
Ultrasound

Ultrasound (US) is the primary initial modality for abdominal imaging in children. It provides multiplanar imaging and has 3-dimensional (3D) capabilities.[1] As smaller pediatric patients with minimal visceral fat, children are well suited to US imaging and can usually be imaged with high-frequency transducers (>7 MHz), which provide excellent resolution. US is also well tolerated in children without sedation or anesthesia; real-time imaging provides ample opportunity to optimize a study with uncooperative patients.

Because sonography does not use ionizing radiation, it is an ideal modality for screening examinations whereby repeated imaging could contribute to a substantial radiation dose over a long interval of screening. Additionally, US is relatively inexpensive in comparison with computed tomography (CT) and MR imaging; among pediatric patients who may need repeated imaging examinations, this can represent a substantial cost savings over a long period.

Newer techniques in US, including 3D sonography, elastography, and US contrast, are rapidly gaining acceptance in clinical practice and have the potential of transforming US. Three-dimensional imaging allows more accurate evaluation of anatomy with improved volumetric measurements. Although most frequently used in adult cardiac and renal imaging, there is untapped potential in pediatric oncology, whereby 3D US could delineate spatial relationships for surgical planning and tumor resection. Elastography estimates the difference in stiffness between tissues by assessing the compressibility of the tissue when subjected to transducer pressure. This technique may contribute to the diagnosis of malignancy by identifying the ways in which tumor alters the mechanical properties of tissues.[2,3]

Finally US contrast agents use microscopic bubbles of air or perfluorocarbon gas bubbles that create backscatter that can be detected by the transducer. Although intravenous (IV) US contrast is not used in pediatric clinical practice in the United States, early research suggests that this contrast may be beneficial in tumor imaging, specifically to identify tumor vascularity.[3]

Computed Tomography

CT should be used judiciously in children because of their radiosensitivities (higher than that of adults) and longer expected life spans, during which radiation-induced neoplasms may manifest.[4] In pediatric patients with tumor-predisposition syndromes, the risk of eventual neoplasm is much higher than the average population; CT should be used sparingly, especially in patients with DNA repair defects. Certainly, US and MR imaging are the preferred modalities for imaging these children.

In acute, life-threatening scenarios, CT can be essential for emergency imaging. It may also provide important information when MR imaging is contraindicated or in clinical settings where US and MR imaging have suboptimal sensitivities, such as in the detection of small lung nodules. When the benefits of CT exceed potential harm, CT usage should be optimized using the principles of ALARA (as low as reasonably achievable) to permit appropriate diagnosis and treatment.

MR Imaging and Whole-Body MR Imaging

MR imaging provides excellent soft tissue contrast without the use of ionizing radiation, rendering it an essential noninvasive tool in the imaging strategy for pediatric patients with tumor predisposition syndromes. The emergence of whole-body MR imaging (WB MR imaging) technology is especially pertinent in the surveillance of pediatric patients with these syndromes, because many of these syndromes are associated with tumors that may span large (extensive) anatomic regions, which may be imaged in a single session with WB MR imaging. WB MR imaging has been used in patients with lymphoma but is also used as a screening tool in patients with neurofibromatosis type 1 and Li-Fraumeni because these syndromes are associated with a high tumor burden that may be scattered throughout discontinuous anatomic areas.[5]

WB MR imaging can be performed within 45 to 60 minutes on both 1.5- and 3.0-T magnets. Sequences can be obtained with continuous table motion, and ever-improving coil technology allows for even shorter examination times. Theoretic advantages of imaging on a 3.0 T-magnet include increased single to noise ratios, improved 3D sequences, and faster acquisition times. However, these advantages are mitigated by the currently lower availability of 3.0-T magnets and by field inhomogeneity that renders assessment of the shoulders and extremities suboptimal. In practice, 1.5-T magnets are used for most whole-body imaging.

Because most tumors and other pathologic lesions demonstrate prolonged T1 and T2 relaxation times, short tau inversion recovery (STIR) sequences are a central component of WB MR imaging. On STIR sequences, pathologic lesions and tumors are hyperintense; this intrinsic high signal within tumor is further accentuated by the excellent fat suppression on STIR sequences. In most WB MR imaging protocols, standard T1- and T2-weighted sequences are also obtained in order to provide basic anatomic and functional information. Functional diffusion-weighted imaging can also be added to assess for restricted diffusion in neoplastic tissues.

Although the large field of view provided by WB MR imaging represents an important diagnostic imaging tool for whole-body tumor detection, intrinsic technical limitations must also be considered. These limitations include small skips in the acquisition, either secondary to technique or patient movement, and obscuration of small lesions, especially those located within the skin and subcutaneous fat. Fusing the coronal images before the conclusion of the examination may aid in the detection of skipped areas, allowing immediate repeated image acquisition in any regions of missed anatomy. Despite this drawback, WB MR imaging is an important imaging modality in disorders, such as neurofibromatosis, Li-Fraumeni, and von Hippel-Lindau syndrome.[6,7]

Whole-Body PET/MR Imaging

Currently, fludeoxyglucose F 18 (^{18}F-FDG) PET/CT is the staging evaluation of choice for many pediatric oncology patients. However, the CT that is used for attenuation correction (and is often non-diagnostic) increases the radiation exposure during the study. Given the superior soft tissue resolution, lack of additional ionizing radiation, and functional imaging capability of MR imaging, PET/MR imaging is currently being explored as a potential alternative to PET/CT in the pediatric population.

Magnetic resonance (MR) could be implemented for PET image reconstruction. Approaches under consideration include either combining PET and MR imaging for simultaneous data acquisition or separate modality acquisitions, which are then subsequently coregistered using appropriate software. Simultaneous data acquisition may be limited by differing acquisition methods of the two modalities. Although many MR sequences are acquired during a breath hold, PET data are acquired over a longer period of free breathing. Coregistration may misalign organs because of a lack of overlap. Sequential, separate imaging may be more straightforward; but challenges include ensuring that the MR equipment is unaffected by PET detectors, which could potentially interfere with the radiofrequency of the magnet or gradient coils and alter image quality.[8,9] Finally, there is some concern over the safety of PET radiotracers in the MR imaging environment, with prior investigations showing that low-frequency magnetic fields have the potential to enhance the carcinogenic potential of ionizing radiation.[10,11]

Certainly, there are technical, cost, and safety barriers that must be overcome before PET/MR imaging can be adopted for widespread clinical use. Once these issues are resolved, the combination of these two dynamic modalities has great potential for tumor screening and surveillance in the pediatric population.

SPECTRUM OF SYNDROMIC DISORDERS IN CHILDREN
Beckwith-Wiedemann Syndrome

Background, genetics, and clinical features
Beckwith-Wiedemann syndrome (BWS), also referred to as congenital overgrowth syndrome, has an incidence of about 1 in 13,700.[12] Approximately 85% of the cases of BWS occur sporadically, whereas the remaining 15% are attributed to familial, dominant inheritance due to alterations in 11p.[13] Five known formative epigenetic and genetic changes at 11p are linked to the syndromic manifestations. As examples, these include overactive expression of insulinlike growth factor 2 (IGF-2), defective copy of CDKN1C (cyclin dependent kinase inhibitor 1C, a cellular proliferation inhibitor), and aberrant DNA methylation of the H19 gene.[14]

BWS demonstrates both clinical and molecular heterogeneity. Physical and laboratory examination findings include abdominal wall defects (eg, omphalocele, umbilical hernia, rectus muscle diastasis), hemihypertrophy, gigantism, macroglossia, and neonatal hypoglycemia. Gigantism may be identified late in pregnancy or early within the first few years of life. Other, less frequent features include midfacial hypoplasia, ear lobe creases or pits, organomegaly (particularly hepatomegaly and nephromegaly), and genitourinary abnormalities.[15–17]

There is an approximately 5% to 20% risk of developing benign or malignant tumors associated with BWS.[13] The risk is higher if both hemihyperplasia and organomegaly (especially nephromegaly) coexist. BWS is associated with increased frequency of embryonal tumors, most commonly Wilms tumor and hepatoblastoma. Others less commonly encountered tumors include pancreatoblastoma, adrenocortical carcinoma, neuroblastoma, and rhabdomyosarcoma.[18,19] Most of these tumors arise before 4 years of age and rarely occur in adulthood. Nonmalignant pathologies are most commonly of renal origin and include hydronephrosis, renal cysts, calyceal diverticula, and nephrolithiasis. Isolated hemihyperplasia that lacks other typical features of BWS is also associated with increased risk of developing embryonal tumors.[20]

Diagnosis and imaging

Several criteria have been proposed for the diagnosis of BWS because of a lack of unifying consensus on critical features. Some of the more widely accepted major and minor criteria are listed in **Box 1**.[12] Diagnosis includes the presence of at least 3 major or 2 major and one minor findings. Although guidelines may vary somewhat by institutions, in general, screening abdominal USs are recommended every 3 months up until 8 years of age (**Box 2** for other screening guidelines).

Up to 93% of cases of Wilms tumor associated with BWS present by 8 years of age and up to 81% by 5 years of age.[21] On US, Wilms tumor typically appears as a round or oval, well-circumscribed mass arising from the kidney, which is commonly hypoechoic to the surrounding renal parenchyma but can be isoechoic to hyperechoic. A claw sign of normal renal parenchyma surrounding the mass can help differentiate it from hepatoblastoma, neuroblastoma, or other abdominal tumors encountered in BWS (**Fig. 1**). Intralesional heterogeneity is usually due to cysts or necrosis. Calcification may be present. It is essential to evaluate the renal veins and inferior vena cava for direct tumor extension and interrogate the other kidney for concurrent bilateral Wilms. CT and MR imaging with IV contrast both demonstrate well-defined masses arising from the kidney that are hypoenhancing relative to the normal renal parenchyma. Metastatic disease occurs most frequently within the lungs, liver, and local lymph nodes.

Hepatoblastomas present as large, solid, encapsulated masses arising from the liver. More than 90% are detectable by increases in serum α-fetoprotein (AFP).[22] Hepatoblastomas often contain lobulations and septations. Calcifications may be present. Most are heterogeneous but may be homogeneous based on the histologic

---

Box 1
Major and minor clinical features of Beckwith-Wiedemann syndrome

Major Features	Minor Features
• Abdominal wall defects	• Pregnancy-related polyhydramnios and prematurity
• Macrosomia	
• Macroglossia	• Neonatal hypoglycemia
• Hemihyperplasia	
• Umbilical hernia or omphalocele	• Vascular skin lesions (head/neck) or hemangiomas
• Childhood embryonal tumors	
○ Wilms	• Cardiomegaly, structural cardiac abnormalities or cardiomyopathy
○ Hepatoblastoma	
○ Neuroblastoma	• Midface abnormalities
○ Rhabdomyosarcoma	
• Organomegaly	• Diastasis recti
• Cytomegaly of fetal adrenal cortex (pathognomonic)	• Advanced bone age
• Anterior ear lobe creases with or without posterior helical pits	
• Renal abnormalities	
• Placental mesenchymal dysplasia	
• Cleft palate	
• (+) Family history	

From Weksberg R, Shuman C, Beckwith JB. Beckwith-Wiedemann syndrome. Eur J Hum Genet 2010;18(1):8–14.

Box 2
Screening guidelines for children with Beckwith-Wiedemann

• Abdominal US every 3 months to 8 years of age

• Measure serum α-fetoprotein level every 3 months to 4 years

• Daily abdominal examination by caretaker

• Physical abdominal examination by physician every 6 months

From Tan TY, Amor DJ. Tumour surveillance in Beckwith-Wiedemann syndrome and hemihyperplasia: a critical review of the evidence and suggested guidelines for local practice. J Paediatr Child Health 2006;42(9):486–90.

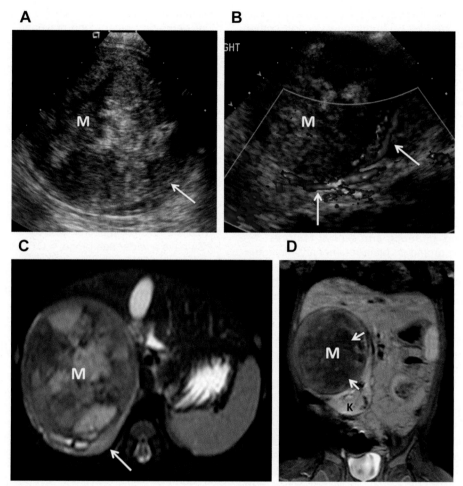

Fig. 1. A 9-month-old boy with Wilms tumor who presented with a palpable abdominal mass. (*A*) Gray-scale longitudinal image of the right kidney demonstrates a well-circumscribed heterogeneous mass (M) that distorts the underlying renal parenchyma (*arrow*). (*B*) Color Doppler longitudinal image of right kidney shows inferior displacement of the right renal vessels (*arrows*) by the large heterogeneous renal mass (M). (*C*) Axial T2-weighted MR image with fat saturation confirms a well-circumscribed heterogeneous mass (M) arising from the upper portion of the right kidney (*arrow*). (*D*) Coronal postcontrast T1-weighted MR image with fat saturation shows a heterogeneously enhancing large mass (M) with areas of hypoenhancement representing underlying cystic and necrotic regions (*arrows*). A normally enhancing inferior portion of the kidney (K) is also seen.

subtype. On US, hepatoblastomas are usually hyperechoic to the surrounding liver. On CT, hepatoblastomas are hypodense to the surrounding liver both on noncontrast and contrast-enhanced CT images with peripheral enhancement seen on arterial phase. On MR imaging, hepatoblastomas tend to be hypointense on T1-weighted sequences and hyperintense on T2-weighted sequences relative to the surrounding liver parenchyma. Hepatoblastomas may invade local vessels (eg, hepatic and portal veins). Metastases most frequently occur to the lung followed by bone, brain, lymph nodes, and rarely the eyes.

Pancreatoblastoma is a slow-growing tumor composed of partially circumscribed lobulated masses with a heterogeneous appearance due to necrosis and calcification. It may secrete adrenocorticotrophic hormone or demonstrate elevation of serum AFP, α_1-antitrypsin, or lactate dehydrogenase.[23] On US, a large multi-lobulated mass with septations is often seen. Septa enhance on contrast-enhanced CT and MR imaging. Frequent peripancreatic tissue invasion into duodenum, adjacent vessels and even perineural tissues is seen. Liver is the most common site of metastatic disease.

Management and treatment

Management and treatment of BWS rests on early detection of the condition and treatment of complications. Neonatal hypoglycemia requires prompt correction. Omphaloceles and other abdominal wall defects often require surgical treatment. Tongue reduction may be necessary in instances of severe macroglossia that impair feeding. Hemihyperplasia and leg length discrepancies may be treated in early adolescents. Nephrology consults are recommended for management of genitourinary issues. Detection of lesions suspicious for tumor on abdominal US necessitates further workup with CT or MR imaging with subsequent surgical resection sometimes in conjunction with chemotherapy.[12,13]

DICER1 Syndrome

Background, genetics, and clinical features

DICER1 syndrome or pleuropulmonary blastoma (PPB)—familial tumor dysplasia syndrome results from a heterozygous loss-of-function mutation in DICER1 found on chromosome 14q followed by second hit leading to loss of both alleles but not necessarily complete loss of function.[24] The result is decreased processing of 5p mature micro-RNA, an RNase endonuclease that regulates gene expression, protein synthesis, cell growth, division, and maturation. Carriers are phenotypically normal.

DICER1 is associated with both benign and malignant lesions, most of which occur during childhood, involving lungs, kidneys, and the endocrine organs (thyroid gland, ovaries, and pituitary gland).[25] Its strongest association is with PPBs, as up to 25% of the patients with PPB carry familial disposition from DICER1 mutation.[26,27] Other associations include renal tumors, specifically multilocular cystic nephroma (CN) and Wilms tumor, and ovarian Sertoli-Leydig tumor.[28] Another less frequent, although highly associated neoplasm is the pituitary blastoma, a very rare, aggressive tumor. Rarer extrapulmonary tumor associations include nasal chondromesenchymal hamartoma, nodular hyperplasia and differentiated carcinoma of thyroid, pineoblastoma, cervical embryonal rhabdomyosarcoma, and ciliary body medulloepithelioma.[29,30]

Diagnosis and imaging

The presence of a cystic lung lesion with cystic renal tumor in a child should be strongly suggestive of DICER1 mutation and concurrent PPB and CN, as literature suggests that, in patients with both pathologically proven PPB and CN, the incidence of DICER1 is nearly 100%.[31] Diagnostic workup includes genetic testing. When cystic lesions are identified on chest radiographs, chest CT and an abdominal or (renal) US should be performed to assess for concurrent PPB and CN, respectively.

Although PPBs are rare entities, they are the most common primary lung malignancy of childhood. PPBs occur in about 10% of the patients with DICER1 mutation and most present by 3 years of age.[25,28,32] The earliest manifestation is usually that of lung cysts, which may be difficult to separate from non-neoplastic cysts. There are 3 types of PPB, which often represent progression from type I to type II and, finally, type III. Certain nonprogressed or regressed cystic PPBs remain type I and are referred to as type I regressed (type Ir).[30] Type I PPBs are cystic and present by 3 years of age. Type II PPBs are a combination of cystic and solid tumors, whereas type III PPBs are solid. Both types II and III present later than type I, after the first year of life. Type Ir PPBs have a wider age range.[30] CT is best suited to diagnose PPBs due to lower sensitivities of chest radiographs. On CT, type I PPBs appear purely cystic with occasional internal septations and pleural effusions. Type II PPBs demonstrate expected mixed cystic and solid components and may contain enhancing nodules. On CT, type III PPBs appear purely solid with heterogeneous solid enhancement (**Fig. 2**).

Types II and III PPBs metastasize to brain, bone, and rarely, liver.[33] Type I PPBs are not associated with metastatic disease and require no additional workup other than assessing for concurrent renal tumors. When type II or III PPBs are present, diagnostic workup includes a CT chest, brain MR imaging, and bone scan. Type III PPBs may invade the great vessels; therefore, echocardiography can be considered for evaluation of mediastinal vascular structures.

Wilms tumor and CN are the two primary renal associations of DICER1. CNs are benign tumors of the kidney and present within the first 2 years of life. On imaging, these appear as multi-loculated cystic masses with several irregular cysts, thin internal septa, and a thick fibrous capsule. There are no solid components or nodules associated with these lesions, which may help differentiate them from Wilms (including cystic Wilms, which often contain solid nodules). Wilms tumor is also associated with DICER1, although to a lesser extent than CN, and is discussed in the BWS section of this review article.

Management and treatment

DICER1 syndrome is a relatively newly identified entity with pleiotropic manifestations and complex penetrance. As such, there are no established screening or management guidelines. In patients with a family history of PPB, screening chest CT to assess for PPB may be beneficial. Otherwise, management is specific to the individual tumors.

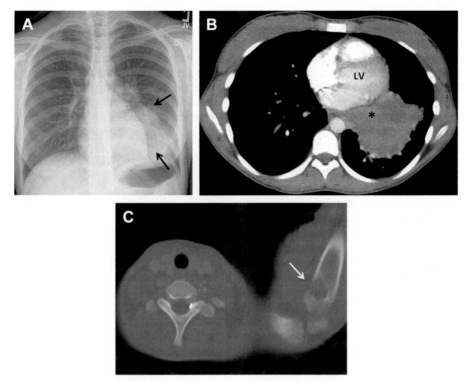

Fig. 2. A 13-year-old girl who presented with left chest pain, diagnosed with pleuropulmonary blastoma. (*A*) Frontal chest radiograph shows a masslike opacity (*arrows*) in the left lower lung zone. (*B*) Axial enhanced CT image shows a mildly heterogeneous soft tissue mass (*asterisk*) with an irregular boarder, abutting the left ventricle (LV). (*C*) Axial bone window CT image shows a lytic lesion (*arrow*) with associated cortical destruction located in the left proximal humeral metaphysis. Findings are consistent with osseous metastatic disease.

When these patients present with PPB, type I PPBs are treated by surgical resection. Because of the metastatic potential of types II and III PPBs, these subtypes undergo surgical resection and adjuvant chemotherapy. There is no clear role for radiation therapy at this time. Cystic nephromas are usually managed surgically with total nephrectomy unless the lesion size is 4.0 cm or less, in which case partial nephrectomy may be preferred.[34,35]

Cowden and Other Phosphatase and Tensin Homolog Hamartoma-Related Syndromes

Background, genetics, and clinical features

Cowden syndrome, also known as multiple hamartoma syndrome, falls within the category of phosphatase and tensin homolog (PTEN) hamartoma syndromes and presents with hamartomas of ectodermal, mesodermal, and endodermal origin. There is increased risk of malignancy of breast, thyroid, and endometrial cancers.[36,37] Other less common PTEN hamartoma syndromes include Bannayan-Riley-Ruvalcaba syndrome (BRRS), PTEN-related Proteus syndrome and Proteus-like

syndrome. The incidence of these Cowden syndromes is roughly 1 in 250,000.[38,39] Initially based on small sample sizes, 80% of the cases of Cowden were attributed to an autosomal dominant mutation in PTEN.[40] PTEN is a tumor suppressor gene on chromosome 10q. Its association with Cowden syndrome has now been lowered to less than 40%, although the PTEN domain may still play a larger role.[37] PTEN mutation is also responsible for roughly 60% of the cases of BRRS.[41] This gene encodes for a phosphatase enzyme that functions in cell cycle regulation and apoptosis, the loss of which in mammalian target of rapamycin (mTOR) cellular proliferation pathway leads to unregulated cell cycle propagation and tumorigenesis.

Manifestations of Cowden disease include facial trichilemmomas, keratotic papules, lipomas, angiolipomas, and vascular anomalies, many of which are present by the second and third decades of life. When papillomas coalesce in the tongue, it leads to a cobblestone appearance of tongue and oral mucosa. Common noncutaneous manifestations include thyroid involvement (goiters, adenomas and carcinomas), breast pathology in up to

50% of the females (ranging from benign to malignant: benign fibrocystic changes, fibroadenomas, ductal papillomas, and invasive carcinomas), and other gynecologic pathologies (also ranging from benign to malignant ovarian cysts, uterine leiomyomas, and endometrial cancer).[39] Perhaps more widely known are the gastrointestinal manifestations, including multiple hamartomatous polyps distributed throughout the gastrointestinal tract (esophagus through large bowel) with rare malignant potential. Other gastrointestinal tumors include lipomas and ganglioneuromas.

Craniomegaly is a more commonly encountered skeletal feature. Others include high-arched palate, kyphoscoliosis, pectus excavatum, and syndactyly. Within the brain, dysplastic cerebellar gangliocytoma is a characteristic finding, whereas other less strongly associated tumors include gliomas and meningiomas.

Diagnosis and imaging

Because of variable mutations, diagnosis of PTEN hamartoma tumor syndromes can be performed with consensus criteria combined with genetic testing. Although there are no formal diagnostic imaging guidelines for pediatric patients with these syndromes, an annual thyroid US should be performed from the time of diagnosis, as rare thyroid cancers have been described in children with PTEN mutations.[42]

Dysplastic cerebellar gangliocytoma or Lhermitte-Duclos is a brain lesion with features of both a hamartoma and a low-grade neoplasm that is highly associated with Cowden syndrome. It is considered a World Health Organization grade 1 tumor that usually presents in young adults but may occur during childhood.[43] On CT, a hypoattenuating mass is usually seen with or without calcification. Occasionally, the tumor is iso-attenuating and nearly imperceptible. Characteristic appearance on MR imaging is that of a striated, tiger-striped folial-patterned cerebellar mass with alternating bands of intensity on both T1- and T2-weighted sequences. These bands are hypointense to isointense on T1-weighted and isointense to hyperintense on T2-weighted MR images (**Fig. 3**). Generally, there is no appreciable enhancement on postcontrast MR images, unless associated with anomalous veins.[44]

Management and treatment

Although dysplastic cerebellar gangliocytomas are low-grade neoplasms, a screening brain MR image is necessary in instances of PTEN mutations because of higher incidences of other tumors, such as gliomas and meningiomas.[45] Dysplastic cerebellar gangliocytomas are surgically resected,

often to decompress mass effect on the posterior fossa and hydrocephalus. Their infiltrative nature and poorly defined margins often preclude complete resection.[46] Other screening and management guidelines for PTEN mutations are largely applicable to adults and are described in **Table 1**. These guidelines include attention to breast and endometrium in females. Renal and dermatology consultations are strongly encouraged.

Neurofibromatosis Types 1 and 2

Neurofibromatosis type 1 (NF1) or von Recklinghausen disease and neurofibromatosis type 2 (NF2) are both autosomal dominant diseases.

Neurofibromatosis type 1

Background, genetics, and clinical features In about 50% of the cases, NF1 occurs in children with a parent affected by NF1, whereas the other remaining 50% occur because of sporadic deletion mutation in the NF1 gene on chromosome 17q.[47,48] The result of the mutation is a truncated form of neurofibromin protein, which is a GTPase-activating protein–related protein. Neurofibromin is a negative regulator of RAS oncogene and deprives RAS proliferation, acting as a tumor suppressor protein. The incidence of NF-1 is about 1 in 3000.[49]

Most common tumors in children affected by NF1 are benign cutaneous neurofibromas and optic nerve gliomas. The disease is also characterized by café-au-lait spots on the skin.[50] Other cutaneous lesions include glomus tumors and juvenile xanthogranulomas. Brainstem and cerebellar gliomas are some of the other central nervous system (CNS) tumors. Leukemia, gastrointestinal stromal tumors, malignant peripheral nerve sheath tumors, pheochromocytoma, rhabdomyosarcoma, neuroblastoma, Wilms tumor, angiomyolipomas, primitive neuroectodermal tumors, and other sarcomas also occur in higher frequencies in children with NF1 than sporadic cases.[51,52]

Nontumor findings of NF1 include iris hamartomas or Lisch nodules, hypertelorism, glaucoma, macrocephaly, sphenoid wing dysplasia, and scoliosis. Affected children may have cognitive impairment and/or predisposition to seizures. Renal hypertension, usually essential, is also associated.

Diagnosis and imaging Diagnosis of NF1 is made by clinical features and genetic testing (**Box 3**). Typically described CT findings of NF1 include small, well-defined neurofibromas within the subcutaneous tissues, focal thoracic scoliosis, scalloping along the posterior aspects of the vertebral bodies, and enlarged neural foramina.[53]

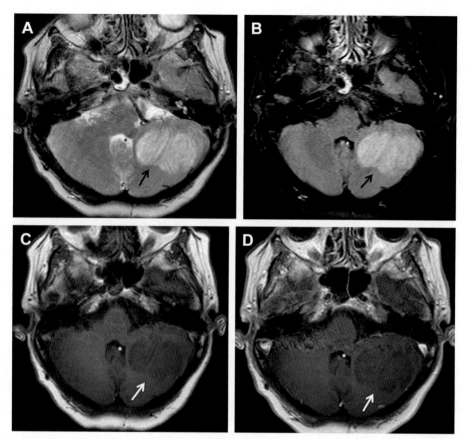

Fig. 3. A 19-year-old woman with Cowden syndrome. Axial T2 (*A*), fluid-attenuated inversion recovery (FLAIR) (*B*), T1 precontrast (*C*), and T1 postcontrast (*D*) MR images demonstrate a T2/FLAIR hyperintense mass (*arrow*) within the left cerebellar hemisphere. The mass expands the left cerebellum, demonstrates mild mass effect on the fourth ventricle (*asterisk*), and has no appreciable postcontrast enhancement. The mass consists of alternating hypointense and hyperintense bands with a tiger-stripe appearance, compatible with Lhermitte-Duclos disease (dysplastic cerebellar gangliocytoma) in this patient with Cowden syndrome.

Peripherally, limb hemihypertrophy, pseudoarthrosis, peripheral nerve neurofibromas, and plexiform neurofibromas are seen.

On CT, neurofibromas are well-defined, low-attenuating, round or ovoid lesions with minimal to no enhancement. On MR imaging, these are hypointense on T1-weighted sequences and hyperintense on T2-weighted sequences with heterogeneous contrast enhancement. A classic targetoid appearance on T2-weighted MR images with a rim of hyperintensity and central low signal is sometimes seen (**Fig. 4**). These lesions may sometimes calcify.

Plexiform neurofibromas are pathognomonic for NF1 and occur early in childhood. These large, conglomerated, multi-lobulated masses demonstrate diffuse involvement of a long segment of a nerve. Imaging features are similar to cutaneous neurofibromas, except plexiform are larger, trans-spatial and sometimes infiltrative. These masses may also calcify.

Management and treatment Patients with NF1 are managed by symptomatology. Optic gliomas and neurofibromas are generally asymptomatic and require no intervention. Optic pathway gliomas should be followed by an experienced ophthalmologist, even if the risk of vision loss is low and rarely require chemotherapy or radiation therapy.[54] Other low-grade CNS gliomas may require surgical debulking when causing obstructive hydrocephalus. Severe scoliosis may require surgical intervention.[53,54]

Because of the risk for malignant transformation of plexiform neurofibromas, surveillance of these lesions with WB MR imaging and/or PET/CT is recommended.[5] Treatment is based on symptoms and concerns for malignancy. PET/CT can help distinguish malignant peripheral nerve sheath tumors from benign neurofibromas.[55] Because of its extensive disease burden, surgery is performed prudently and may even be necessary in benign lesions with bulky

Table 1
Screening and surveillance guidelines for Cowden and other phosphatase and tensin homolog hamartoma syndromes

- Children <18 y old
- Adults
- Women at 30 y old
- Adult men and women
- Family history of early onset cancer of any type

- Annual thyroid US and dermatologic examinations
- Yearly thyroid US and dermatologic examinations
- Monthly breast self-examinations, annual breast cancer screening, transvaginal US or endometrial biopsy
- Colonoscopy beginning at 35 y old and frequency determined by degree of polyposis present
- Starting at 40 y old, renal imaging (CT/MR imaging) every 2 y
- Screening 5–10 y before youngest age of onset

disease burden due to mass effect, pain, and severe disfiguring.

Neurofibromatosis type 2

Background, genetics, and clinical features NF2 primarily affects the skin, nervous, and musculoskeletal systems. It occurs because of a mutation on chromosome 22. Tumor associations with NF2 can be recalled with the acronym MISME: multiple

Box 3
Clinical features in the diagnosis of neurofibromatosis type 1: at least 2 features should be present to make diagnosis

- *6 or more* café-au-lait macules (>5 mm kids; >15 mm adults)
- 2 or more cutaneous or subcutaneous neurofibromas or 1 plexiform neurofibroma
- Axillary or inguinal freckling
- Optic pathway glioma
- 2 or more Lisch nodules
- Bone dysplasia
- First-degree relative with neurofibromatosis type 1

inherited schwannomas, meningiomas, and ependymomas. Affected pediatric patients also may develop posterior subcapsular lenticular opacities and cutaneous schwannomas, which may give the false appearance of skin tags. Café au lait spots are rare, and cutaneous neurofibromas typically encountered in NF1 are not seen.

Diagnosis and imaging When multiple spinal neurofibromas are seen without accompanying cutaneous lesions, the leading diagnosis should be NF2. This can be tested genetically. Once established, screening of pediatric patients with NF2 should entail a brain MR imaging to assess for vestibular schwannomas, which are seen in up to 95% of the cases and are often bilateral.[56] Trigeminal schwannomas are much less common. A spine MR imaging should also be performed due to high association with other CNS tumors, namely meningiomas and ependymomas. These NF2 associated tumors have typical imaging findings seen with sporadic brain tumors.

Management and treatment After diagnosis of NF2 is established, a comprehensive brain and full spine MR imaging are recommended to prognosticate. Audiometry and brainstem auditory evoked responses should be tested when there are concerns for hearing loss.[54] Vestibular schwannomas should be managed by physicians particularly skilled in NF2 management. Small tumors limited within the internal auditory canal may undergo full resection, while larger are usually debulked.[56,57] Other cranial and spinal tumors such as meningiomas and ependymomas, and nonvestibular schwannomas can be monitored by imaging until symptomology necessitates intervention. Radiation therapy should only be used cautiously due to controversy that its implementation may accelerate or transform preexisting benign tumors into aggressive, malignant entities.[58]

Multiple Endocrine Neoplasia: Types 1 and 2

Increased tumor susceptibility to both endocrine and nonendocrine tumors are seen in both Multiple endocrine neoplasia 1 (MEN 1) and MEN 2 in the pediatric population.

Multiple endocrine neoplasia type 1

Background, genetics, and clinical features MEN 1, also known as Wermer syndrome, is an autosomal dominant syndrome with high penetrance due to a germline mutation in MEN 1 on chromosome 11q. This portion of the genome encodes the tumor suppressor protein menin, which plays

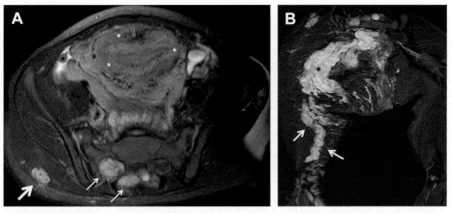

Fig. 4. A 2-year-old boy with NF1 and leg asymmetry. (*A*) Axial T2-weighted MR image with fat-saturated through the pelvis demonstrate a typical targetoid appearance of right gluteal neurofibromas, with peripheral T2 hyperintensity and a T2 hypointense center (*thick arrow*). Abnormal tissue seen in right upper sacral foramina corresponds to a large plexiform neurofibroma (*thin arrows; B*). Diffuse bladder wall thickening (*asterisks*) reflects a biopsy-proven infiltrating ganglioneuroma. (*B*) Coronal STIR MR image through bilateral thighs demonstrates a large hyperintense mass that arises from and extends along the right S1-S4 nerve roots (*asterisk*), compatible with a plexiform neurofibroma. The mass extends along the course of the sciatic nerve into the popliteal region (*arrows*).

a role in gene transcription, cell proliferation, apoptosis, and stability of the genome.

MEN 1 tumors include the 3 *Ps*: parathyroid adenomas (65%–90%), pancreatic neuroendocrine tumors (50%–70%), and anterior pituitary gland adenomas (most microadenomas).[59,60]

Diagnosis is based on 2 of these tumors occurring within same individual. Pituitary adenomas, in decreasing order of frequency, include prolactinomas, growth hormone-secreting tumors, nonfunctional adenomas, and rarely an adrenocorticotropic hormone or thyroid-stimulating hormone secreting tumors. The most common pancreatic neuroendocrine tumor are gastrinomas; insulinomas and glucagonomas are seen more rarely. Other less commonly encountered tumors include adrenocortical carcinomas, carcinoids, lipomatous tumors, and collagenomas. Roughly 85% to 90% of the affected pediatric patients have facial angiofibromas.[61] Mortality in this cohort is most commonly attributed to malignant pancreatic tumors. Further clinical features are described in **Table 2**.

Diagnosis and imaging Screening recommendations for MEN 1 are discussed in **Table 3**.[62] In MEN 1, greater than 95% of affected patients have primary hyperparathyroidism, usually multiglandular.[59,63] US is the first-line modality for diagnosing parathyroid adenomas, which appear as oval, well-defined hypoechoic masses posterior to thyroid gland. These masses are sometimes large, multi-lobulated with echogenic areas. Technetium-99m sestamibi (^{99m}Tc-MIBI) planar

imaging is another modality that is sensitive for detection of parathyroid adenomas and is performed both early (approximately 15 minutes after tracer injection) and delayed (approximately 2 hours after tracer injection). Standard of practice is a combination of US with scintigraphy. MR imaging has a higher sensitivity to visualize these adenomas over CT but is not routinely used. When incidentally detected, these tumors are hyperintense on T2-weighted sequences.

Most MEN 1–associated pancreatic tumors are functional and have less malignant potential than sporadically occurring pancreatic tumors. When gastrinomas are present (approximately 60%), it

Table 2 Summary of tumors and features of multiple endocrine neoplasia type 1	
Major tumors and features	• Parathyroid hyperplasia or adenomas • Pancreatic islet cell tumors • Pituitary tumors (anterior portion of gland)
Other more minor tumors and features	• Facial angiofibromas • Collagenomas • Adrenocortical tumors • Lipomas • Foregut carcinoids

Table 3 Screening recommendations for multiple endocrine neoplasia type 1	
Patients with MEN 1 and asymptomatic gene carriers older than 25 y	• Screening starting around 10 y old for asymptomatic children • Measure: fasting glucose, calcium, parathyroid hormone, insulin, prolactin, & IGF-1 levels • Annual pancreatic, liver, and adrenal US • Chest and abdominal CT or MR imaging every 3–5 y for carcinoid and pancreas • Pituitary MR imaging every 3–5 y

From Burgess J. How should the patient with multiple endocrine neoplasia type 1 (MEN 1) be followed? Clin Endocrinol (Oxf) 2010;72(1):13–6.

is not uncommon to encounter Zollinger-Ellison syndrome. About 30% of the pancreatic tumors are insulinomas and may coexist with gastrinomas.[64,65] Diagnostic imaging localization can be performed with US, CT, MR imaging, somatostatin receptor scintigraphy (SRS), and PET. Venous sampling can also be performed for diagnosis of these pancreatic tumors.

Transabdominal US is widely considered first line for imaging evaluation of pancreatic neuroendocrine tumors, although it has a lower sensitivity than invasive endoscopic US. When detected, these pancreatic tumors are homogeneously hypoechoic on US. CT is more sensitive for detecting tumors less than 2 cm of size, although multiphasic imaging may be necessary as these tumors are iso-attenuating on unenhanced CT. They avidly enhance in arterial phase (about 25 seconds after injection) and may washout on delayed images (50 seconds or more) (**Fig. 5**). Water may be used as a neutral enteric contrast to detect periampullary lesions. MR imaging has greater sensitivity for smaller tumors, with neuroendocrine neoplasms demonstrating low signal on T1-weighted sequences and higher signal on

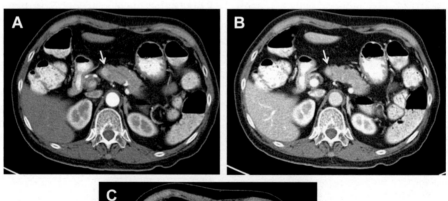

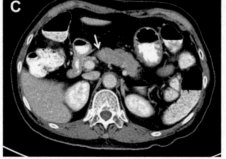

Fig. 5. A 70-year-old woman with MEN 1 and episodes of hypoglycemia. Multiphase enhanced CT images at the level of pancreas demonstrate a well-defined lesion at the pancreatic head-neck junction (*arrow*) that shows early homogeneous hyperenhancement relative to the pancreas at 25 seconds (*A*). Subsequent delayed phases at 40 (*B*) and 70 (*C*) seconds demonstrate relative washout of the lesion, which becomes slightly hypodense in relation to the normal pancreatic parenchyma. The appearance of this lesion is compatible with a neuroendocrine tumor. The patient was subsequently diagnosed with an insulinoma.

T2-weighted sequences relative to the remainder of the gland. Higher signal on T1-weighted sequences is related to higher quantities of collagen within the tumor. SRS detection with indium 111 (¹¹¹In)-octreotide can also be performed.

About 30% of the anterior pituitary adenomas associated with MEN 1 are functioning, typically secreting prolactin (60%), growth hormone (<25%), or adrenocorticotrophic hormone (5%).[63,66] These adenomas are diagnosed by dedicated pituitary MR imaging protocols that use a small field of view and thin multiplanar cuts. Intravenous contrast is necessary to detect small adenomas, and most are hypointense relative to normal pituitary gland on both the precontrast and postcontrast sequences. Other imaging findings include erosive changes of the sellar floor, abnormal convexity or bulge at upper margin of the gland, and deviation of the pituitary stalk (Fig. 6).

Adrenal adenomas occur in 40% in MEN 1 and are generally nonfunctional. Either CT or MR imaging is the first-line modality for diagnosis and requires identification of intracellular lipid for imaging diagnosis. Rarely adrenocortical carcinomas are seen, but these are generally large

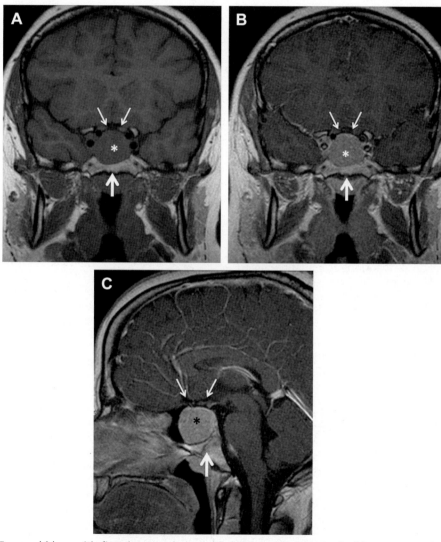

Fig. 6. A 17-year-old boy with first-degree relative with MEN 1 who presented with gynecomastia. Coronal T1 precontrast (A) and coronal (B) and sagittal (C) T1 postcontrast MR images demonstrate a well-defined lobulated mass (asterisk) centered in the pituitary gland. The mass extends into the right cavernous sinus and suprasellar space (thin arrows), bowing the sellar floor (thick arrow), and displaying mild diffuse enhancement. Findings are compatible with a pituitary macroadenoma in this patient with known MEN 1. Laboratory studies revealed a prolactinoma.

heterogeneous masses with hemorrhage and necrosis. Adrenocortical carcinomas may also contain calcification.

Carcinoids are generally found distributed in the foregut structures, including the thymus, bronchi, stomach, and duodenum. Almost all are hormonally inactive but may be locally invasive, particularly in the thymus.

Management and treatment Treatment of hyperparathyroidism associated with MEN 1 is localization of the lesion and parathyroidectomy. Treatment of the other MEN 1–associated tumors is more challenging as these may be multiple, more likely to present with occult metastatic disease, and may be larger and more aggressive than the sporadic forms.[65] For instance, functioning pancreatic neuroendocrine tumors often tend to be multiple; but this does not preclude attempting surgical resection. Treatment of pituitary lesions in MEN 1 includes medical therapy for endocrinopathy and/or transsphenoidal surgery. If the pituitary tumor is unresectable, radiation therapy can be attempted. At the time of parathyroidectomy, patients with MEN 1 should undergo a prophylactic thymectomy to reduce risk of carcinoid tumors.

Multiple endocrine neoplasia type 2
Background, genetics, and clinical features Mutations in MEN 2 involve the RET proto-oncogene on chromosome 10q, which codes for a member of the tyrosine kinase family. The mutated version of this gene is phosphorylated and activated, resulting in a gain-of-function effect. MEN 2 is subclassified into MEN 2A and -2B, but both manifestations are due to errors in the RET proto-oncogene.[67] MEN 2B is rarer and usually occurs from a new mutation rather than family history. Pathognomonic traits for MEN 2 include a tall, marfanoid-type appearance and mucosal neuromas.

MEN 2 encompasses both MEN 2A and -2B as well as familial medullary thyroid carcinoma. All these entities share complete penetrance of medullary thyroid cancer in affected individuals. MEN 2A presents with medullary thyroid carcinoma, pheochromocytoma, and either parathyroid hyperplasia or adenomas. MEN 2B is characterized by medullary thyroid carcinoma, pheochromocytoma, multiple mucosal neuromas, and intestinal ganglioneuromas. Rarer association with Hirschsprung disease is also seen.[68]

Diagnosis and imaging Table 4 reviews common screening guidelines for MEN 2.[59] Because of the universal development of medullary thyroid carcinoma (MTC) in this cohort, careful evaluation of

Table 4
Screening guidelines and recommendations for multiple endocrine neoplasia type 2

Biochemical screening:	• Serum calcitonin • Serum calcium & parathyroid hormone • Urinary catecholamines
Recommendations	• Early genetic screening • MEN2 gene carriers undergo prophylactic thyroidectomy[73–75] (before 5 y of age in MEN 2A & before 6 mo of age in MEN 2B)

the thyroid gland is crucial for surveillance. MEN 2 associated thyroid cancers present earlier than the sporadic forms and may produce ectopic thyroid hormones or elevate serum calcitonin levels. Local invasion is common with nodal spread to neck and mediastinum. Sites of distant metastases include liver, lung, and bone.[69]

On imaging, these are solid-appearing tumors, which may contain calcifications. Neuroendocrine radioisotopes, such as Iodine-123 metaiodobenzylguanidine (^{123}I-MIBG), and somatostatin analogues (eg, Indium-111 octreotide or ^{111}In-octreotide) often demonstrate uptake into these tumors. PET can be used to detect nodal disease. A more novel technique using ^{18}F-dihydroxyphenylalanine tracer for PET may have higher sensitivity than FDG PET.[70]

Pheochromocytomas are the second most common tumors in MEN 2, seen in approximately 50% of the cases.[71] In 50% of cases, these are bilateral; nearly all affected pediatric patients manifest biochemical abnormalities. These pheochromocytomas are rarely malignant and may be seen in the context of adrenal medullary hyperplasia. Optimal imaging evaluation involves CT or MR imaging. These lesions are generally well-defined ovoid lesions, which may be homogeneous or heterogeneous secondary to hemorrhage or necrosis. CT may detect speckled calcifications in just more than 10% of cases.[72] Historical concerns of hypertensive crises precipitated by the administration of ionic intravenous contrast have been resolved by near-universal use of nonionic intravenous contrast; on postcontrast images, pheochromocytomas are avidly enhancing masses. On MR imaging, T2-weighted MR imaging shows markedly T2 hyperintense lesions, in the absence of significant intralesional hemorrhage (**Fig. 7**). Radiolabeled whole-body MIBG scintigraphy has sensitivity near 90% for primary and metastatic disease.[70]

Management and treatment MTC is treated with total thyroidectomy and radical lymph node dissection. Surveillance can be performed with biannual or annual measurements of serum calcitonin. Adrenal surveillance is also important to detect pheochromocytomas. Some institutions treat MEN 2 with bilateral adrenalectomies (see **Table 4**).[73–75]

Li-Fraumeni Syndrome

Background, genetics, and clinical features

Li-Fraumeni syndrome (LFS) is one of the most widely recognized autosomal dominant familial cancer syndromes. In about 75% of the cases, it is caused by a loss-of-function mutation in the TP53 gene, which encodes the p53 tumor suppressor protein. The remaining 25% of cases occur through unknown genetic causes, potentially through other genes that stabilize the p53 suppressor pathway but are not yet authenticated.[76,77]

LFS is associated with lifelong risk of osteosarcoma, soft tissue sarcomas, leukemia, breast cancer, brain tumors, melanoma and adrenocortical tumors.[76] Overall, females have a 93% lifetime risk and males have 75% lifetime risk of developing cancer.[78] Individuals have up to 50% chance of developing invasive cancer by 30 years of age and 90% chance by 60 years of age.[79]

Clinical diagnostic criteria of LFS include a proband with sarcoma diagnosed before 45 years of age and a first-degree or second-degree relative with any cancer diagnosed before 45 years of age or sarcoma at any age; proband of multiple tumors (exclusion of multiple breast tumors), 2 of which must belong within the LFS spectrum and first occurring before 46 years of age; irrespective of any family history, a patient who presents with both adrenocortical carcinoma or choroid plexus tumor. In particular, when a child presents with adrenocortical carcinoma, underlying TP53 germline mutation should be strongly considered.

Diagnosis and imaging

After genetic diagnosis is established, surveillance is paramount in pediatric patients with LFS. Proposed screening guidelines are summarized in **Table 5**.[6]

Osteosarcoma is one of the more common tumors associated with LFS. Findings of osteosarcoma in children with LFS include an aggressive, destructive osseous lesion with a permeative or lytic appearance, aggressive periosteal reaction,

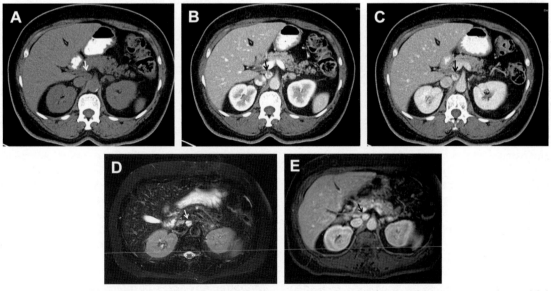

Fig. 7. A 53-year-old woman with suspected MEN 2, receiving screening CT for possible tumor. Unenhanced (*A*), early arterial (*B*; 25 seconds), and delayed (*C*; 70 seconds) axial CT images through the upper abdomen demonstrate a round well-defined mass (*arrow*) in the aortocaval region with early peripheral enhancement that subsequently fills in on more delayed images. (*D*) Axial T2-weighted fat-suppressed MR image demonstrates hyperintense signal characteristics within the mass (*arrow*). (*E*) Postcontrast axial T1-weighted fat-suppressed MR image demonstrates diffuse enhancement of the lesion (*arrow*) at 70 seconds. Resection of the mass revealed a pheochromocytoma.

Table 5
Proposed surveillance for patients with germline TP53 mutations

Children (birth to 18 y/o) and adults (>18–40 y/o) Screening for adrenocortical carcinoma	• Abdomen and pelvis US every 3–4 mo • Blood tests every 3–4 mo (17-OH-progesterone, total testosterone, DHEA, androstenedione) • 24-h urine cortisol
Children (birth to 18 y/o) and adults (>18 y/o) Screening for brain tumor	• Annual brain MR imaging
Children (birth to 18 y/o) Screening for soft tissue and bone sarcomas	• Annual rapid WB MR imaging
Adults (>18 y/o) Screening for soft tissue and bone sarcomas	• Annual rapid WB MR imaging • Abdomen and pelvis US every 3–4 mo
Children (birth to 18 y/o) and adults (>18 y/o) Screening for leukemia/lymphoma	• Blood tests every 3–4 mo (CBC, ESR, LDH)
Children (birth to 18 y/o) General assessment	• Complete physical examination every 3–4 mo (growth curve) • Assess for signs of virilization • Full neurological assessment
Adults (>18 y/o) Breast cancer	• Monthly breast self-examination (18 y/o onward) • Clinical breast examination twice a year (20–25 y/o onward or 5–10 y before earliest known breast cancer within family) • Annual mammography and breast MR imaging screening (aged 20–75 y or 5–10 y before earliest known breast cancer within family) • Consider risk-reducing bilateral mastectomy
Adults (>18 y/o) Colorectal cancer	• Colonoscopy every 2 y (start 25 y/o or 10 y before earliest known colon cancer)
Adults (>18 y/o) Melanoma	• Annual dermatologic examination
Adults (>18 y/o) General assessment	• Complete physical examination every 3–4 mo

Abbreviations: CBC, complete blood count; DHEA, dehydroepiandrosterone sulfate; ESR, erythrocyte sedimentation rate; LDH, lactate dehydrogenase; y/o, years old.

From Villani A, Shore A, Wasserman JD, et al. Biochemical and imaging surveillance in germline TP53 mutation carriers with Li-Fraumeni syndrome: 11 year follow-up of a prospective observational study. Lancet Oncol 2016;17(9):1295–305.

and osteoid matrix. Enhancing components are seen on MR imaging, and T2 hyperintense signal is often seen in nonmineralized soft tissue components. There is often peri-tumoral edema. The anatomic coverage of MR imaging should include the entire bone of origin to assess for skip lesions. Staging requires both chest CT and bone scan to assess for lung nodules as well as metastatic or synchronous osseous lesions (**Fig. 8**).

Adrenocortical carcinoma is typically evaluated by CT or MR imaging. When small, these tumors may appear homogeneous. However, affected pediatric patients generally present with a large, well-defined, heterogeneous suprarenal mass. Tumors may demonstrate internal cystic changes, hemorrhage, necrosis, and sometimes calcification (up to

30%).[80] These tumors enhance heterogeneously, often at the periphery. As extension into the renal veins and IVC occurs in up to 40% of the cases, contrast-enhanced studies are essential for assessing vascular invasion. Sites of metastatic disease include local lymph nodes, lung, liver, and bone. Liver metastases are often hypervascular.[80]

Management and treatment
As emphasized earlier, whole-body tumor surveillance is crucial in pediatric patients diagnosed with LFS. To minimize radiation, this is feasible with WB MR imaging.[6,81] Treatment of osteosarcoma, adrenocortical carcinomas, and many of the other invasive solid tumors in pediatric patients

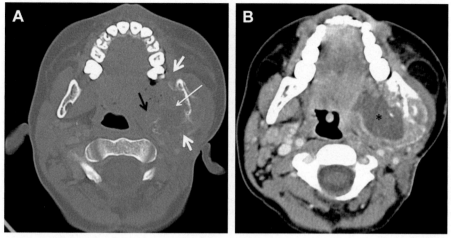

Fig. 8. An 11-year-old girl with Li-Fraumeni syndrome and facial asymmetry. Axial contrast-enhanced images in bone (*A*) and soft tissue (*B*) algorithms through the level of the jaw demonstrate a destructive left mandibular lesion involving the ramus and body of the left mandible with an associated soft tissue mass (*thick white arrows*). There is aggressive periosteal reaction (*thin white arrow*) with osteoid matrix (*black arrow*). Low density within the soft tissue portion (*asterisk*) is compatible with necrosis. Biopsy of this lesion demonstrated osteosarcoma.

with LFS includes surgery, often with adjuvant chemotherapy and radiation in advanced disease.

Von Hippel-Lindau

Background, genetics, and clinical features

Von Hippel-Lindau (VHL) syndrome is a genetic disorder with autosomal dominant inheritance, due to a mutation in VHL tumor suppressor gene on chromosome 3p that inactivates one of the VHL alleles. A subsequent second allele-inactivating event then occurs with complete functional loss of tumor suppression, resulting in overexpression of proteins that mediate neo-angiogenesis and tumorigenesis (such as vascular endothelial growth factor, platelet-derived growth factor B, erythropoietin, and so forth).[82,83] The syndrome has high penetrance and variable expression.[84,85]

VHL has a prevalence of roughly 1 in 36,000.[86] Associated tumors are endocrine and nonendocrine in cause. These tumors include hemangioblastomas, endolymphatic sac tumors, clear cell renal cell carcinoma (RCC), adrenal pheochromocytomas, and islet cell tumors. The syndrome is also associated with renal and pancreatic cysts and tumors and epididymal cystadenoma.[87] CNS and ocular hemangioblastomas are characteristic tumors in VHL, especially cerebellar hemangioblastomas, which are seen in 35% to 79% of the cases.[84,88] Spinal cord hemangioblastomas occur at a younger age and have a worse prognosis than isolated hemangioblastomas. Roughly 50% of affected patients also have retinal hemangioblastomas, often multiple and bilateral.[89]

Diagnosis and imaging

Clinical criteria in patients with known family history include presence of single retinal or cerebellar hemangioblastoma, RCC, or pheochromocytoma. Individuals without a known family history are diagnosed when 2 or more retinal or cerebellar hemangioblastomas or a single hemangioblastoma and one other characteristic lesion are present.[90]

Given varied types of tumors and diversity of organ involvement, imaging evaluation may involve US, CT, MR imaging, and nuclear scintigraphy. On imaging, hemangioblastomas are highly vascular and demonstrate robust enhancement. The most characteristic appearance is a cystic lesion with enhancing solid mural nodule. However, entirely cystic, solid, hemorrhagic, or mixed lesions are also seen. Large lesions often have prominent peripheral feeding/draining vessels that may appear as flow voids on MR imaging (**Fig. 9**). Spinal lesions may have an associated syrinx.

VHL is the most common cause of hereditary kidney cancer, with bilateral multicentric RCC presenting by the third or fourth decade of life.[87] Screening includes serum or urine catecholamine for early detection of pheochromocytomas. Recommended imaging guidelines are variable by institutions, but an example is provided in **Table 6**.[91,92]

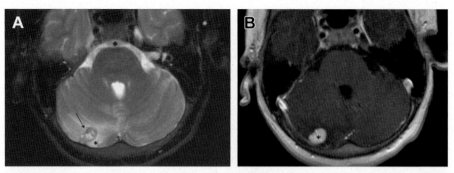

Fig. 9. A 12-year-old boy with von-Hippel Lindau and multiple intracranial hemangioblastomas. (A) Axial T2-weighted fat-suppressed MR image through the posterior fossa demonstrates a right cerebellar lesion with a subtle flow void (*arrow*) and heterogeneous central areas of T2 hyperintensity. Surrounding T2 hyperintensity (*asterisk*) is compatible with edema. (B) Postcontrast axial T1-weighted MR image demonstrates an avidly enhancing mass (*asterisk*) abutting the pial surface. (*Courtesy of* Jennifer Vaughn, MD, Boston, MA.)

Management and treatment

Two largest contributors to morbidity and mortality in VHL are hemangioblastomas and RCC. Early detection and appropriate surgical resection and treatment are the mainstays of management.[93] Hemangioblastomas are treated by resection, although given the hypervascular nature of the tumor, preoperative arterial embolization may be beneficial. Treatment of CNS hemangioblastomas entails significant perioperative and postoperative risk.[94]

Tuberous Sclerosis

Background, genetics, and clinical features

Also known as Bourneville disease, tuberous sclerosis (TS) is an autosomal dominant disease that occurs in 1 in 10,000 people.[95] There are 2 mutations attributed to this disease including TSC1 on

Table 6
Proposed surveillance scheme of von Hippel-Lindau

For retinal hemangiomas	• Annual ophthalmologic evaluation and visual field testing starting around age 2 y old
For CNS hemangioblastomas	• MR imaging of brain and spine every 2 y starting early adolescence
Renal pathology	• Annual abdominal US starting at 5 y old
Pancreatic cancer	• Abdominal CT or MR imaging starting at 20 y old
Pheochromocytomas	• Frequent blood pressure monitoring and measurement of urinary catecholamine levels or plasma metanephrine levels every 1–2 y starting at 2 y old

Adapted from Frantzen C, Klasson TD, Links TP, et al. Von Hippel-Lindau syndrome BTI. GeneReviews(R); and Maher ER. Von Hippel-Lindau disease. (1566–5240 (Print)).

Table 7
Various clinical manifestations of tuberous sclerosis

Ocular	• Retinal hamartomas
Neuro	• Subependymal nodules • Cortical tubers • Intracranial calcifications • Cognitive impairment
Dental	• Gingival fibromas • Enamel pits
Pulmonary	• Lymphangioleiomyomatosis • Multifocal micronodular pneumocyte hyperplasia
Cardiovascular	• Myocardial rhabdomyomas
Renal	• Angiomyolipomas • Renal cysts
Cutaneous	• Facial angiofibromas • Ash-leaf spots (hypomelanotic macules), earliest manifestation, seen at birth • Nevi • Periungual fibromas • Café-au-lait macules

chromosome 9, which encodes the hamartin protein, and TSC2 on chromosome 16, which encodes the tuberin protein. Both hamartin and tuberin work together to hydrolyze GTP → GDP, which then inhibits GTPase proteins Rab and Rheb to prevent activation of the mTOR pathway. Both hamartin and tuberin function as tumor suppressor proteins.[96–98]

There are several manifestations with loss of these tumor suppressor proteins demonstrated in **Table 7**. The major findings include pulmonary lymphangioleiomyomatosis, intracranial subependymal nodules and cortical tubers, cardiac rhabdomyomas, and renal angiomyolipomas. In patients with the TSC2 gene deletion, multiple renal cysts may also be present, as the

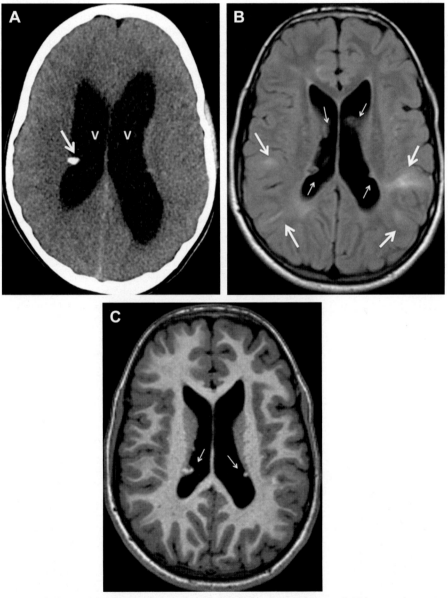

Fig. 10. A 17-year-old boy with known tuberous sclerosis. (*A*) Axial unenhanced CT image demonstrates ventriculomegaly (V) and a calcified right subependymal nodule (*arrow*). Axial fluid-attenuated inversion recovery (FLAIR) (*B*) and postcontrast axial T1-weighted (*C*) MR images demonstrate multiple bilateral cortical tubers (*thick arrows*) and subependymal nodules (*thin arrows*). Cortical tubers are most apparent on FLAIR-weighted sequences.

polycystic kidney disease gene is contiguously located on chromosome 16.[99] More variable abdominal findings include gastrointestinal polyps, fibrous tumors, vascular malformations, and leiomyomas.

Diagnosis and imaging

Given the varied clinical features and manifestations, there is no critical clinical finding that is diagnostic for TS. Imaging can play an important role in the diagnosis of pediatric patients with TS. When cortical or subependymal tubers are found with cardiac rhabdomyomas, and renal AMLs, TS can be diagnosed by imaging.

Cortical tubers and subependymal nodules are amongst the most frequent CNS imaging findings in pediatric patients with TS. Most cortical tubers occur in frontal lobes and are hypointense on T1-weighted sequences and hyperintense on T2-weighted sequences. Approximately 10% of cortical tubers show enhancement.[100] In older children and adults, these may become more iso-intense to surrounding gray matter. Subependymal nodules are hamartomatous lesions that are often multiple. These lesions are associated with calcification and appear hyperintense on T1-weighted sequences and iso-intense to hyperintense on T2-weighted sequences (**Fig. 10**). TS is also associated with subependymal giant cell astroycytomas (SEGA). Although these lesions are benign, they most frequently occur at the foramen of Monro and can present with obstructive hydrocephalus. SEGA are hyperattenuating on unenhanced CT.

Cardiac rhabdomyomas are benign muscular tumors. Most of these neoplasms (75%) present before 1 year of age, but most regress and even disappear by 4 years of age.[101,102]

Pulmonary lymphangioleiomyomatosis (LAM) is seen in approximately one-third of female patients with TS and is a rare entity exclusively affecting females.[103] Secondary to diffuse interstitial proliferation and cystic changes, thin-section CT demonstrates diffuse, multiple round, thin-walled cysts that vary in size and morphology (**Fig. 11**). LAM is often complicated by frequent pneumothoraces and chylous pleural effusions or ascites. When multiple, tiny subcentimeter nodules are scattered in random distribution throughout the lungs in a woman with TS, a rarer pulmonary association of TS, multifocal micronodular pneumocyte hyperplasia (MMPH), should be considered.[98]

Renal angiomyolipomas (AMLs) are the most common TS-associated tumor of the kidney. These tumors are composed of an abnormal collection of blood vessels and immature fat and smooth muscle cells. Although also occurring sporadically, AML in patients with TS occur at younger ages and tend to be bilateral, multiple, and larger, with demonstrable growth. On US, AMLs are typically echogenic masses with through transmission, although the presence of hemorrhage may yield a more heterogeneous appearance (**Fig. 12**). On CT, the presence of intralesional macroscopic fat is diagnostic for AML. In a minority of AMLs, the intratumoral fat is occult on CT. These lipid-poor AMLs are diagnostically challenging to separate from RCC, although the incidence of RCC in pediatric patients with TS may be the same as the general population. Renal guidelines for patients with TS are summarized in **Table 8**.

Management and treatment

Renal-related complications are the largest cause of morbidity in patients with TS. Renal AML may

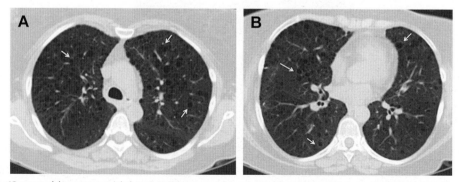

Fig. 11. A 43-year-old woman with known tuberous sclerosis and lymphangioleiomyomatosis. Axial noncontrast CT images through the upper (A) and lower (B) lungs demonstrate multiple thin-walled and rounded cysts of various sizes (arrows), uniformly scattered throughout both lungs. Appearance of the lungs is consistent with lymphangioleiomyomatosis.

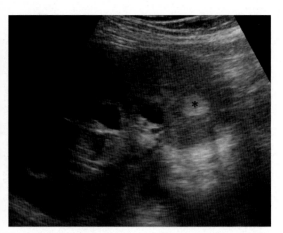

Fig. 12. An 18-year-old boy with known tuberous sclerosis and angiomyolipoma. Long-axis gray-scale US image of left kidney demonstrates a round and homogeneously echogenic lesion (*asterisk*), compatible with an angiomyolipoma.

lead to chronic kidney disease or life-threatening hemorrhage. Recently, use of mTOR inhibitors has been proposed for management of asymptomatic AMLs that are larger than 3 cm.[104,105] Second-line treatment involves selective embolization or kidney-sparing resection of these AMLs.

Although SEGA represent slow-growing CNS tumors, these may cause noncommunicating hydrocephalus at the level of foramen of Monro and can also be managed by mTOR inhibitors or surgery.[106] Efficaciously, mTOR inhibitors also seem to play a role in mitigating seizures and cognitive impairment in children with TS.[107]

Table 8 Renal guidelines for patients with tuberous sclerosis (International Tuberous Sclerosis Complex Consensus Group)	
Renal guidelines for patients with TS	• Renal US or MR imaging every 1–3 y if no renal lesions • Renal US biannually if known AML

Adapted from Northrup H, Krueger DA; International Tuberous Sclerosis Complex Consensus Group. Tuberous sclerosis complex diagnostic criteria update: recommendations of the 2012 international tuberous sclerosis complex consensus conference. Pediatr Neurol 2013;49: 243–54; and Krueger DA, Northrup H; International Tuberous Sclerosis Complex Consensus Group. Tuberous sclerosis complex surveillance and management: recommendations of the 2012 International Tuberous Sclerosis Complex Consensus Conference. Pediatric Neurol 2013;49:255–65.

SUMMARY

Although it is not possible to discuss all pediatric abnormalities with tumor associations, recognizing that cancers in children may be syndromic in higher incidences than in the adult population, especially when associated with multiple tumors or other benign pathologies (such as hamartomatous lesions), may provide a unique opportunity for the astute radiologist to potentially alter the life and course of a patient's treatment. Early diagnosis, detection, and screening under the care of a multidisciplinary approach are imperative to optimal patient care. Imaging evaluation plays a central role, and the potential risks associated with ionizing radiation may be further minimized in the future with highly anticipated advancements in WB MR imaging and PET/MR imaging.

REFERENCES

1. Riccabona M. Pediatric three-dimensional ultrasound: basics and potential clinical value. J Clin Imaging 2005;29:1–5.
2. Lyshchik A, Higashi T, Asato R, et al. Thyroid gland tumor diagnosis at US elastography. Radiology 2005;237(1):202–11.
3. Stenzel M, Mentzel HJ. Ultrasound elastography and contrast-enhanced ultrasound in infants, children and adolescents. Eur J Radiol 2014;83(9):1560–9.
4. Smith-Bindman R, Lipson J, Marcus R, et al. Radiation dose associated with common computed tomography examinations and the associated lifetime attributable risk of cancer. Arch Intern Med 2009;169(22):2078–86.
5. Ahlawat S, Fayad LM, Khan MS, et al. Current whole-body MRI applications in the neurofibromatoses. Neurology 2016;87(Suppl 1):S31–9.
6. Villani A, Shore A, Wasserman JD, et al. Biochemical and imaging surveillance in germline TP53 mutation carriers with Li-Fraumeni syndrome: 11 year follow-up of a prospective observational study. Lancet Oncol 2016;17(9):1295–305.
7. Kruizinga RC, Sluiter WJ, de Vries EGE, et al. Calculating optimal surveillance for detection of von Hippel-Lindau-related manifestations. Endocr Relat Cancer 2013;21(1):63–71.
8. Torigian DA, Zaidi H, Kwee TC, et al. PET/MR imaging: technical aspects and potential clinical applications. Radiology 2013;267(1):26–44.
9. Aghighi M, Pisani LJ, Sun Z, et al. Speeding up PET/MR for cancer staging of children and young adults. Eur Radiol 2016;26(12):4239–48.
10. Brix G, Nekolla EA, Nosske D, et al. Risks and safety aspects related to PET/MR examinations. Eur J Nucl Med Mol Imaging 2009;36(Suppl 1):S131–8.

11. Miyakoshi J, Yoshida M, Shibuya K, et al. Exposure to strong magnetic fields at power frequency potentiates X-ray-induced DNA strand breaks. J Radiat Res 2000;41(3):293–302.

12. Weksberg R, Shuman C, Beckwith JB. Beckwith-Wiedemann syndrome. Eur J Hum Genet 2010; 18(1):8–14.

13. Shuman C, Beckwith JB, Weksberg R. Beckwith-Wiedemann syndrome. Gene Rev 2000.

14. Soejima H, Higashimoto K. Epigenetic and genetic alterations of the imprinting disorder Beckwith-Wiedemann syndrome and related disorders. J Hum Genet 2013;58:402–9.

15. Cohen MM Jr. Overgrowth syndromes: an update. Adv Pediatr 1999;46:441–91.

16. Elliott M, Bayly R, Cole T, et al. Clinical features and natural history of Beckwith-Wiedemann syndrome: presentation of 74 new cases. Clin Genet 1994; 46(2):168–74.

17. Bates DG, Faerber EN, Hernanz-Schulman M, et al. Caffey's pediatric diagnostic imaging. 12th edition. Philadelphia: Elsevier Saunders; 2013.

18. Tan TY, Amor DJ. Tumour surveillance in Beckwith-Wiedemann syndrome and hemihyperplasia: a critical review of the evidence and suggested guidelines for local practice. J Paediatr Child Health 2006;42(9):486–90.

19. Lapunzina P. Risk of tumorigenesis in overgrowth syndromes: a comprehensive review. Am J Med Genet C Semin Med Genet 2005;137C(1):53–71.

20. Hoyme HE, Seaver LH, Jones KL, et al. Isolated hemihyperplasia (hemihypertrophy): report of a prospective multicenter study of the incidence of neoplasia and review. Am J Med Genet 1998; 79(4):274–8.

21. Beckwith J. Nephrogenic rests and the pathogenesis of Wilms tumor: developmental and clinical considerations. Am J Med Genet 1998;79:268–73.

22. Chung EM, Lattin GE Jr, Cube R, et al. From the archives of the AFIP: pediatric liver masses: radiologic-pathologic correlation part 2. Malignant tumors. RadioGraphics 2011;31:483–507.

23. Montemarano H, Lonergan GJ, Bulas DI, et al. Pancreatoblastoma: imaging findings in 10 patients and review of the literature. Radiology 2000;214: 476–82.

24. Pugh TJ, Yu W, Yang J, et al. Exome sequencing of pleuropulmonary blastoma reveals frequent biallelic loss of TP53 and two hits in DICER1 resulting in retention of 5p-derived miRNA hairpin loop sequences. Oncogene 2014;33:5295–302.

25. Hill DA, Ivanovich J, Priest JR, et al. DICER1 mutations in familial pleuropulmonary blastoma. Science 2009;325:965.

26. Foulkes WD, Priest JR, Duchaine TF. DICER1: mutations, microRNAs and mechanisms. Nat Rev Cancer 2014;14(10):662–72.

27. Priest JR, Watterson J, Strong L, et al. Pleuropulmonary blastoma: a marker for familial disease. J Pediatr 1996;128:220–4.

28. Slade I, Bacchelli C, Davies H, et al. DICER1 syndrome: clarifying the diagnosis, clinical features and management implications of a pleiotropic tumor predisposition syndrome. J Med Genet 2011; 48:273–8.

29. Dehner LP, Messinger YH, Schultz KA, et al. Pleuropulmonary blastoma: evolution of an entity as an entry into familial tumor predisposition syndrome. Pediatr Developmental Pathol 2015;18(6):504–11.

30. Messinger YH, Stewart DR, Priest JR, et al. Pleuropulmonary blastoma: a report on 350 central pathology-confirmed pleuropulmonary blastoma cases by the international pleuropulmonary blastoma registry. Cancer 2015;121(2):276–85.

31. Doros LA, Rossi CT, Yang J, et al. DICER1 mutations in childhood cystic nephroma and its relationship to DICER1-renal sarcoma. Mod Pathol 2014; 27:1267–80.

32. Bahubeshi A, Bal N, Rio Frio T, et al. Germline DICER1 mutations and familial cystic nephroma. J Med Genet 2010;47(12):863–6.

33. Priest JR, McDermott MB, Bhatia S, et al. Pleuropulmonary blastoma: a clinicopathologic study of 50 cases. Cancer 1997;80(1):147–61.

34. Han HH, Choi KH, Oh YT, et al. Differential diagnosis of complex renal cysts based on lesion size along with the Bosniak renal cyst classification. Yonsei Med J 2012;53:729–33.

35. Granja MF, O'Brien AT, Trujillo S, et al. Multilocular cystic nephroma: a systematic literature review of the radiologic and clinical findings. AJR 2015; 205:1188–93.

36. Eng C. Will the real Cowden syndrome please stand up: revised diagnostic criteria. J Med Genet 2000;37:828–30.

37. Pilarski R, Burt R, Kohlman W, et al. Cowden syndrome and the PTEN hamartoma tumor syndrome: systemic review and revised diagnostic criteria. J Natl Cancer Inst 2013;105:1607–16.

38. Barnard J. Screening and surveillance recommendations for pediatric gastrointestinal polyposis syndromes. J Pediatr Gastroenterol Nutr 2009; 48(Suppl 2):S75–8.

39. Farooq A, Walker LJ, Bowling J. Cowden syndrome. Cancer Treat Rev 2010;36:577–83.

40. Liaw D, Marsh DJ, Li J, et al. Germline mutations of the PTEN gene in Cowden disease, an inherited breast and thyroid cancer syndrome. Nat Genet 1997;16(1):64–7.

41. Marsh DJ, Kum JB, Lunetta KL, et al. PTEN mutation spectrum and genotype-phenotype correlations in Bannaya-Riley Ruvalcaba syndrome suggest a single entity with Cowden syndrome. Hum Mol Genet 1999;8:1461–72.

42. Smith JR, Marqusee E, Webb S, et al. Thyroid nodules and cancer in children with PTEN hamartoma tumor syndrome. J Clin Endocrinol Metab 2011; 96(1):34–7.

43. Vieco PT, del Carpio-O'Donovan R, Melanson D, et al. Dysplastic gangliocytoma (Lhermitte-Duclos disease): CT and MRI imaging. Pediatr Radiol 1992;22:366–9.

44. Awwad EE, Levy E, Martin DS, et al. Atypical MR appearance of Lhermitte-Duclos disease with contrast enhancement. Am J Neuroradiol 1995; 16:1719–20.

45. Shinagare AB, Patil NK, Sorte SZ. Case 144: dysplastic cerebellar gangliocytoma (Lhermitte-Duclos disease). Radiology 2009;251:298–303.

46. Vantomme N, Van Calenbergh F, Goffin J, et al. Lhermitte-Duclos disease is a clinical manifestation of Cowden's syndrome. Surg Neurol 2001;56(3):201–4.

47. Fahsold R, Hoffmeyer S, Mischung C, et al. Minor lesion mutational spectrum of the entire NF1 gene does not explain its high mutability but points to a functional domain upstream of the gap-related domain. Am J Hum Genet 2000;66(3):790–818.

48. Ars E, Kruyer H, Morell M. Recurrent mutations in the NF1 gene are common among neurofibromatosis type 1 patients. J Med Genet 2003;40:e82.

49. Williams VC, Lucas J, Babcock MA, et al. Neurofibromatosis type 1 revisited. Pediatrics 2009; 123(1):124–33.

50. Riccardi VM. Von Recklinghausen neurofibromatosis. N Engl J Med 1981;305:1617–27.

51. Brems H, Beert E, de Ravel T, et al. Mechanisms in the pathogenesis of malignant tumors in neurofibromatosis type 1. Lancet Oncol 2009;10:508–15.

52. Ferrari A, Bisogno G, Macaluso A, et al. Soft-tissue sarcomas in children and adolescents with neurofibromatosis type 1. Cancer 2007;109(7):1406–12.

53. Fortman BJ, Kuszyk BS, Urban BA, et al. Neurofibromatosis type 1: a diagnostic mimicker at CT. Radiographics 2001;21:601–12.

54. Gutmann DH, Aylsworth A, Carey JC. The diagnostic evaluation and multidisciplinary management of neurofibromatosis 1 and neurofibromatosis 2. JAMA 1997;278:51–7.

55. Karabatsou K, Kiehl TR, Wilson DM, et al. Potential role of 18fluorodexoyglucose-positron emission tomography/computed tomography in differentiating benign neurofibroma from malignant peripheral nerve sheath tumor associated with neurofibromatosis 1. Neurosurgery 2009;65:A160–70.

56. Briggs RJS, Brackmann DE, Baser ME, et al. Comprehensive management of bilateral acoustic neuromas. Arch Otolaryngol Head Neck Surg 1994;120:1307–14.

57. Miyamoto R, Campbell RL, Fritsch M, et al. Preservation of hearing in neurofibromatosis 2. Otolaryngol Head Neck Surg 1990;103:619–24.

58. Liu A, Kuhn EN, Lucas JT Jr, et al. Gamma Knife radiosurgery for meningiomas in patients with neurofibromatosis type 2. J Neurosurg 2015;122: 536–42.

59. Brandi ML, Gagel RF, Angeli A, et al. Guidelines for diagnosis and therapy of MEN type 1 and type 2. J Clin Endocrinol Metab 2001;86:5658–71.

60. Glascock MJ, Carty SE. Multiple endocrine neoplasia type 1: fresh perspective on clinical features and penetrance. Surg Oncol 2002;11(3): 143–50.

61. Darling TN, Skarulis MC, Steinberg SM, et al. Multiple facial angiofibromas and collagenomas in patients with multiple endocrine neoplasia type 1. Arch Dermatol 1997;133:853–7.

62. Burgess J. How should the patient with multiple endocrine neoplasia type 1 (MEN 1) be followed? Clin Endocrinol (Oxf) 2010;72(1):13–6.

63. Benson L, Ljunghall S, Akerstrom G, et al. Hyperparathyroidism presenting as the first lesion in multiple endocrine neoplasia type 1. Am J Med 1987; 82:731–7.

64. Thakker RV. Multiple endocrine neoplasia type 1. Endocrinol Metbl Clin North Am 2000;29:541–67.

65. Thakker RV. Multiple endocrine neoplasia type 1 (MEN1) and type 4 (MEN4). Mol Cell Endocrinol 2014;386:2–15.

66. Marx S, Spiegel AM, Skarulis MC, et al. Multiple endocrine neoplasia type 1: clinical and genetic topics. Ann Int Med 1998;129:484–94.

67. Scarsbrook AF, Thakker RV, Wass JAH, et al. Multiple endocrine neoplasia: spectrum of radiologic appearances and discussion of a multitechnique imaging approach. RadioGraphics 2006; 26:433–51.

68. Romeo G, Ceccherini I, Celli J, et al. Association of multiple endocrine neoplasia type 2 and Hirschsprung disease. J Intern Med 1998;243:515–20.

69. Szakall S, Esik O, Bajzik G, et al. 18F-FDG PET detection of lymph node metastases in medullary thyroid carcinoma. J Nucl Med 2002;43:66–71.

70. Hoegerle S, Nitzsche E, Altehoefer C, et al. Pheochromocytomas: detection with 18F DOPA whole body PET - initial results. Radiology 2002;222: 507–12.

71. Turner HE, Wass J. Multiple endocrine neoplasia. Oxford handbook of endocrinology and diabetes. Oxford (United Kingdom): Oxford University Press; 2002. p. 718–30.

72. Pacak K, Ilias I, Adams KT, et al. Biochemical diagnosis, localization and management of pheochromocytoma: focus on multiple endocrine neoplasia type 2 in relation to other hereditary syndromes and sporadic forms of the tumour. J Intern Med 2005;257:60–8.

73. de Graaf JS, Dullaart RP, Zwierstra P. Complications after bilateral adrenalectomy for

phaeochromocytoma in multiple endocrine neoplasia type 2–a plea to conserve adrenal function. Eur J Surg 1999;165(9):843–6.

74. Moore SW, Appfelstaedt J, Zaahl MG. Familial medullary carcinoma prevention, risk evaluation, and RET in children of families with MEN2. J Pediatr Surg 2007;42(2):326–32.

75. Toledo SP, dos Santos MA, Toledo Rde A, et al. Impact of RET proto-oncogene analysis on the clinical management of multiple endocrine neoplasia type 2. Clinics (Sao Paulo) 2006; 61(1):59–70.

76. Nichols KE, Malkin D, Garber JE, et al. Germ-line p53 mutations predispose to wide spectrum of early-onset cancers. Cancer Epidemiol Biomarkers Prev 2001;10(2):83–7.

77. Varley J. TP53, hChk2, and the Li-Fraumeni syndrome. Methods Mol Biol 2003;222:117–29.

78. Monslave J, Kapur J, Malkin D, et al. Imaging of cancer predisposition syndromes in children. RadioGraphics 2011;31(1):263–80.

79. Shinagare AB, Giardino AA, Jagannathan JP, et al. Hereditary cancer syndromes: a radiologist's perspective. AJR Am J Roentgenol 2011;197: W1001–7.

80. Johnson PT, Horton KM, Fishman EK. Adrenal mass imaging with multidetector CT: pathologic conditions, pearls, and pitfalls. Radiographics 2009;29(5):1333–51.

81. Ballinger ML, Mitchell G, Thomas DM. Surveillance recommendations for patients with germline TP53 mutations. Curr Opin Oncol 2015;27(4): 332–7.

82. Kaelin W. Von Hippel-Lindau disease. Annu Rev Pathol 2007;2:145–73.

83. Shehata BM, Stockwell CA, Castellano-Sanchez AA, et al. Von Hippel-Lindau (VHL) disease: an update on the clinico-pathologic and genetic aspects. Adv Anat Pathol 2008;15(3):165–71.

84. Maher ER, Iselius L, Yates JR, et al. von Hippel-Lindau disease: a genetic study. J Med Genet 1991;28(7):443–7.

85. Neumann HP, Wiestler OD. Clustering of features and genetics of von Hippel-Lindau syndrome. Lancet 1991;338:258.

86. Shanbhogue KP, Hoch M, Ftterpaker G, et al. von Hippel-Lindau disease: review of genetics and imaging. Radiol Clin North Am 2016;54(3): 409–22.

87. Leung RS, Biswas SV, Ducan M, et al. Imaging features of von Hippel-Lindau disease. RadioGraphics 2008;28:65–79.

88. Maher ER, Yates JR, Ferguson-Smith MA. Statistical analysis of the two stage mutation model in von Hippel-Lindau disease, and in sporadic cerebellar haemangioblastoma and renal cell carcinoma. J Med Genet 1990;27:311–4.

89. Choyke PL, Glenn GM, Walther MM, et al. Von Hippel Lindau disease: genetic clinical and imaging features. Radiology 1995;194(3):629–42.

90. Couch V, Lindor NM, Karnes PS, et al. von Hippel-Lindau disease. Mayo Clin Proc 2000; 75(3):265–72.

91. Frantzen C, Klasson TD, Links TP, et al. Von Hippel-Lindau syndrome. Gene Rev 2000.

92. Maher ER. Von Hippel-Lindau disease. Curr Mol Med 2004;4:833–42.

93. Binderup ML, Jensen AM, Budtz-Jorgensen E, et al. Survival and causes of death in patients with von Hippel-Lindau disease. J Med Genet 2017;54(1): 11–8.

94. Feletti A, Anglani M, Scarpa B, et al. Von Hippel-Lindau disease: an evaluation of natural history and functional disability. Neuro Oncol 2016;18: 1011–20.

95. Baron Y, Barkovich AJ. MR imaging of tuberous sclerosis in neonates and young infants. Am J Neuroradiol 1999;20:907–16.

96. Kandt RS, Haines JL, Smith M, et al. Linkage of an important gene locus for tuberous sclerosis to a chromosome 16 marker for polycystic kidney disease. Nat Genet 1992;2:37–41.

97. van Slegtenhorst M, de Hoogt R, Hermans C, et al. Identification of the tuberous sclerosis gene TSC1 on chromosome 9q34. Science 1997;277:805–8.

98. Umeoka S, Koyama T, Miki Y, et al. Pictorial review of tuberous sclerosis in various organs. RadioGraphics 2008;28(7):e32.

99. Brook-Carter PT, Peral B, Ward CJ, et al. Deletion of the TSC2 and PKD1 genes associated with severe infantile polycystic kidney disease - a contiguous gene syndrome. Nat Genet 1994;8:328–32.

100. Evans JC, Curtis J. The radiological appearances of tuberous sclerosis. Br J Radiol 2000;73:91–8.

101. Nir A, Tajik AJ, Freeman WK, et al. Tuberous sclerosis and cardiac rhabdomyoma. Am J Cardiol 1995;76:419–21.

102. Smith HC, Watson GH, Patel RG, et al. Cardiac rhabdomyomata in tuberous sclerosis: their course and diagnostic value. Arch Dis Child 1989;64:196–200.

103. Ristagno RL, Biddinger PW, Pina EM, et al. Multifocal micronodular pneumocyte hyperplasia in tuberous sclerosis. Am J Roentgenol 2005;184: S37–9.

104. Northrup H, Krueger DA, International Tuberous Sclerosis Complex Consensus Group. Tuberous sclerosis complex diagnostic criteria update: recommendations of the 2012 International Tuberous Sclerosis Complex Consensus Conference. Pediatr Neurol 2013;49:243–54.

105. Krueger DA, Northrup H, International Tuberous Sclerosis Complex Consensus Group. Tuberous Sclerosis complex surveillance and management: recommendations of the 2012 International

Tuberous Sclerosis Complex Consensus Conference. Pediatr Neurol 2013;49:255–65.

106. Roach ES. Applying the lessons of tuberous sclerosis: the 2015 Hower award lecture. Pediatr Neurol 2016;63:6–22.

107. Jozwiak S, Kotulska K, Domanska-Pakiela D, et al. Antiepileptic treatment before the onset of seizures reduces epilepsy severity and risk of mental retardation in infants with tuberous sclerosis complex. Eur J Paediatr Neurol 2011;15:424–31.

Index

Note: Page numbers of article titles are in **boldface** type.

Radiol Clin N Am 55 (2017) 895–904
http://dx.doi.org/10.1016/S0033-8389(17)30071-4
0033-8389/17

Moving?

Make sure your subscription moves with you!

To notify us of your new address, find your **Clinics Account Number** (located on your mailing label above your name), and contact customer service at:

Email: journalscustomerservice-usa@elsevier.com

800-654-2452 (subscribers in the U.S. & Canada)
314-447-8871 (subscribers outside of the U.S. & Canada)

Fax number: 314-447-8029

Elsevier Health Sciences Division
Subscription Customer Service
3251 Riverport Lane
Maryland Heights, MO 63043

*To ensure uninterrupted delivery of your subscription, please notify us at least 4 weeks in advance of move.

ELSEVIER